Management Strategies in Antithrombotic Therapy

Management Strategies in Antithrombotic Therapy

By

ARMAN T. ASKARI
Cleveland Clinic Foundation, Cleveland, Ohio, USA

ADRIAN W. MESSERLI
St. Joseph's Hospital, Lexington, Kentucky, USA

A. MICHAEL LINCOFF
Cleveland Clinic Foundation, Cleveland, Ohio, USA

BICENTENNIAL 1807 WILEY 2007

John Wiley & Sons, Ltd

Telephone (+44) 1243 779777

Email (for orders and customer service enquiries): cs-books@wiley.co.uk
Visit our Home Page on www.wiley.com

Other Wiley Editorial Offices

John Wiley & Sons Inc., 111 River Street, Hoboken, NJ 07030, USA

Jossey-Bass, 989 Market Street, San Francisco, CA 94103-1741, USA

Wiley-VCH Verlag GmbH, Boschstr. 12, D-69469 Weinheim, Germany

John Wiley & Sons Australia Ltd, 33 Park Road, Milton, Queensland 4064, Australia

John Wiley & Sons (Asia) Pte Ltd, 2 Clementi Loop #02-01, Jin Xing Distripark, Singapore 129809

John Wiley & Sons Canada Ltd, 6045 Freemont Blvd, Mississauga, Ontario, L5R 4J3, Canada

Wiley also publishes its books in a variety of electronic formats. Some content that appears in print may not be available in electronic books.

Anniversary Logo Design: Richard J. Pacifico

Library of Congress Cataloging in Publication Data

Askari, Arman.
Management strategies in antithrombotic therapy / by Arman Askari and Michael Lincoff.
p. ; cm.
Includes bibliographical references and index.
ISBN 978-0-470-31938-3 (alk. paper)
1. Thrombolytic therapy. 2. Thrombosis—Treatment. 3. Fibrinolytic agents. I. Lincoff, A. Michael. II. Messerli, Adrian W. III. Title.
[DNLM: 1. Coronary Thrombosis—drug therapy. 2. Heart Diseases—drug therapy. 3. Fibrinolytic Agents—therapeutic use. WG 300 A834m 2007]
RC694.3.A77 2007
616.1′42—dc22

2007024176

British Library Cataloguing in Publication Data

A catalogue record for this book is available from the British Library

ISBN 978-0-470-31938-3

Typeset in 10/12pt Times by Integra Software Services Pvt. Ltd, Pondicherry, India
Printed and bound in Great Britain by Antony Rowe Ltd, Chippenham, Wiltshire
This book is printed on acid-free paper responsibly manufactured from sustainable forestry in which at least two trees are planted for each one used for paper production.

To my wife Jamie, and my children, Alexa, Amanda, and Jacob and to my parents Ali and Houri for their unwavering support.

Arman T. Askari, M.D.

To Marco...for coming.

Adrian W. Messerli, M.D.

To my wife, Debra, and my children, Gabrielle, Aaron, and Jacob - for their support and understanding.

A. Michael Lincoff, M.D.

Contents

Abbreviations and Acronyms

ABBREVIATIONS

AA	arachidonic acid
ACC	American College of Cardiology
ACE	angiotensin-converting enzyme
ACS	acute coronary syndrome(s)
ACT	activated clotting time
ADP	adenosine diphosphate
AHA	American Heart Association
AIVR	accelerated idioventricular rhythm
APSAC	antistreplase
aPTT	activated partial thromboplastin time
ASA	acetylsalicylic acid
AT	antithrombin
AUC	area under the curve
CABG	coronary artery bypass graft
CKD	chronic kidney disease
COX-1	cyclooygenase-1
CRP	C-reactive protein
CV	cardiovascular
CVD	cardiovascular disease
CYP	cytochrome P450
DES	drug-eluting stents
DTI	direct thrombin inhibitors
DVT	deep vein thrombosis
EC	endothelial cell
ELISA	enzyme-linked immunosorbent assay
fVIIa/TF	serine protease factor VIIa
FDA	[US] Food and Drug Administration
GI	gastro-intestinal
HACA	human anti-chimeric antibody
HAT	heparin-associated thrombocytopenia
HCII	heparin cofactor II
HF	heart failure
HIPA	heparin-induced platelet aggregation
HIT	heparin-induced thrombocytopenia
HITTS	HIT with thrombosis syndrome
HMG CoA	hydroxymethylglutaryl-coenzyme A
HUVEC	human umbilical vein EC
ICAM	intracellular adhesion molecule

ICH	intracranial hemorrhage
IHD	ischemic heart disease
IL-1	interleukin-1
IL-8	interleukin-8
INR	international normalized ratio
IRA	infarct-related artery
IV	intravenous
IVIG	intravenous gamma globulin
LMWH	low-molecular-weight heparin
LTA	light transmittance platelet aggregation
LV	left ventricular
MI	myocardial infarction
NAP-2	neutrophil-activating-peptide-2
NPH	neutral protein Hagedorn
NSAID	non-steroidal anti-inflammatory drug
NSTE ACS	UA or NSTEMI
NSTEMI	non-ST-segment-elevation myocardial infarction
OPCAB	off-pump coronary artery bypass
PAD	peripheral arterial disease
PAI-1	plasminogen activator inhibitor-1
PAR	protease-activated receptor
PCI	percutaneous coronary intervention
PE	pulmonary embolism
PECAM-1	platelet–endothelial cell adhesion molecule 1
PF	platelet factor
PRP	platelet-rich plasma
PVD	peripheral vascular disease
RCT	randomized controlled trial
rNAPc2	recombinant nematode anticoagulant protein c2
r-PA	reteplase
rt-PA	recombinant tissue plasminogen activator
RR	relative risk
SAT	subacute thrombosis
SC	subcutaneous
SK	streptokinase
SRA	serotonin release assay
STEMI	ST-segment-elevation myocardial infarction
TEG	thrombelastography
TFPI	tissue factor pathway inhibitor
TIA	transient ischemia attack
TIMI	Thrombolysis in Myocardial Infarction
TNF	tumor necrosis factor
TNK	tenecteplase
t-PA	tissue plasminogen activator (alteplase)
TTP	thrombotic thrombocytopenic purpura
UA	unstable angina
UH	unfractionated heparin

UK	urokinase
VCAM	vascular adhesion molecule
VKA	vitamin K antagonist
VTE	venous thromboembolism
vWF	von Willebrand factor

TRIAL/STUDY ACRONYMS

In the text trials and studies are referred to by their acronyms, which are collected here for convenience.

ACUITY	A Randomized Trial of Angiomax versus Clexane in Patients Undergoing Early Invasive Management in Acute Coronary Syndromes without ST Elevation
ADMIRAL	Abciximab before Direct Angioplasty and Stenting in Myocardial Infarction Regarding Acute and Long-term Follow-up
ALBION	Assessment of the best Loading dose of clopidogrel to Blunt platelet activation, Inflammation and Ongoing Necrosis
ARMYDA-2	Antiplatelet therapy for Reduction of Myocardial Damage during Angioplasty
AT-BAT	Anticoagulant Therapy with Bivalirudin to Assist in PCI
BAT	Bivalirudin Angioplasty Trial
CADILLAC	Controlled Abciximab and Device Investigation to Lower Late Angioplasty Complications
CAPRIE	Clopidogrel versus Aspirin in Patients at Risk of Ischemic Events
CAPTURE	c7E3 Fab Anti-Platelet Therapy in Unstable Refractory Angina
CATS	Canadian American Ticlopidine Study
CLARITY	Clopidogrel as Adjunctive Reperfusion TherapY trial
CLASSICS	Clopidogrel Aspirin Stent International Cooperative Study
COMMIT	Clopidogrel Metoprolol Myocardial Infarction trial
CREDO	Clopidogrel for the Reduction of Events During Observation
CURE	Clopidogrel in Unstable Angina to Prevent Recurrent Events
EPIC	Evaluation of c7E3 for Prevention of Ischemic Complications
EPILOG	Evaluation in PTCA to Improve Long-term Outcome with Abciximab GP IIb/IIIa Blockade
EPISTENT	Evaluation of Platelet Inhibition in Stenting
ESPRIT	Enhanced Suppression of the Platelet IIb/IIIa Receptor with Integrilin Therapy
ESSENCE	Efficacy and Safety of Subcutaneous Enoxaparin in Unstable Angina and Non-Q-wave Myocardial Infarction
FANTASTIC	Full ANTicoagulation versus ASpirin and TIClopidine
GRACE	Global Registry of Acute Coronary Events
ISAR-REACT	Intracoronary Stenting and Antithrombotic Regimen: Rapid Early Action for Coronary Treatment
ISAR-CHOICE	Intracoronary Stenting and Antithrombotic Regimen: Choose Between 3 High Oral Doses for Immediate Clopidogrel Effect

MATTIS	Multicenter Aspirin and Ticlopidine Trial after Intracoronary Stenting
NICE	National Investigators Collaborating on Enoxaparin
PCI-CURE	Percutaneous Coronary Intervention-Clopidogrel in Unstable Angina to Prevent Recurrent Events trials
PURSUIT	Platelet IIb/IIIa in Unstable angina: Receptor Suppression Using Integrilin Therapy
REPLACE-2	Randomized Evaluation in PCI Linking Angiomax to Reduced Clinical Events
STARS	Stent Anticoagulation Restenosis Study
STIMS	Swedish Ticlopidine Multicentre Study
STEEPLE	Safety and Efficacy of Enoxaparin in PCI Patients; an International Randomized Evaluation
TASS	Ticlopidine Aspirin Stroke Study
TIMI	Thrombolysis in Myocardial Infarction
TISS	Ticlopidine Indobufen Stroke Study

Preface

It has become well-established that there is an enormous cost, both clinical and economic, associated with intravascular thrombosis. Understanding the central role of thrombosis in the pathogenesis of the acute coronary syndromes, ischemic complications of percutaneous coronary intervention, and venous thromboembolic disease has facilitated the rapid expansion of available antithrombotic therapies to treat these potentially life-threatening conditions. Furthermore, investigation focusing on the use of fibrinolytic therapy, antiplatelet therapy (aspirin, the thieneopyridines, glycoprotein IIb/IIIa inhibitors) and antithrombin therapy (unfractionated heparin, low-molecular-weight heparins, direct thrombin inhibitors) as well as novel combinations of these agents has resulted in a marked improvement in outcomes for patients stricken with a thrombotic event. Despite the improvement in outcomes, the burden of thrombosis remains, as does the search for improved antithrombotic therapies.

Given the burgeoning field of antithrombotic therapies, it is appropriate to develop a resource that not only presents the evidence supporting the various agents but also synthesizes the data in a clinically useful manner. *Management Strategies in Antithrombotic Therapy* provides an in-depth look at the various categories of antithrombotic therapies. Unique to *Management Strategies in Antithrombotic Therapy* are the comprehensive tables in each chapter that provide top-line results of the seminal work supporting the various antithrombotic agents. Coupled with an algorithmic approach to the treatment of patients with ACS, *Management Strategies in Antithrombotic Therapy* provides a clinically useful reference for healthcare providers ranging from medical students, residents, and fellows to attending physicians and the integral nursing staff involved in caring for these patients.

Following a brief introduction *Management Strategies in Antithrombotic Therapy* is divided into two major sections. The first section consists of 8 chapters that focus on commonly used antiplatelet, antithrombin, and fibrinolytic agents. Chapters 2-4 provide detailed data about the pharmacology and clinical utility of aspirin, the thieneopyridines, and glycoprotein IIb/IIIa inhibitors. Chapters 5, 6, and 7 discuss unfractionated heparin, the low-molecular-weight heparins, and the direct thrombin inhibitors, respectively, while chapter 8 focuses on fibrinolytic agents.

The second section of *Management Strategies in Antithrombotic Therapy* discusses the contemporary management of acute coronary and venous thromboembolic disease as well as a potentially lethal complication of heparin therapy. Chapters 9, 10, and 11 discuss ST-segment-elevation myocardial infarction, non-ST-segment-elevation myocardial infarction, and percutaneous coronary interventions, respectively. Chapter 12 focuses on the prevention and treatment of venous thromboembolic disease. The final chapter is dedicated to the dreaded complication of unfractionated heparin exposure, heparin-induced thrombocytopenia.

Management Strategies in Antithrombotic Therapy will definitely be an asset to any healthcare provider who must treat patients with vascular thrombosis.

Arman T. Askari, M.D.
Adrian W. Messerli, M.D.
Michael Lincoff, M.D.

1 Thrombosis and Antithrombotics in Vascular Disease

1.1 THE BURDEN OF THROMBOSIS

Intravascular thrombus formation presents the greatest challenge in the field of cardiovascular disease. Within the arterial tree, it is the culprit inducing clinical presentation in the majority of patients presenting with acute coronary syndromes (ACS), including unstable angina (UA) and non-ST-segment elevation myocardial infarction (NSTEMI) and ST-segment elevation myocardial infarction (STEMI). In the United States alone, approximately 1 million individuals will be stricken with an acute myocardial infarction (MI) and approximately 700,000 will undergo a percutaneous coronary intervention (PCI). Although already staggering, these numbers are increasing for several reasons, including an increasingly aged population, a growing burden of chronic risk factors such as diabetes, obesity and sedentary behavior, and improvements in early recognition and intervention.

Thrombus formation within the venous circuit also results in substantial morbidity and mortality. Despite significant advances in prevention and treatment of venous thromboembolism (VTE), pulmonary embolism (PE) remains a common preventable cause of hospital deaths. Although mortality from VTE has decreased over the past 10 to 20 years, it remains a major national health problem in the United States, being responsible for 150,000 to 200,000 deaths annually [1, 2]. Given the spectrum and diversity of disease processes associated with and resulting from thrombus formation, an appreciation of the underlying pathophysiology is essential in order to comprehend the various therapeutic regimens that have been developed targeted at either arterial or venous thrombosis.

1.2 ESSENTIAL COMPONENTS OF THROMBOSIS

Normal hemostasis is the result of a set of well-regulated processes that accomplish two important functions: (1) maintenance of blood in a fluid, clot-free state in normal vessels; and (2) induction of a rapid and localized hemostatic plug at a site of vascular injury. In contrast, thrombosis can be considered an inappropriate activation of normal hemostatic processes, such as the formation of a thrombus in uninjured vasculature or thrombotic occlusion of a vessel after relatively minor injury. Our current understanding of the pathogenesis of vascular thrombosis was first outlined by Virchow more than 150 years ago. He proposed that thrombotic disorders were associated with a triad of abnormalities: those involving the endothelium/endocardium ('abnormal vessel wall'), those involving hemorheology and turbulence at bifurcations, including atheroma at the vessel wall ('abnormal blood flow')

Management Strategies in Antithrombotic Therapy Arman T. Askari, Adrian W. Messerli and A. Michael Lincoff

and those involving platelets and the coagulation and fibrinolytic pathways ('abnormal blood constituents'). In addition, he proposed that abnormalities in this triad are found in patients with arterial or venous thromboembolism. Since this initial association, our understanding of contributors to thrombogenesis has evolved; however, Virchow's triad remains at the epicenter of pathogenesis.

THE ENDOTHELIUM

The endothelium serves to modulate two, diametrically opposed processes (Table 1.1). On the one hand, the endothelium facilitates normal blood flow through its many antiplatelet, anticoagulant and fibrinolytic properties. Endothelial cell-surface heparan sulfate and thrombomodulin are potent modulators of thrombin activity [3]. In addition, endothelial cells produce prostacyclin and nitric oxide, effective vasodilators and, importantly, inhibitors of platelet aggregation [4]. Furthermore, the vessel wall serves to modulate fibrin deposition [3].

On the other hand, after damage induced by direct trauma, or perturbation by exposure to endotoxin, inflammatory cytokines such as interleukin-1 (IL-1) and tumor necrosis factor (TNF), thrombin or low oxygen tension, the endothelium exhibits several prothrombotic properties. Perturbed endothelial cells synthesize tissue factor and plasminogen activator

Table 1.1 Antithrombotic and prothrombotic products of the endothelium

Product	Product type	Properties
Antithrombotic		
Heparan sulfate	Surface-expressed	Catalyzes the inhibition of thrombin and factor Xa by antithrombin
Thrombomodulin	Surface-expressed	Binds to and regulates the activity of thrombin. Once bound to thrombomodulin, thrombin not only loses its prothrombotic activity but, by activating protein C, triggers a potent antithrombotic pathway
Prostacyclin	Secreted	Potent vasodilator and inhibitor of platelet aggregation
Nitric oxide	Secreted	Inhibits platelet adhesion and aggregation. Potent vasodilator
t-PA	Stored and secreted	Activates bound plasminogen to plasmin. Potent inhibitor of fibrin deposition.
Ectonucleotidases	Surface-expressed	Enzymes that regulate the breakdown of prothrombotic nucleotides
Prothrombotic		
PAI-1	Secreted, circulating, matrix-bound	Inhibits the actions of t-PA allowing for fibrin deposition during thrombosis
PAF	Secreted and surface-expressed	Potent platelet and leukocyte stimulant
TF	Surface-expressed on activated endothelium	Potent prothrombotic. Activates the extrinsic coagulation cascade
vWF	Stored and secreted	Cofactor for platelet adhesion

PAF = platelet activating factor; TF = tissue factor

inhibitor-1 (PAI-1) and internalize thrombomodulin – changes that promote thrombogenesis. Furthermore, damaged endothelial cells produce less t-PA, the principal activator of fibrinolysis. In addition to these effects, the endothelial cells express surface receptors for many different ligands. Coupled with interactions with the cellular constituents of blood, these serve as the substrate for thrombus formation.

THE PLATELET

At the site of arterial injury, platelets adhere, almost instantaneously, to exposed collagen, von Willebrand factor (vWF), and fibrinogen. Adherent platelets are then activated by several mechanisms including collagen, thrombin, serotonin and adenosine diphosphate (ADP). Activated platelets degranulate, prompting secretion of vasoactive amines, clotting factors and chemotaxins, promoting more thrombin generation and additional platelet accumulation: a cycle of thrombosis (Table 1.2). With activation, the final common pathway of platelet aggregation, the glycoprotein (GP) IIb/IIIa receptor undergoes a conformational change and becomes receptive to ligand binding [5]. Platelet aggregation culminates in a large platelet core at the site of vascular injury: an ideal milieu for thrombus formation.

Table 1.2 Products of platelet secretion

Location in platelet	Product
Alpha granules	– PDGF – TGF-β – PF4 – vWF – Factor V – Fibrinogen – Thrombospondin – β-Thromboglobulin – Fibronectin – Vitronectin – β_2-Macroglobulin – α_1-Proteinase inhibitor – Albumin – P-selectin
Dense granules	– Serotonin – Histamine – Calcium – ATP – ADP – Epinephrine
Lysosomes	– PF3 – Acid phosphatase – Glucose-6 phosphatase – α-Arabinosidase – β-*N*-Acetyl-galactosominidase

ATP = adenosine triphosphate; TGF = transforming growth factor

The Coagulation Cascade

Although platelets are the first line of thrombus formation, until it is reinforced by the fibrin cross-linking induced by the coagulation cascade, the platelet thrombus is quite unstable and can be easily dislodged. Thus, both platelets and fibrin are essential for stable thrombus formation.

The coagulation cascade is essentially a series of enzymatic conversions, turning inactive proenzymes into activated enzymes and culminating in the formation of thrombin (Figure 1.1). Thrombin then converts the soluble plasma protein fibrinogen precursor into the insoluble fibrous protein fibrin. While the coagulation cascade has traditionally been divided into intrinsic and extrinsic pathways, these pathways reflect the way coagulation is measured in the laboratory. *In vivo*, however, coagulation is initiated almost exclusively by the tissue factor pathway. In this pathway, a proportion of the circulating activated factor VII – factor VIIa – binds to tissue factor at sites of vascular injury. The tissue factor–factor VIIa complex then activates both factor IX and factor X. Factor Xa completes the coagulation cascade by converting prothrombin to thrombin in the presence of activated factor V, phospholipid and calcium. Thrombin then converts fibrinogen to fibrin, activates platelets and activates factor XIII, which, in the presence of calcium, cross-links the fibrin, thereby stabilizing the clot. To ensure continuous generation of thrombin, thrombin and factor Xa activate factors VIII and V, markedly accelerating the coagulation reactions involving these two cofactors, and thrombin activates factor XI, which in turn activates additional factor IX, establishing a positive feedback loop.

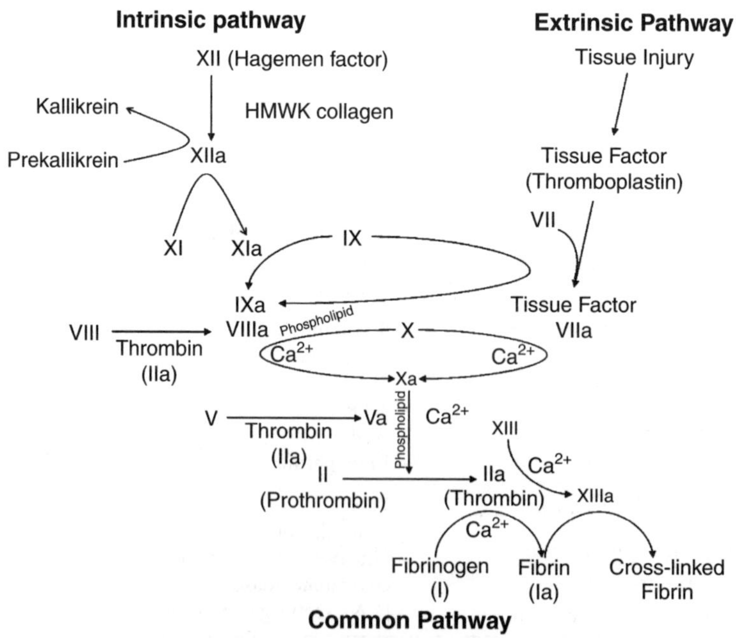

Figure 1.1 The coagulation cascade

Thrombosis occurs once the coagulation cascade and platelet activation are almost simultaneously activated by an inciting event that results in vascular damage or perturbation. With the understanding that thrombin plays a pivotal role in coordinating and regulating hemostasis, numerous investigations across the spectrum of cardiovascular diseases including STEMI, NSTEMI and UA, as well as venous thromboembolic disease, have assessed the efficacy of various antithrombotic regimens. Despite remarkable progress within the arena of vascular pharmacotherapeutics, the currently available agents remain less than perfect. Thus the search for the ideal antithrombotic agent continues.

1.3 THROMBOSIS IN THE ACUTE ISCHEMIC SYNDROMES

The initiating event of acute ischemic syndromes involves erosion or rupture of an atherosclerotic plaque and subsequent local thrombosis which either sub-totally (UA/NSTEMI) or totally (STEMI) occludes antegrade myocardial perfusion. Similar pathophysiology is present during PCI, which is essentially an iatrogenic plaque rupture. By targeting the three essential components of thrombus formation, platelets, fibrin and thrombin, various regimens, combining antiplatelet agents (e.g. aspirin, clopidogrel, GP IIb/IIIa inhibitors), anti-thrombotics (e.g. heparin, LMWH (enoxaparin), DTI (Bivalirudin)), and either fibrinolysis or PCI, have improved outcomes following acute ischemic syndromes. The agents currently used for the treatment of acute ischemic syndromes depend on the presenting syndrome, the use of PCI and on certain patient characteristics.

STEMI

The mainstay of therapy for STEMI centers around an approach that focuses on prompt and complete reperfusion, either pharmacologic or mechanical. In addition, a multi-pronged approach to the thrombotic process has led to the lowest mortality rates following STEMI to date [6, 7].

Despite the recently demonstrated improved outcomes, a substantial morbidity and mortality persists. Incomplete reperfusion and recurrent ischemia and re-occlusion continue to thwart improvement in outcomes for these patients [8]. Furthermore, a considerable proportion of patients who do achieve normal (TIMI 3) coronary blood flow fail to achieve microvascular, or tissue-level, reperfusion, manifested by persistent ST-segment elevation [9]. The hope had been that combination chemotherapy for acute STEMI would improve early patency and, ultimately, survival. Unfortunately this has not been the case, as demonstrated by recent trials of 'enhanced' fibrinolytics [6, 7, 10–12]. Furthermore, some regimens have been associated with increased bleeding rates [7].

Currently used pharmacologic therapies include aspirin, heparin and a fibrinolytic such as reteplase or tenecteplase. Recent data suggests that the low-molecular-weight heparin (LMWH) enoxaparin is safe and effective when combined with full dose fibrinolytics. These alternative regimens, including combined GP IIb/IIIa inhibitors with half-dose fibrinolytics, have resulted in limitations similar to those of the standard therapies for patients with STEMI. What has improved outcomes for these patients is the use of early PCI. In addition, routine PCI following full-dose fibrinolysis has suggested improved outcomes in the stent era [13]; however, the data remain controversial. Interestingly, the treatments for acute STEMI are moving away from 'stand-alone' pharmacologic regimens to various pharmaco-invasive reperfusion hybrids: a 'facilitated' PCI approach.

NSTEMI/UA

NSTEMI and UA are positioned on the continuum of acute ischemic syndromes. However, their management has traditionally been slightly different than that of STEMI. Fibrinolytics have been associated with worse outcomes in this patient population [14]. Traditional therapeutic approaches have employed the antiplatelet aspirin, the antithrombotic heparin, and agents used to decrease myocardial oxygen demand such as nitroglycerin and beta blockers. Recent data suggest that newer antithrombotic agents such as enoxaparin may be associated with improved outcomes [15]. In the current era of early invasive therapy for these patients, enoxaparin has been demonstrated to be noninferior to unfractionated heparin [16].

The ability of aspirin to reduce both mortality and nonfatal events across the spectrum of acute coronary syndromes is well known. In addition, the newest antiplatelet agent, the thienopyridine clopidogrel, has exhibited benefit in these patients when combined with aspirin and heparin [17]. Furthermore, by targeting the final common pathway of platelet aggregation with GP IIb/IIIa inhibitors, outcomes have been incrementally improved. On further analyses of this last class of agents, however, it has become apparent that the majority of benefit imparted by the GP IIb/IIIa inhibitors relates to patients who actually have serologic evidence of increased risk (elevated troponin, CD40L or myeloperoxidase) or undergo early PCI. Similar to trends in STEMI, it has become apparent that high-risk patients with NSTEMI/UA benefit from an early, invasive approach to their management [18].

Direct thrombin inhibitors (DTI) have also been evaluated as an alternative to heparin in patients undergoing PCI. The primary agent, bivalirudin, has demonstrated noninferiority to heparin in unstable [19] and stable [20] patients undergoing PCI. In addition, bivalirudin has been associated with fewer hemorrhagic complications, making it an attractive agent for patients at increased risk of bleeding.

Unfortunately, no single antithrombotic agent has optimized outcomes while minimizing complications across the spectrum of acute ischemic syndromes. Thus, the continued search for improved agents or regimens continues and will continue as long as thrombosis continues to result in such devastating consequences.

1.4 VENOUS THROMBOEMBOLIC DISEASE

Several variables need to be considered before optimal prevention and treatment of VTE can be implemented. These include the underlying clinical disease state, severity of illness, concomitant co-morbidities (i.e. chronic kidney disease, pregnancy, morbid obesity, etc.), and characteristics of the currently available antithrombotic agents. In addition, optimal timing and duration of the administration of each antithrombotic agent for the purposes of prevention and treatment of VTE are essential. An understanding of these issues will better arm the clinician with ammunition to prevent and treat the formidable foe of VTE.

PREVENTION OF VTE

Unfractionated heparin (UH) is indicated for prophylaxis of VTE. However, with the demonstration that LMWHs are easier to administer, do not require monitoring, are associated with fewer bleeding complications and impart a lower risk for developing heparin-induced thrombocytopenia (HIT), these agents have become the antithrombotics of choice for this indication. Nevertheless, a role for UH remains.

LMWHs have been shown to be efficacious in the prophylaxis of VTE, and a number of these agents are approved for this indication (Chapter 6). The attraction of LMWHs for VTE prophylaxis is that they can be administered once or twice daily at a constant dose without laboratory monitoring. In addition, a substantially lower risk of HIT with LMWH compared with UH has been suggested.

The development of new anticoagulants has been pursued with the aim of finding more effective, safer and/or more convenient therapies. Thrombin is a central regulator in the coagulation and inflammation process and several direct thrombin inhibitors with distinct pharmacological profiles, as well as pharmacological differences from conventional anticoagulants, are currently in clinical use for certain indications or are under development. Despite the efficacy of the oral direct thrombin inhibitors, the lack of safety with the most-well-studied agent, ximelagatran, has contributed to the current, experimental status within the United States.

The primary prophylactic measure employed depends on the risk category of the individual patient and the clinical situation. In general, LMWHs have become the antithrombotic agents of choice for the prevention of VTE. Effective alternative agents remain low-dose UH (5000 U subcutaneous every 8–12 h) and oral anticoagulation with warfarin (following major orthopedic surgery). That the currently approved agents for VTE prophylaxis cannot be applied to patients across the spectrum of VTE risk has fostered a continued search for improved alternatives. As an example, the newer agent fondaparinux has demonstrated promise as an effective prophylactic agent, especially within the realm of management for patients with hip fractures. However, more research needs to be conducted before replacement of the current standards occurs.

TREATMENT OF VTE

Antithrombotic therapy remains the principal treatment for deep vein thrombosis (DVT) and PE. The anticoagulant regimen used to treat these VTE disorders has continued to evolve. Whereas therapy for both entities historically has been with IV UH simultaneously initiated with oral warfarin in an inpatient setting, the development of strategies aimed at reducing costs without sacrificing safety and efficacy has challenged this dogma. However, owing to the potential morbidity and mortality associated with PE, initial treatment is delivered in a closely monitored setting in all but the most stable cases. Integral to the move towards a less-intensive approach to both DVT and PE has been the appearance of newer antithrombotic agents such as the LMWH class of anticoagulants (Chapter 6). The need for improving the efficacy of antithrombotic therapy for the treatment of VTE without increasing the risk of bleeding has fostered continued expansion of the range of available antithrombotic agents. In addition, the optimal duration of therapy continues to be elucidated for specific clinical conditions in order to decrease the risk of recurrent VTE while minimizing the risk of bleeding complications.

Table 1.3 Currently available antithrombotic agents

Agent	Antithrombotic class	$T_{1/2}$	Delivery	Labeled indications
			Antithrombin agents	
Bivalirudin (Angiomax)	DTI	25 min	IV	Anticoagulant in UA patients undergoing PCI who receive concomitant aspirin
Argatroban (Argatroban)	DTI	39–51 min	IV; requires monitoring of aPTT/ACT	Anticoagulant for prophylaxis or treatment of thrombosis in patients with HIT
Desirudin (Iprivask)	DTI	2–3 h	SC	Prophylaxis of DVT in patients undergoing elective hip replacement surgery
Lepirudin (Refludan)	DTI	1.3 h*	IV; requires monitoring of aPTT	Anticoagulation in patients with HIT and associated thromboembolic disease
Dalteparin sodium (Fragmin)	LMWH	1.5–2.5 h	SC	1) VTE prophylaxis in patients undergoing hip and abdominal surgery 2) Prevention of ischemic complications in UA and NSTEMI
Enoxaparin (Lovenox, Clexane 40, Clexane Forte, Klexane)	LMWH	4.5 h	SC	1) Prophylaxis and treatment of DVT in patients undergoing hip or knee replacement surgery, in patients undergoing abdominal surgery, and in medical patients with acute illness 2) Inpatient treatment DVT with or without PE, when administered in conjunction with warfarin 3) Outpatient treatment of acute DVT without PE 4) Prophylaxis of ischemic complications of UA and NSTEMI when administered with aspirin
Tinzaparin sodium (Innohep or Logiparin)	LMWH	3–4 h	SC	Treatment of DVT with or without PE, when administered in conjunction with warfarin
Ardeparin (Normiflo)	LMWH	3–4 h	SC	DVT prophylaxis

Heparin	UH	~30 min	SC, IV	Prevention and treatment of various thromboembolic disorders
Fondaparinux sodium (Arixtra)	Selective factor Xa inhibitor	17–21 h	SC	Prophylaxis of VTE following hip fracture surgery
Warfarin sodium (Coumadin; others)	Vitamin K antagonist	~40 h (20–60)	Oral; requires INR monitoring	Prophylaxis and treatment ofvarious thromboembolic disorders, including patients with mechanical heart valves, VHD, MI, atrial fibrillation, and low EF
			Antiplatelet Agents	
Abciximab (ReoPro)	GP IIb/IIIa inhibitor	30 min	IV	1) Adjunct to PCI for prevention of acute ischemic complications in patients undergoing PCI 2) UA patients refractory to conventional medical therapy when PCI is planned in 24h
Eptifibatide (Integrilin)	GP IIb/IIIa inhibitor	25 h	IV	Treatment of ACS; including medically managed patients and those undergoing PCI
Tirofiban (Aggrastat)	GP IIb/IIIa inhibitor	~2 h	IV	Treatment of ACS; including medically managed patients and those undergoing PCI or atherectomy
Aspirin	Cyclooxygenase inhibitor	~20 min	Oral	1) Prophylaxis against recurrent TIAs or strokes in men 2) MI and death prophylaxis in UA or prior MI patients
Clopidogrel bisulfate (Plavix)	Thienopyridine	8 h	Oral	CVD risk reduction in patients at high risk of recurrent events
Ticlopidine HCL (Ticlid)	Thienopyridine	12.6 h	Oral	Stroke prevention in patients with prior cerebrovascular disease
			Fibrinolytics	
Alteplase (Activase)	Fibrinolytic	<5 min	IV	Acute MI, acute ischemic stroke, acute massive PE
Tenecteplase (TNK)	Fibrinolytic	20–24 min	IV	Acute MI
Reteplase (Retavase)	Fibrinolytic	13–16 min	IV	Acute MI

EF = ejection fraction; VHD = valvular heart disease

1.5 THE IDEAL ANTITHROMBOTIC AGENT

The splendor of clinical medicine rests, in part, with the continuous investigation for mechanisms that not only enhance our understanding of disease states but also foster the development of novel therapeutics, with the goal being improved patient outcomes. The agents available in today's armoury, although the most efficacious to date, possess several limitations. For example, although clopidogrel may incrementally improve outcomes in patients with ACS or those undergoing PCI, its use has been associated with a substantial risk of bleeding in patients who require emergent coronary artery bypass graft surgery. With respect to antithrombotic agents, enoxaparin may improve outcomes in patients with ACS and VTE but is difficult to reverse in patients with bleeding complications. The cardiovascular community would welcome an agent that possessed both improved efficacy compared with the currently available anticoagulants together with an improved safety profile.

Characteristics that an ideal anticoagulant should possess include the following:

- It should be easy to administer, either intravenously, orally, or subcutaneously.
- It should possess a predictable pharmacodynamic profile making monitoring unnecessary.
- It should not require dose adjustments.
- It should not interact with other adjunctive medicines commonly used.
- It should possess a potent antithrombotic effect.
- It should be readily reversible.

The art of anticoagulation across the spectrum of cardiovascular (CV) disease lies in selecting a regimen that has the ability to optimize the management of patients from presentation through ultimate treatment plan completion. An 'ideal' agent that can accomplish this remains to be discovered. The goal of this book is to acquaint readers with the data behind the commonly used antithrombotic agents and to assist them in formulating a sound, evidence-based therapeutic strategy. The currently available antithrombotic agents are listed in Table 1.3.

REFERENCES

[1] Horlander, K.T., Mannino, D.M., Leeper, K.V., (2003) Pulmonary embolism mortality in the United States, 1979–1998: an analysis using multiple-cause mortality data. *Arch Intern Med*, 163(14): 1711–17.

[2] Lilienfeld, D.E., (2000) Decreasing mortality from pulmonary embolism in the United States, 1979–1996. *Int J Epidemiol*, 29(3):465–9.

[3] Esmon, C.T., (1987) The regulation of natural anticoagulant pathways. *Science*, 235(4794): 1348–52.

[4] Moncada, S., Herman, A.G., Higgs, E.A., *et al.*, (1977) Differential formation of prostacyclin (PGX or PGI2) by layers of the arterial wall. An explanation for the anti-thrombotic properties of vascular endothelium. *Thromb Res*, 11(3):323–44.

[5] Lefkovits, J., Plow, E.F., Topol, E.J., (1995) Platelet glycoprotein IIb/IIIa receptors in cardiovascular medicine. *N Eng J Med*, 332:1553–9.

[6] The GUSTO V Investigators, (2001) Reperfusion therapy for acute myocardial infarction with fibrinolytic therapy or combination reduced fibrinolytic therapy and platelet glycoprotein IIb/IIIa inhibition: the GUSTO V randomized trial. *Lancet*, 357:1905–14.

[7] Efficacy and safety of tenecteplase in combination with enoxaparin, abciximab, or unfractionated heparin: the ASSENT-3 randomised trial in acute myocardial infarction. (2001) *Lancet*, 358(9282):605–13.

[8] Hudson, M.P., Granger, C.B., Topol, E.J., *et al.*, (2001) Early reinfarction after fibrinolysis: experience from the global utilization of streptokinase and tissue plasminogen activator (alteplase) for occluded coronary arteries (GUSTO I) and global use of strategies to open occluded coronary arteries (GUSTO III) trials. *Circulation*, 104(11):1229–35.

[9] de Lemos, J.A., Antman, E.M., Giugliano, R.P., *et al.*, (2000) ST segment resolution and infarct-related artery patency and flow after thrombolytic therapy. Thrombolysis in Myocardial Infarction (TIMI) 14 investigators. *Am J Cardiol*, 85(3):299–304.

[10] Brener, S.J., Zeymer U., Adgey, A.A., *et al.*, (2002) Eptifibatide and low-dose tissue plasminogen activator in acute myocardial infarction: the integrilin and low-dose thrombolysis in acute myocardial infarction (INTRO AMI) trial. *J Am Coll Cardiol*, 39(3):377–86.

[11] The Strategies for Patency Enhancement in the Emergency Department (SPEED) Group. (2000) Trial of abciximab with and without low-dose reteplase for acute myocardial infarction. *Circulation*, 101(24):2788–94.

[12] Antman, E.M., Giugliano, R.P., Gibson, C.M., *et al.*, (1999) Abciximab facilitates the rate and extent of thrombolysis: results of the thrombolysis in myocardial infarction (TIMI) 14 trial. The TIMI 14 Investigators. *Circulation*, 99(21):2720–32.

[13] Fernandez-Aviles F., Alonso, J.J., Castro-Beiras A, *et al.*, (2004) Routine invasive strategy within 24 hours of thrombolysis versus ischaemia-guided conservative approach for acute myocardial infarction with ST-segment elevation (GRACIA-1): a randomised controlled trial. *Lancet*, 364(9439):1045–53.

[14] Effects of tissue plasminogen activator and a comparison of early invasive and conservative strategies in unstable angina and non-Q-wave myocardial infarction. Results of the TIMI IIIB Trial. Thrombolysis in Myocardial Ischemia (1994) *Circulation*, 89(4):1545–56.

[15] Antman, E.M., Cohen, M., Radley, D., *et al.*, (1999) Assessment of the treatment effect of enoxaparin for unstable angina/non-Q-wave myocardial infarction. TIMI 11B-ESSENCE meta-analysis. *Circulation*, 100(15):1602–8.

[16] Ferguson, J.J., Califf, R.M., Antman, E.M., *et al.*, (2004) Enoxaparin vs unfractionated heparin in high-risk patients with non-ST-segment elevation acute coronary syndromes managed with an intended early invasive strategy: primary results of the SYNERGY randomized trial. *JAMA*, 292(1):45–54.

[17] Yusuf, S., Zhao, F., Mehta, S.R., *et al.*, (2001) Effects of clopidogrel in addition to aspirin in patients with acute coronary syndromes without ST-segment elevation. *N Eng J Med*, 345(7): 494–502.

[18] Cannon, C.P., Weintraub, W.S., Demopoulos, L.A., *et al.*, (2001) Comparison of early invasive and conservative strategies in patients with unstable coronary syndromes treated with the glycoprotein IIb/IIIa inhibitor tirofiban. *N Eng J Med*, 344(25):1879–87.

[19] Bittl, J.A., Feit, F., (1998) A randomized comparison of bivalirudin and heparin in patients undergoing coronary angioplasty for postinfarction angina. Hirulog Angioplasty Study Investigators. *Am J Cardiol*, 82(8B):43P–9P.

[20] Lincoff, A.M., Bittl, J.A., Harrington, R.A., *et al.*, (2003) Bivalirudin and provisional glycoprotein IIb/IIIa blockade compared with heparin and planned glycoprotein IIb/IIIa blockade during percutaneous coronary intervention: REPLACE-2 randomized trial. *JAMA*, 289(7):853–63.

2 Aspirin

2.1 INTRODUCTION

Cardiovascular disease (CVD), which includes ischemic heart disease (IHD), peripheral vascular disease (PVD) and stroke, remains the leading cause of morbidity and mortality in developed countries. Platelets are central to the pathogenesis of these arterial atherothrombotic disorders. It is therefore not surprising that the original antiplatelet agent, aspirin, has been demonstrated to be of benefit in these disorders from the time of its discovery in the late 1800s. The efficacy of aspirin in decreasing the risk of CVD has been seen in primary prevention of first myocardial infarction (MI); in secondary prevention in patients after acute MI, strokes, stable coronary disease and after coronary artery bypass graft (CABG) surgery; in the management of acute coronary syndromes; as an adjunctive agent after PCI; and in the management of acute stroke. Even with these data, the utilization of aspirin has been less than uniform. In addition, the optimal dose of aspirin that confers the greatest benefit with the lowest risk has yet to be fully defined.

The vast experience with aspirin in patients with CVD has revealed that, in addition to its beneficial effects, aspirin is associated with several limitations that have prompted a search for a more 'optimal' antiplatelet agent. Aspirin at higher doses is associated with significant gastro-intestinal (GI) toxicity. In addition, the entity of aspirin resistance and its associated increased risk of adverse events have been gaining more attention, especially as the number of alternative oral antiplatelet agents continues to grow. This chapter will serve to review the mechanism of action of aspirin, its utility across the spectrum of CVD and its potential limitations.

2.2 PHARMACOLOGY

MECHANISM OF ACTION

Anti-thrombotic effects

The most likely mechanism of aspirin's beneficial effects in CVD relates to its ability to irreversibly inhibit cyclooxygenase (COX-1 and COX-2), the enzyme associated with platelet aggregability, reducing the risk of intravascular thrombosis [1]. COX catalyzes the first step in the synthesis of prostaglandins: the conversion of arachidonate to prostaglandin H_2 [2]. COX-1 is constitutively expressed in most tissues and in platelets and is involved in the synthesis of the prostaglandins and thromboxane involved in mediating platelet–endothelium interactions. Thromboxane A_2 is synthesized and released by platelets in response to a variety of stimuli including thrombin, collagen and ADP, and in turn induces irreversible platelet

Management Strategies in Antithrombotic Therapy Arman T. Askari, Adrian W. Messerli and A. Michael Lincoff

aggregation [3–5] providing a mechanism for amplification of the platelet response to such diverse agonists. Aspirin selectively acetylates the hydroxyl group of a single serine residue at position 529 within the polypeptide chain of platelet COX-1 [6, 7], causing the irreversible loss of its cyclooxygenase activity. The result is decreased conversion of arachidonate to prostaglandin G_2 and ultimately of prostaglandin H_2 and thromboxane A_2 production for the life of the platelet.

Aspirin is a much more potent inhibitor of COX-1 than of COX-2 [8]. The irreversible inhibition of COX-1 appears to be complete at low doses of aspirin as demonstrated by a lack of additional inhibition with increasing doses. In addition, very high doses have been postulated to be deleterious owing to concomitant inhibition of endothelial cell synthesis of prostacyclin (a vasodilator and inhibitor of platelet aggregation) [9], although the clinical relevance of relative prostacyclin sparing has not been clearly demonstrated.

ADDITIONAL BENEFICIAL EFFECTS OF ASPIRIN IN CVD

The emergence of the 'era of inflammation,' with respect to atherothrombosis has resulted in closer attention to and attempted treatment of a patient's inflammatory burden as assessed by C-reactive protein (CRP) [10]. In addition to its antiplatelet activity, aspirin may have additional beneficial effects in patients with CVD and, in particular, on inflammation. In a randomized study of patients with chronic stable angina and elevated pro-inflammatory cytokines and CRP the daily administration of aspirin for six weeks appeared to be anti-inflammatory [11]. This beneficial effect of aspirin appears to extend to apparently healthy men, albeit in those with higher baseline CRP levels [12], and to those presenting with unstable coronary syndromes [13].

PHARMACOKINETICS AND PHARMACODYNAMICS

Although no 'gold standard' measurement of aspirin's pharmacodynamics exists, the clinical pharmacology of aspirin has been delineated through measurements of serum Thromboxane B2 (the stable metabolite of Thromboxane A2), and urinary excretion of thromboxane metabolites [14–16]. Single oral doses of aspirin ranging from 5 mg to 100 mg impart a dose-dependent inhibition of platelet COX-1 with near complete inhibition using doses as low as 100 mg [17]. Aspirin is readily absorbed in the stomach and upper intestine, achieving peak plasma concentrations within 30 min [18]. Despite a relatively low systemic bioavailability, 46% to 51% following single oral doses of between 20 and 1300 mg [18], the inhibitory effect of aspirin is evident after 1 h, probably as a result of irreversible inhibition of platelet COX-1 in the portal circulation [18]. Because platelet COX-1 is acetylated in the presystemic circulation, the antiplatelet effect of aspirin is largely independent of its systemic bioavailability. An understanding of these pharmacokinetics has spawned the development of alternative formulations of aspirin with negligible systemic bioavailability in order to selectively inhibit thromboxane A2 synthesis without interfering with prostacyclin formation [9, 19]. The utility of these formulations has not been fully evaluated, however.

Aspirin is metabolized to salicylate through hydrolysis by esterases located in the GI mucosa, red blood cells, synovial fluid and blood. Excretion occurs primarily in the urine. Although the elimination half-life of aspirin is quite rapid, ranging from 15 to 20 min, aspirin has been shown to be fully effective as an antiplatelet agent with once-daily dosing. This can be explained by the absence of the biosynthetic machinery to replenish COX-1 in platelets combined with the irreversible nature of aspirin's effect. Because of this permanent effect on platelets, the inhibitory effect of low daily doses of aspirin is cumulative, with complete inhibition of platelet thromboxane biosynthesis within 7 to 10 days [14, 15]. Ultimately, aspirin's effects persist for the lifespan of the platelet, 7–10 days, with slow recovery of COX-1 activity as a function of platelet turnover [20].

2.3 CLINICAL USES OF ASPIRIN

The efficacy and safety of aspirin across the spectrum of atherothrombotic diseases has been documented in a myriad of clinical trials, accumulating hundreds of thousands of patients. In addition, the beneficial effects of aspirin have been observed with variable lengths of administration. Uniformly, the beneficial effect of aspirin in preventing fatal and non-fatal vascular events has been demonstrated in these trials; however, the magnitude of the effects and the absolute benefit of aspirin remain somewhat heterogeneous in the different clinical settings and different patient subsets.

PRIMARY PREVENTION OF CARDIOVASCULAR DISEASE

That the regular administration of aspirin is associated with a decreased risk of coronary events in men has been suggested by observational trials dating back to the 1970s [21, 22]. More recently, an analysis of the Nurses' Health Study suggested that aspirin use reduced the risk of MI in apparently healthy women [23]. In this study, women who reported taking between one and six aspirins per week experienced a 32% relative risk reduction of a first MI. The beneficial effects of aspirin were seen primarily in women older than 50. Importantly, these observational data have since been somewhat supported by randomized controlled trials in various populations of patients.

There have been seven major randomized trials of aspirin for the primary prevention of coronary events (Table 2.1). With the exception of one trial, the British Doctors' trial [24], these trials have provided the main support for the use of aspirin to prevent coronary events in a broad range of patients including healthy men [25], high-risk men and women [26, 27], hypertensive patients [28], and patients with chronic stable angina [29]. The beneficial effect of aspirin was shown to be primarily related to the prevention of first MI, with the reduction in relative risk ranging between 4% and 44%. Notably, none of these trials demonstrated a reduction in the risk of death or of stroke; however, none of these trials was designed to do so. In addition, women were grossly under-represented in these trials, making the interpretation of the effect of aspirin for the primary prevention of vascular events difficult in these patients.

A recent analysis of the Women's Health Study has shed some light on the utility of aspirin for the primary prevention of vascular event in women [30]. In this trial of 39,876 healthy women, randomized to receive 100 mg of aspirin or placebo every other day, a non-significant reduction in the relative risk of major cardiovascular events was seen after 10 years of aspirin use (RR 0.91; 95% CI, 0.80–1.03, p-value = 0.13). However, unlike the situation in men, aspirin use was associated with a significant 17% reduction in the risk of stroke in women. Subgroup analysis also suggested a beneficial effect of aspirin on the incidence of a major CV event, ischemic stroke or MI in women older than 65. These

Table 2.1 Primary prevention trials of aspirin in ICD

Trial	*N*	Patient population	Aspirin dose (mg)	Follow up (yr)	Placebo event rate (%/yr)	Comment
British Doctors' Trial [24]	5,139	Healthy men	500 daily	5.8	1.4	No significant effects of 500 mg of aspirin on CV event rates
Physicians' Health Study [25]	22,071	Healthy men	325 qod	5.0	0.7	Aspirin at 325 mg qod was associated with a 44% reduction in risk of first MI
Thrombosis Prevention Trial [26]	5,085	High-risk men	75 daily	6.3	1.6	Aspirin associated with a 20% reduction in risk of total IHD primarily related to a 32% reduction in risk of non-fatal MI
Primary Prevention Project [27]	4,495	High-risk men and women	100 daily	3.6	0.8	Aspirin was associated with a 28% relative risk reduction in any CV event
Hypertension Optimal Treatment [28]	18,790	Hypertensives	75 daily	3.8	1.1	Aspirin was associated with a reduction in the risk of CV events by 15% and all MIs by 36%
Swedish Angina Pectoris Aspirin Trial [29]	2,035	Chronic stable angina	75 daily	4.2	3.7	Aspirin was associated with a 34% relative RR in the primary endpoint of sudden death and MI
WHS [30]	39,876	Healthy women	100 qod	10	0.26	Aspirin (100 mg qod) resulted in a non-significant 9% decrease in the RR of major CV events in apparently healthy women. A significant 17% decrease in the RR of stroke was noted. Women over 65 years of age appeared to benefit from ASA with respect to CV endpoints

qod = every other day

data provide evidence for the beneficial effects of aspirin in women and highlight gender differences, the mechanisms of which require further investigation.

Unfortunately, the beneficial effects of aspirin were not without risk. The majority of these trials also revealed an increase in hemorrhagic events with aspirin at the doses used in these trials [31]. These event ranged from minor episodes of epistaxis and easy bruising to major GI bleeds. An increase, albeit non-significant, in the risk of strokes was also seen. Despite the increased risk of hemorrhagic events, the utility of aspirin for primary prevention of cardiovascular events is evident in those at greatest risk.

That the magnitude of benefit with the use of aspirin is directly correlated with the baseline risk of cardiovascular events is evident in recent meta-analyses of these trials [31, 32]. Whereas the reduction in the absolute risk with aspirin use is only 0.08% per year with a baseline risk of MI of 0.5% per year, it increases to 0.4% per year when the baseline risk of MI increases to 1.5% per year [31]. A more inclusive meta-analysis further supported this theme of maximum benefit with minimal adverse events in patients at the highest baseline risk [32]. For 1000 patients with a 5% risk for coronary heart disease events over five years, aspirin would prevent 6 to 20 myocardial infarctions but would cause 0 to 2 hemorrhagic strokes and 2 to 4 major GI bleeding events. For patients with a risk of 1% over five years, aspirin would prevent 1 to 4 myocardial infarctions but would cause 0 to 2 hemorrhagic strokes and 2 to 4 major GI bleeding events. Coupled with data in other populations of patients including those with diabetes mellitus [33], the use of aspirin for the primary prevention of cardiovascular events should be based on baseline risk for coronary events. Those at highest risk will derive the most net benefit with the use of aspirin.

SECONDARY PREVENTION CARDIOVASCULAR DISEASE

Long-term aspirin therapy reduces the risk of subsequent MI, stroke, and vascular death among patients with a wide range of prior manifestations of cardiovascular disease. The magnitude and range of benefit was illustrated in the Antithrombotic Trialists' Collaboration overview, which analyzed the results of 195 studies of antiplatelet therapy among more than 135,000 high-risk patients with prior evidence of CVD, including prior or acute MI, prior or acute stroke or transient ischemia attacks (TIA), and other high-risk groups such as patients with UA, stable angina, peripheral vascular disease, CABG, PCI, atrial fibrillation and valvular disease [33]. Although other antiplatelet agents were included in this analysis, the majority of trials assessed the efficacy of aspirin.

Overall, allocation to antiplatelet therapy reduced the combined outcome of any serious vascular event by about 22% [33]. The proportional benefit of aspirin in reducing the risk of non-fatal MI, non-fatal stroke, and vascular mortality was relatively consistent and ranged between 20% and 30%. Antiplatelet therapy led to the avoidance of 36 vascular events per 1000 patients with a previous MI treated for two years; 38 events per 1000 patients with an acute myocardial infarction treated for one month; 36 events per 1000 patients with a previous stroke or TIA treated for two years; 9 events per 1000 patients with acute stroke treated for three weeks; and 22 events per 1000 patients with other high-risk features, including stable angina and peripheral arterial disease treated for two years. Despite an increase in hemorrhagic endpoints with antiplatelet therapy, the absolute benefits substantially outweighed the absolute risks of major extracranial bleeding.

Further support for aspirin use following an acute ischemic event, acute MI or UA can be derived from the evaluation of the Multicenter Myocardial Ischemia Research Group [34].

In this study of 936 patients one to six months after an acute MI (651) or UA (285), aspirin use was associated with reduced all-cause mortality (2.5% vs 6.5%) and cardiac death (1.6% vs 5.4%) compared with non-users. These differences were not explained by imbalances in predictors of postinfarction risk or therapy other than aspirin and they persisted at least two years after enrollment.

Given its designation as a coronary disease equivalent [35], the presence of diabetes mellitus is of sufficient risk to warrant the use of long-term aspirin therapy especially for patients with known CV disease. Long-term treatment with aspirin has been associated with a significant, 5% absolute reduction in cardiac mortality in patients with diabetes and a 2% absolute reduction for non-diabetic patients with coronary artery disease compared with non-aspirin users [36].

The long-term clinical benefit derived from aspirin appears to be relatively independent of dose. In the Antithrombotic Trialists' Collaboration, the most widely tested regimen in the secondary prevention trials was 'medium dose' aspirin (75–325 mg/day). Neither higher aspirin doses nor other antiplatelet drugs were more effective than daily aspirin in this dose range [33]. Aspirin at a dose of 75–150 mg/day was as effective as a dose of 150–325 mg/day. It is noteworthy that lower dose aspirin also facilitates safer long-term use.

Cerebrovascular disease

The Antiplatelet Trialists' Collaboration evaluated the efficacy of antiplatelet therapy, primarily with aspirin, in 21 randomized trials involving 18,270 patients with a prior stroke or TIA [33]. Antiplatelet therapy resulted in the avoidance of 36 events per 1000 patients with a previous stroke or TIA treated for two years. This benefit of aspirin was similar to that seen in a previous meta-analysis that assessed low- (50–100 mg), medium- (250–500 mg) and high-dose (>1000 mg) aspirin in patients with a prior stroke or TIA [37]. A 13% relative risk reduction in vascular events was seen in patients on aspirin, irrespective of the daily dose. Consistent with the observations in patients with CVD taking aspirin for secondary prevention, higher doses were associated with greater toxicity.

Peripheral arterial disease

Patients with peripheral arterial disease are considered to be at high risk for future vascular events [38]. Thus, it is not surprising that the use of antiplatelet therapy in this patient population is associated with decreased risk of future vascular events. Overall, among 9214 patients with peripheral arterial disease in 42 trials there was a proportional reduction of 23% in serious vascular events (p-value = 0.004), with similar benefits among patients with intermittent claudication, those having peripheral grafting and those having peripheral angioplasty [33].

MANAGEMENT OF ACUTE ATHEROTHROMBOTIC DISORDERS

Aspirin use for PCI

Since the initial percutaneous intervention in the late 1970s, PCI has evolved at a dramatic pace. Through advances in technology, together with improved availability and an enhanced understanding of adjunctive medicines, PCI has evolved into the treatment of choice for obstructive CAD. The use of antiplatelet and antithrombotic agents during PCI serves to prevent complications at the site of PCI and, ultimately, to improve the clinical outcome. Aspirin has maintained an important role as a key antiplatelet agent during the evolution of PCI.

Although unsuccessful in achieving its original goal, to reduce restenosis following PCI [39–41], the use of aspirin has evolved mainly to decrease the incidence of peri-procedural ischemic complications [40, 42] and to improve overall prognosis in those patients with CAD [43] (Table 2.2). In a study of 376 patients undergoing elective PCI, aspirin (990 mg/day) combined with dipyridamole (225 mg/day) had no significant effect on the primary endpoint of restenosis [39]. However, a significant decrease in peri-procedural MI was noted. That the addition of an outmoded therapy, dipyridamole, to aspirin did not improve clinical outcomes in patients undergoing elective PCI [44] contributed to the elimination of dipyridamole from the adjunctive armamentarium. However, the benefit of dual antiplatelet therapy following PCI in the present era has been unequivocally demonstrated when aspirin is combined with a thienopyridine (Chapter 3).

Aspirin Use for Acute STEMI

Rupture of an atherosclerotic plaque with the resultant adhesion of circulating platelets, elaboration of coagulants such as thrombin, and the generation of cross-linked fibrin can culminate in occlusion of the coronary artery, clinically represented by acute STEMI. The essential feature of the management of STEMI is rapid and complete restoration of antegrade blood flow. In order to achieve this, the three integral components of an occlusive thrombus, platelets, thrombin and fibrin, need to be adequately targeted. Fibrinolytic therapy, however, targets only one of these components, fibrin, and is therefore incapable of restoring antegrade blood flow in a substantial proportion of patients. In addition, these agents release clot-bound thrombin, accentuating the prothrombotic milieu via platelet activation [45]. Given this prothrombotic milieu, adjunctive therapies targeting both thrombin and platelets seem essential [46]. Aspirin has served as an integral adjunct to reperfusion therapy of acute STEMI.

The pivotal role of aspirin in the management of patients with acute STEMI was established in the ISIS-II trial [47]. Compared to placebo, aspirin (160 mg/day for 30 days) reduced mortality five weeks after MI by 23%, a risk reduction similar to that of streptokinase (SK) alone (25% reduction). Furthermore, the combination of aspirin and SK appeared to have an additive benefit on mortality (42% reduction). The beneficial effect of aspirin in this setting also resides in its ability to decrease the risk of re-occlusion following fibrinolytic therapy [48]. These data have contributed to establishing aspirin as the backbone of antiplatelet therapy for the treatment of STEMI.

The importance of aspirin in the treatment of acute STEMI can be emphasized by an understanding of its benefits in the Antiplatelet Trialists' Collaboration overview [33]. Allocation to a mean duration of one month of antiplatelet therapy resulted in 38 fewer serious vascular events per 1000 treated patients in 19,288 patients with suspected acute MI in 15 trials. This reflects large and highly significant reductions in non-fatal reinfarction (13 fewer/1000; p-value <0.0001) and in vascular death (23 fewer/1000; p-value <0.0001), together with

Table 2.2 Selected trials of the effect of antiplatelet therapy on outcomes after PCI

Study	Study type	*N*	Patient population	Treatment	Outcome assessed	Placebo event rate (%)	Treatment event rate (%)	*p*-value	Comment
Schwartz *et al.* [39]	RCT	187	Elective PCI	Aspirin, 330 mg tid + dipyridamole, 75 mg tid	Restenosis (primary endpoint)	38.6	37.7	NS	The benefit of peri-procedural antiplatelet therapy was seen with less MI
		189		Placebo	Peri-procedural MI	6.9	1.6	0.0113	
Barnathan *et al.* [90]	Observational study	121	All patients undergoing PCI	No aspirin	Clinically significant thrombosis at PCI	10.7			The lack of adequate antiplatelet therapy was most closely related to the formation of clinically significant thrombus
		110		Aspirin			1.8	0.005	
		32		Aspirin + dipyridamole			0	0.04	
White *et al.* [91]	RCT	110	Elective PCI	Placebo	Immediate procedural complications: Abrupt closure, thrombosis, major dissection	14		< 0.005	Study published in abstract form
		111		Aspirin 325 mg bid + dipyridamole 75 mg tid			5		
		112		Ticlopidine 250 mg tid			2		

Lembo *et al.* [44]	RCT	115	Elective PCI	Aspirin 325 mg tid (G1)	Q-wave MI	NA	1.7 (G1)	4.3 (G2)	NS	Addition of dipyridamole to aspirin as pretreatment of patients undergoing PTCA did not significantly reduce acute complica- tions compared to aspirin alone
					Emergency CABG		2.6 (G1)	6.1 (G2)	(LNS)	
		117		Aspirin 325 mg tid + dipyridamole 75 mg tid (G2)	D		$n = 1$ (G2)			
Knudtson *et al.* [92]	RCT	136	Elective PCI	Placebo	Restenosis (primary endpoint)	32	27		NS	All patients received aspirin plus dipyridamole
		134		Prostacyclin × 48 h	Acute vessel closure	10.3	3.0		<0.01	
					Ventricular arrhythmias	3.4	0		<0.05	

Table 2.2 (*Continued*)

Study	Study type	*N*	Patient population	Treatment	Outcome assessed	Placebo event rate (%)	Treatment event rate (%)	*p*-value	Comment
Taylor *et al.* [93]	RCT	216	Elective PCI	Placebo	Restenosis at 6 months	43	35	NS	Restenosis occurred in 42 of 168 (25%) aspirin- and 51 of 135 (38%) placebo-treated lesions (p-value <0.025)
				Aspirin 100 mg daily					
Savage *et al.* [40]	RCT	752	Elective PCI	Placebo	D/MI/Restenosis with RA or need for revascularization at 6 months	41			Neither active treatment differed significantly from placebo in the rate of angiographic restenosis: 39% (73 of 188) in the aspirin-assigned group, 53% (100 of 189) in the sulotroban group, and 43% (85 of 196) in the placebo group
				Aspirin 325 mg daily			30	0.046	
				Sulotroban 800 mg qid			44		

bid = twice daily; D = death; G1 = group 1; G2 = group 2; NA = not applicable; PTCA = percutaneous transluminal coronary angioplasty; qid = four times daily; RA = refractory angina; tid = three times daily a small but significant reduction in non-fatal stroke (2 fewer/1000; p-value = 0.02). The net benefit was substantially larger than the excess risk of major extracranial bleeding.

The beneficial effects of aspirin have also been shown to be durable over the long term as demonstrated by the decrease of 36 vascular events per 1000 patients with a prior MI treated over a mean of two years [33]. This benefit was also achieved over a range of aspirin doses, the most widely used being between 75 mg and 325 mg daily. However, a dose of 75 mg to 150 mg per day may afford optimal benefit while limiting toxicity [33] which, in the company of potent anticoagulants, can be devastating.

Aspirin Use for Acute Coronary Syndromes

Four randomized trials have evaluated the efficacy of aspirin in the management of patients with UA/NSTEMI (Table 2.3). Several observations regarding the use of aspirin in this setting can be made.

- Short-term aspirin use provides a readily evident and durable benefit in patients with UA/NSTEMI [49].
- Long-term aspirin use following presentation with an ACS is safe and effective.
- Aspirin combined with UH given by continuous intravenous infusion provides an additive benefit with a slightly increased risk of bleeding [52].
- The benefit of aspirin use combined with UH relates to the attenuation of reactivation events that occur following cessation of UH therapy [52].

When analyzed in totality, antiplatelet therapy, primarily with aspirin, is associated with a significant 46% reduction in the combined endpoint of subsequent non-fatal MI, non-fatal stroke or vascular death (8.0% vs 13.3% in patients without antiplatelet therapy) [33]. Recent data suggest that combined therapy with clopidogrel may be more beneficial than aspirin therapy alone (Chapter 3) [53].

As with the use of aspirin in other atherothrombotic disorders, the optimal dose of aspirin for the treatment of UA/NSTEMI remains incompletely defined. However, based on the available data, an initial loading dose of 162 mg to 325 mg should be given as soon as possible to these patients [54]. Thereafter, a dose of 75 mg to 150 mg daily may provide optimal efficacy with limited toxicity [33].

Given the pervasive nature of atherothrombotic disorders and the associated beneficial effects of aspirin, it is very common to encounter patients presenting with an ACS who are already taking aspirin. In these cases, the prior use of aspirin has been associated with both favorable and unfavorable effects. A non-randomized evaluation of more than 11,000 patients with and without a history of CAD enrolled in the Global Registry of Acute Coronary Events (GRACE) revealed a lower likelihood of presenting with a STEMI as well as reductions in in-hospital mortality (3.1% vs 7.1%) and the development of heart failure or pulmonary edema (15.7% vs 22%) with prior aspirin use [55]. Similarly, in a careful review of 539 consecutive patients admitted for an ACS, the 214 who were taking aspirin were significantly less likely to have an MI (24% vs 54% in those not taking aspirin) and, among those who had an MI, were less likely to have a STEMI (62% vs 76%) [56]. A proposed mechanism for these beneficial effects has been a lower thrombus burden at the site of plaque rupture with prior aspirin use.

Table 2.3 Trials of aspirin in ACS

Study	*N*	Study type	Treatment	Outcome assessed	Placebo event rate (%)	Treatment event rate (%)	*p*-value	Comment
VA Cooperative Study [49]	1266	RCT	Placebo Aspirin 324 mg daily × 12 weeks	Death and MI	10.1	5.0	0.0005	The reduction in mortality in the aspirin group was also 51% (1.6% vs 3.3%, *p*-value = 0.054). No difference in GI toxicity or bleeding. Mortality benefit of aspirin persisted at 1 year (5.5% vs 9.6%, *p*-value = 0.008)
Canadian Multicenter Trial [50]	555	RCT	Placebo Aspirin 325 mg qid Sulfinpyrazone 200 mg qid Aspirin 325 mg + sulfinpyrazone 200 mg qid	Death and MI	17.0	8.6 (for groups receiving aspirin)	0.008	Patients were followed for 2 years. There was no observed benefit of sulfinpyrazone for any outcome event, and there was no evidence of an interaction between sulfinpyrazone and aspirin
RISC Group [51]	796	RCT	Placebo Aspirin 75 mg daily IV UH qid × 5 days Aspirin 75 mg daily + IV UH qid × 5 days	Death and MI	17.1	6.5	<0.0001	The risk of MI and death was reduced by aspirin. After 5 days the risk ratio was 0.43 (confidence intervals, 0.21–0.91), at 1 month 0.31 (0.18–0.53), and at 3 months 0.36 (0.23–0.57). The combination of aspirin and UH had the same benefit as aspirin alone. Benefits persisted with continued aspirin for 1 year

Theroux [52]	479	RCT	Placebo	RA	23.0			There were too few deaths overall to permit evaluation of the effect of treatment on this endpoint. The combination of aspirin and heparin had no greater protective effect than heparin alone but was associated with slightly more serious bleeding (3.3% vs 1.7%)
			Aspirin 325 mg bid	MI	11.9	3.0 (Aspirin)	0.012	
						0.8 (UH)	<0.001	
			UH 1000 U/h			1.6 (Aspirin + UH)	0.003	
			Aspirin 325 mg bid + UH 1000 U/h	Death	1.7			

bid = twice daily; GI = gastrointestinal; qid = four times daily

In contrast to the studies mentioned above, non-randomized comparisons from clinical trials of patients with UA/NSTEMI have also found an increased risk of adverse events with recent (within seven days of the incident) aspirin use [57, 58]. Although less likely to have an enrollment MI, prior aspirin users enrolled in the Platelet IIb/IIIa in Unstable angina: Receptor Suppression Using Integrilin Therapy (PURSUIT) trial were more likely to have death or MI at 30 days (16.1% vs 13.0%, p-value = 0.001) and at 6 months (19.9% vs 15.9%, p-value = 0.001) [57]. The effect of prior aspirin use is also one of the seven adverse predictors in the Thrombolysis in Myocardial Infarction (TIMI) risk score in these patients [59].

The most likely explanation for the observed higher rate of adverse events in some studies is that development of an acute coronary syndrome *despite* ongoing aspirin use may be a sign of more severe underlying vascular disease in these patients. One retrospective study of patients presenting with UA/NSTEMI revealed a higher likelihood of a prior MI (59% vs 30%) and of prior coronary revascularization (49% vs 23%) in patients taking aspirin [60].

Aspirin Use for Acute Stroke

When initiated within 48 hours of presentation with an acute stroke, aspirin therapy has been associated with improved outcomes and a decrease in the recurrence of ischemic stroke. Two large randomized trials provide the majority of the insight with respect to aspirin use in this setting [61, 62]. The Chinese Acute Stroke Trial (CAST) was a large randomized, placebo-controlled trial of the effects of aspirin treatment (160 mg/day) started early after the onset of suspected acute ischemic stroke and continued in hospital for up to four weeks [62]. A significant 14% reduction in the primary endpoint of death from any cause during the four-week treatment period was evident in the 21,106 patients with acute ischemic stroke enrolled in this study. Significantly fewer recurrent ischemic strokes were noted in those allocated to aspirin (1.6% vs 2.1%, $2p = 0.01$) at the expense of a trend towards more hemorrhagic strokes (1.1% vs 0.9%, $2p = \text{NS}$). Ultimately, the other primary endpoint of death or dependency at hospital discharge was slightly reduced by the use of aspirin.

How aspirin and UH would fare in the management of acute stroke was assessed in the International Stroke Trial (IST) [61]. In the IST, 19,435 patients were randomized to aspirin (300 mg/day), subcutaneous UH (5000 or 12,500 U bid), both treatments, or neither, within 48 hours of the onset of symptoms of an acute ischemic stroke. Aspirin-treated patients experienced significant reductions in the 14-day recurrence of ischemic stroke (2.8% vs 3.9%) and in the combined outcome of non-fatal stroke or death (11.3% vs 12.4%). Taken together, CAST and the similarly large IST show reliably that aspirin started early in hospital produces a small but definite net benefit, with about 9 fewer deaths or non-fatal strokes per 1000 in the first few weeks ($2p = 0.001$), and with 13 fewer dead or dependent per 1000 after several weeks to six months of follow-up.

Aspirin use for venous thromboembolic disease

Although a beneficial effect of aspirin in the prophylaxis of DVT after major orthopedic procedures has been suggested [63], further insight into the efficacy of aspirin has revealed a greater risk of VTE with aspirin compared with warfarin [64] or LMWH [65]. Therefore, the use of aspirin as the sole agent for the prophylaxis of VTE cannot be recommended, especially with the availability of safe and effective alternatives.

CLINICAL CONSIDERATIONS

Despite being one of the most comprehensively studied medications available today, understanding of the nuances associated with aspirin use and its beneficial effects in atherothrombotic diseases continues to evolve. Advances in the understanding of several areas relating to the use of aspirin in the prevention and treatment of atherothrombotic disorders continue to surface even after more than 100 years of use. Importantly in the cardiovascular arena, the issues of 'aspirin resistance,' optimal dosing strategies, toxicity and potential drug interactions remains active research interests.

Aspirin Resistance

Although aspirin use has been associated with a reduction in the risk of vascular events across a broad range of 'high-risk' patients, its beneficial effects are less than uniform [33]. Aspirin fails to prevent the majority of vascular events in patients with symptomatic atherothrombosis. Given the multifactorial nature of atherothrombosis and the possibility that platelet-mediated thrombosis may not be responsible for all vascular events, it is not surprising that only a fraction (~25%) of all vascular complications can be prevented by any single preventive strategy. Although the mechanisms involved in aspirin resistance are not well understood, plausible explanations for this 'treatment failure,' ranging from suboptimal prescribing of aspirin to good-candidate patients, patient non-compliance and a non-atherothrombotic etiology of the vascular events to alternative pathways of platelet activation and aberrant genetic mechanisms, have been proposed (Table 2.4). Despite a still-evolving correlation with clinical outcomes, the phenomenon of 'aspirin resistance' appears to be a multifactorial entity.

Laboratory tests of platelet function

A definition of aspirin resistance has been the inability of aspirin to produce a specific effect on tests of platelet function (Table 2.5). Although the interpatient variability of aspirin's effects on each of these laboratory tests has been demonstrated, the clinical significance of this 'biochemical' aspirin resistance has yet to be assessed in a prospective randomized trial with an appropriate control arm (e.g. other antiplatelet medications). Nevertheless, information regarding some specific characteristics of aspirin resistance has been gleaned from these laboratory evaluations of platelet function. 'A number of studies have suggested that the laboratory techniques assessing the effects of aspirin on platelet function – the optical platelet aggregation study [66], the semi-automated Accumetrics® device [67] and a test that assesses thromboxane generation (urinary 11-dehydrothromboxane B2) [68] – are useful.'

Association of aspirin resistance and clinical outcomes

The correlation between *ex vivo* aspirin responsiveness and clinical outcomes has identified a broad prevalence (5% to 75%) of biochemically aspirin-resistant patients and has been met with varied clinical correlations. Variable platelet responsiveness to aspirin has been seen in patients with cerebrovascular disease, with recurrent events more likely to occur in those who develop aspirin resistance over time, despite increased doses [69, 70]. However,

Table 2.4 Possible explanations for a diminished benefit of aspirin therapy

Potential explanation
Non-atherothrombotic causes of vascular events
Embolic phenomena
Arteritis
Arterial Dissection (rare)
Patient non-compliance – Not taking aspirin
Inadequate aspirin dose
Co-ingestion of drugs that interfere with the antithrombotic effects of aspirin
Ibuprofen [77]
Alternate pathways of platelet activation
Erythrocyte-induced platelet activation [94, 95]
Increased sensitivity of platelets to collagen and ADP [96]
Enhanced platelet aggregation with increased levels of catecholamines [97, 98]
Extra-platelet production of TXA2 (monocyte/macrophage COX-2) [99]
Smoking
Increased platelet turnover (e.g. post-operative states)
Genetic polymorphisms
COX-1 [100]
COX-2 up-regulation [101]
PLA1/A2 [102]

PLA1/A2 = GP IIIa receptor polymorphism; TXA2 = thromboxane A2

in patients with cerebral ischemia a 40 mg dose of aspirin was found to suppress platelet aggregation responses to the extent observed with higher dosage aspirin [71]. Furthermore, 75 mg aspirin daily resulted in consistently reduced platelet aggregation without attenuation during long-term treatment in patients with ACS [72]. The discrepancy in the findings can be partially related to the limitations of the various biochemical tests used to identify the 'aspirin-resistant' patients in each trial (Table 2.5).

That aspirin-resistant thromboxane biosynthesis [68] and optical platelet aggregation [66] could be used to identify aspirin-resistant patients has been demonstrated. Although an independent and significant linear association was seen between increasing baseline urinary concentrations of 11-dehydrothromboxane B2 (a marker of *in vivo* thromboxane generation) and increasing risk of future MI or cardiovascular death in patients at high vascular risk treated with aspirin [68], this study was limited by an incomplete assessment of compliance with aspirin therapy as well as a lack of information on potential drug interactions that could contribute to aspirin resistance.

In a study designed to determine the association of aspirin resistance with clinical events, Gum and colleagues assessed aspirin sensitivity by optical platelet aggregation using ADP and arachidonic acid (AA) in 326 stable cardiovascular patients on aspirin (325 mg/day for $\geq$7 days) [66]. Although this study was limited by few endpoint events, the 5% of the patients who were deemed aspirin resistant were more likely to experience a clinical ischemic event over almost two years of follow-up.

Although clinical data continue to accrue relating aspirin resistance, assessed by currently available laboratory tests [73], with increased adverse events, the lack of a uniformly reliable test and adequate treatments limit the diagnostic and management options. These limitations preclude the routine assessment of patients for their responsiveness to aspirin.

Table 2.5 Selected laboratory tests of aspirin's effects on platelets

Laboratory test	Advantages	Limitations
Platelet aggregation		
Optical platelet aggregation	Widely available Correlated with clinical events [66]	Labor intensive Operator dependent Interpreter dependent Lacks specificity Not highly reproducible
Semi-automated platelet aggregation (PFA-100, Ultegra RPFA)	Rapid Easy to perform Correlated with clinical events [67, 103]	Lacks specificity Not highly reproducible
Skin bleeding time	Easy to perform Widely available	Lacks sensitivity and specificity Not strongly correlated with clinical events Not highly reproducible Operator dependent
Thromboxane generation	Linear correlation with clinical events [68]	Not widely available Sensitivity and specificity remain suboptimally evaluated

Optimal dose of aspirin

A key issue in the use of aspirin relates to the optimal dosing for various clinical situations. The results of biochemical studies on its mechanism of action, the lack of a dose–response relationship in clinical studies evaluating its antithrombotic effects and the dose dependence of its side effects all support the use of as low a dose of aspirin as has been found to be effective in the treatment of various thromboembolic disorders [74–76] (Table 2.6).

It has been suggested that aspirin doses lower than 75 mg daily may have a greater protective effect as a result of prostacyclin sparing [15]. However, when doses less than 75 mg and those greater than or equal to 75 mg were compared in 3570 patients, no significant

Table 2.6 Clinical conditions and minimum effective dose of aspirin studied. Adapted from Patrono *et al.* [104]

Clinical condition	Aspirin dose (mg)	Higher doses more effective? (Y/N)
High-risk men	75	NA
Hypertension	75	NA
Stable angina	75	NA
ACS	75	N
STEMI	160	NA
History of TIA or stroke	50	N
Acute ischemic stroke	160	N
Carotid artery disease	75	N

NA = not assessed

Table 2.7A Direct comparison of the effects of different doses of aspirin on vascular events in high-risk patients. Adapted from Antiplatelet Trialists' Collaboration [33]

Aspirin dose compared (mg)	*N*	Number of trials	Odds reduction (%)
500–1500 vs 75–325	3197	7	3 ± 10
$\geq$75 vs <75	3570	3	-8 ± 10
Subtotal	6767	10	-3 ± 7

p-value = NS for all comparisons

Table 2.7B Odds reduction of vascular events in high-risk patients with different doses of aspirin: indirect comparison. Adapted from Antiplatelet Trialists' Collaboration [33]

Aspirin dose (mg)	*N*	Number of trials	Odds reduction (%)
500–1500	22,451	34	19 ± 3
160–325	26,513	19	26 ± 3
75–150	6,676	12	32 ± 6
<75	3,655	3	19 ± 8*
Any aspirin	58,395	65	23 ± 2

**p*-value = NS

differences in outcomes were observed (Table 2.7A) [33]. One caveat regarding the actual efficacy of dosing regimens less than 75 mg daily rests with the fact that this regimen has been infrequently assessed and therefore some uncertainty remains with respect to these extremely low doses.

Both direct comparisons of high-versus low-dose aspirin (Table 2.7A) and indirect comparisons of high-versus low-dose aspirin in trials with patients allocated to aspirin or placebo (Table 2.7B) have failed to demonstrate a benefit of high-dose aspirin and have revealed higher bleeding rates [33]. Thus, use of the lowest effective dose of aspirin (i.e. 50 to 150 mg daily for long-term treatment) will optimize the beneficial effects and minimize the toxicity of aspirin.

Selected drug interactions

Interaction with Ibuprofen

The potential interaction between aspirin and ibuprofen was assessed by administering aspirin two hours before ibuprofen or the same medications in reverse order [77]. Serum thromboxane B2 levels (an index of COX-1 activity in platelets) were higher and platelet aggregation was not inhibited when ibuprofen was administered prior to aspirin. On the contrary, thromboxane B2 levels and platelet aggregation were maximally inhibited 24 hours after the administration of aspirin in the subjects who took aspirin before a single daily dose of acetaminophen, diclofenac, or rofecoxib (selective COX-2 inhibitor).

That concomitant treatment with ibuprofen may limit the cardioprotective effects of aspirin was assessed in 7107 patients discharged on low-dose aspirin (<325 mg/day) after their first hospital admission for CV disease [78]. Compared with those who used aspirin alone, patients taking aspirin plus ibuprofen had an increased risk of all-cause mortality (adjusted hazard ratio 1.93, 95% CI 1.30–2.87, p-value = 0.0011) and cardiovascular mortality (1.73, 1.05–2.84, p-value = 0.0305). More recent data casts some doubt on the adverse interaction between ibuprofen and aspirin [79, 80]. Among 70, 316 patients discharged after admission for an MI, 66,739 were discharged on aspirin alone, 844 (1.2%) were discharged on aspirin and ibuprofen and 2733 (3.9%) were discharged on aspirin and another NSAID. Multivariable modeling revealed a similar risk of death among patients regardless of discharge regimen. A recent nested case-control study further supports the lack of an adverse interaction between ibuprofen, other non-steroidal anti-inflammatory drugs (NSAID), and aspirin [80].

Although the mechanism of ibuprofen's adverse interaction is incompletely understood, the available data suggests that it may interfere with aspirin's interaction with its target site on cyclooxygenase. This interaction appears to occur primarily when ibuprofen is administered prior to aspirin and not vice versa, although with chronic ibuprofen therapy interaction may occur regardless of the sequence of dosing. Despite the conflicting data regarding the aspirin/ibuprofen interaction, it seems prudent to use an alternative NSAID to ibuprofen if needed in patients at high risk of vascular events.

Interaction with ACE inhibitors

IHD remains the most common underlying cause of congestive heart failure, and thus aspirin and ACE inhibitors are commonly used together for treatment in this setting. Currently, it is perceived that a significant component of the beneficial effect of ACE inhibitors is related to augmentation of bradykinin levels, which among other effects stimulate the release of prostacyclin [81]. The prostaglandins play an important vasodilatory role and counteract the enhanced peripheral vasoconstriction state in congestive heart failure. Aspirin, on the other hand, inhibits the production of prostacyclin by blocking cyclooxygenase. Although the mechanism of an adverse interaction between ACE inhibitors and aspirin has been thought to be related to the counteracting effect of aspirin on the augmentation of prostacyclin synthesis by ACE inhibitors, a recent study has called this into question by demonstrating no effect on the vasodilator response to bradykinin or substance P with concomitant therapy [82].

The issue of possible attenuation of the effect of angiotensin-converting enzyme (ACE) inhibitors by ASA has been an area of intense debate. Whereas several animal [83] and human [84, 85] studies have demonstrated an attenuation of the beneficial effects of ACE inhibitors with concomitant aspirin use, an equal number refute the interaction [86–88]. A systematic review of over 22,000 patients revealed that the beneficial effects of ACE inhibitor use in patients with CV disease were more evident in patients given concomitant aspirin [89]. Thus, in order to optimize patient outcomes, both ACE inhibitors and aspirin should be prescribed in the absence of contraindications.

2.4 CONCLUSIONS

Since its synthesis in 1897, aspirin has been one of the most thoroughly researched pharmaceutical agents. However, numerous questions have been born out of this research relating to the pharmacology of aspirin, the optimal dosing of aspirin, and to potential interactions with other therapeutic agents. Despite these unanswered questions, aspirin has remained an integral component in the anti-atherothrombotic armamentarium. Nevertheless, there exists a burgeoning field of anti-platelet agents, including but not limited to the thienopyridines (Chapter 3), which target alternative pathways of platelet activation. These agents are being studied as additions and/or alternatives to aspirin in the management of various atherothrombotic diseases. Hopefully, another 100 years won't leave us still asking questions.

REFERENCES

[1] Vane, J.R., (1971) Inhibition of prostaglandin synthesis as a mechanism of action for aspirin-like drugs. *Nat New Biol*, 231(25): 232–5.

[2] Smith, W.L., (1992) Prostanoid biosynthesis and mechanisms of action. *Am J Physiol*, 263(2 Pt 2): F181–91.

[3] FitzGerald, G.A., (1991) Mechanisms of platelet activation: thromboxane A2 as an amplifying signal for other agonists. *Am J Cardiol* 68(7): 11B-15B.

[4] Polgar, J., *et al.*, (1998) Adenosine diphosphate (ADP) and ADP receptor play a major role in platelet activation/aggregation induced by sera from heparin-induced thrombocytopenia patients. *Blood*, 91(2): 549–54.

[5] Roberts, D.E., McNicol, A., Bose, R., (2004) Mechanism of collagen activation in human platelets. *J Biol Chem*, 279(19): 19421–30.

[6] Roth, G.J., Stanford, N., Majerus, P.W., (1975) Acetylation of prostaglandin synthase by aspirin. *Proc Natl Acad Sci USA*, 72(8): 3073–6.

[7] Hoak, J.C., (1983) Mechanisms of action: aspirin. *Thromb Res* Suppl, 4: 47–51.

[8] Mitchell, J.A., *et al.*, (1993) Selectivity of nonsteroidal antiinflammatory drugs as inhibitors of constitutive and inducible cyclooxygenase. *Proc Natl Acad Sci USA*, 90(24): 11693–7.

[9] Clarke, R.J., *et al.*, (1991) Suppression of thromboxane A_2 but not of systemic prostacyclin by controlled-release aspirin. *N Eng J Med*, 325: 1137–41.

[10] Ridker, P.M., *et al.*, (2005) C-reactive protein levels and outcomes after statin therapy. *N Eng J Med*, 352(1): 20–8.

[11] Ikonomidis, I., *et al.*, (1999) Increased proinflammatory cytokines in patients with chronic stable angina and their reduction by aspirin. *Circulation*, 100: 793–8.

[12] Ridker, P.M., *et al.*, (1997) Inflammation, aspirin, and the risk of cardiovascular disease in apparently healthy men. *N Eng J Med*, 336: 973–9.

[13] Kennon, S., *et al.*, (2001) The effect of aspirin on C-reactive protein as a marker of risk in unstable angina. *J Am Coll Cardiol*, 37(5): 1266–70.

[14] Patrignani, P., Filabozzi, P., Patrono, C., (1982) Selective cumulative inhibition of platelet thromboxane production by low-dose aspirin in healthy subjects. *J Clin Invest*, 69(6): 1366–72.

[15] Patrono, C., *et al.*, (1985) Clinical pharmacology of platelet cyclooxygenase inhibition. *Circulation*, 72(6): 1177–84.

[16] Patrono, C., *et al.*, (1986) Estimated rate of thromboxane secretion into the circulation of normal humans. *J Clin Invest*, 77(2): 590–4.

[17] Weksler, B.B., *et al.*, (1983) Differential inhibition by aspirin of vascular and platelet prostaglandin synthesis in atherosclerotic patients. *N Eng J Med*, 308(14): 800–5.

[18] Pedersen, A.K., FitzGerald, A., (1984) Dose-related kinetics of aspirin. Presystemic acetylation of platelet cyclooxygenase. *N Eng J Med*, 311(19): 1206–11.

[19] McAdam, B., *et al.*, (1996) Transdermal modification of platelet function: an aspirin patch system results in marked suppression of platelet cyclooxygenase. *J Pharmacol Exp Ther*, 277(2): 559–64.

[20] Burch, J.W., Stanford, N., Majerus, P.W., (1978) Inhibition of platelet prostaglandin synthetase by oral aspirin. *J Clin Invest*, 61(2): 314–19.

[21] Hammond, E.C., Garfinkel, L., (1975) Aspirin and coronary heart disease: findings of a prospective study. *Br Med J*, 2(5965): 269–71.

[22] Jick, H., Miettinen, O.S., (1976) Regular aspirin use and myocardial infarction. *Br Med J*, 1(6017): 1057.

[23] Manson, J.E., *et al.*, (1991) A prospective study of aspirin use and primary prevention of cardiovascular disease in women. *JAMA*, 266(4): 521–7.

[24] Peto, R., *et al.*, (1988) Randomised trial of prophylactic daily aspirin in British male doctors. *Br Med J* (Clin Res Ed), 296(6618): 313–16.

[25] Steering Committee of the Physicians' Health Study Research Group. (1989) Final report on the aspirin component of the ongoing Physicians' Health Study. *N Eng J Med*, 321(3): 129–35.

[26] Antithrombotic Trialists' Collaboration, (1998) Thrombosis prevention trial: randomised trial of low-intensity oral anticoagulation with warfarin and low-dose aspirin in the primary prevention of ischaemic heart disease in men at increased risk. The Medical Research Council's General Practice Research Framework. *Lancet*, 351(9098): 233–41.

[27] de Gaetano, G., (2001) Low-dose aspirin and vitamin E in people at cardiovascular risk: a randomised trial in general practice. Collaborative Group of the Primary Prevention Project. *Lancet*, 357(9250): 89–95.

[28] Hansson, L., *et al.*, (1998) Effects of intensive blood-pressure lowering and low-dose aspirin in patients with hypertension: principal results of the Hypertension Optimal Treatment (HOT) randomised trial. HOT Study Group. *Lancet*, 351(9118): 1755–62.

[29] Juul-Moller, S., *et al.*, (1992) Double-blind trial of aspirin in primary prevention of myocardial infarction in patients with stable chronic angina pectoris. The Swedish Angina Pectoris Aspirin Trial (SAPAT) Group. *Lancet*, 340(8833): 1421–5.

[30] Ridker, P.M., *et al.*, (2005) A Randomized Trial of Low-Dose Aspirin in the Primary Prevention of Cardiovascular Disease in Women. *N Eng J Med*, 352 (13):1293–304

[31] Sanmuganathan, P.S., *et al.*, (2001) Aspirin for primary prevention of coronary heart disease: safety and absolute benefit related to coronary risk derived from meta-analysis of randomised trials. *Heart*, 85(3): 265–71.

[32] Hayden, M., *et al.*, (2002) Aspirin for the primary prevention of cardiovascular events: a summary of the evidence for the U.S. Preventive Services Task Force. *Ann Intern Med*, 136(2): 161–72.

[33] Collaborative meta-analysis of randomised trials of antiplatelet therapy for prevention of death, myocardial infarction, and stroke in high risk patients, (2002) *Br Med J*, 324(7329): 71–86.

[34] Goldstein, R.E., *et al.*, (1996) Marked reduction in long-term cardiac deaths with aspirin after a coronary event. Multicenter Myocardial Ischemia Research Group. *J Am Coll Cardiol*, 28(2): 326–30.

[35] The National Cholesterol Education Program (NCEP) Expert Panel, (2001) Executive Summary of The Third Report of The National Cholesterol Education Program (NCEP) Expert Panel on Detection, Evaluation, And Treatment of High Blood Cholesterol In Adults (Adult Treatment Panel III). *JAMA*, 285(19): 2486–97.

[36] Harpaz, D., *et al.*, (1998) Effects of aspirin treatment on survival in non-insulin-dependent diabetic patients with coronary artery disease. Israeli Bezafibrate Infarction Prevention Study Group. *Am J Med*, 105(6): 494–9.

[37] Tijssen, J.G., (1998) Low-dose and high-dose acetylsalicylic acid, with and without dipyridamole: a review of clinical trial results. *Neurology*, 51(3 Suppl 3): S15–16.

[38] Chiu, J.H., *et al.*, (2003) Peripheral vascular disease and one-year mortality following percutaneous coronary revascularization. *Am J Cardiol*, 92(5): 582–3.

[39] Schwartz, L., *et al.*, (1988) Aspirin and dipyridamole in the prevention of restenosis after percutaneous transluminal coronary angioplasty. *N Eng J Med*, 318(26): 1714–9.

[40] Savage, M.P., *et al.*, (1995) Effect of thromboxane A2 blockade on clinical outcome and restenosis after successful coronary angioplasty. Multi-Hospital Eastern Atlantic Restenosis Trial (M-HEART II). *Circulation*, 92(11): 3194–200.

[41] Kastrati, A., *et al.*, (1997) Restenosis after coronary stent placement and randomization to a 4–week combined antiplatelet or anticoagulant therapy: six-month angiographic follow-up of the Intracoronary Stenting and Antithrombotic Regimen (ISAR) Trial. *Circulation*, 96(2): 462–7.

[42] Barry, W.L., Sarembock, I.J., (1994) Antiplatelet and anticoagulant therapy in patients undergoing percutaneous transluminal coronary angioplasty. Cardiol Clin, 12(3): 517–35.

[43] Wallentin, L.C., (1991) Aspirin (75 mg/day) after an episode of unstable coronary artery disease: long-term effects on the risk for myocardial infarction, occurrence of severe angina and the need for revascularization. Research Group on Instability in Coronary Artery Disease in Southeast Sweden. *J Am Coll Cardiol*, 18(7): 1587–93.

[44] Lembo, N.J., *et al.*, (1990) Effect of pretreatment with aspirin versus aspirin plus dipyridamole on frequency and type of acute complications of percutaneous transluminal coronary angioplasty. *Am J Cardiol*, 65(7): 422–6.
[45] Coulter, S.A., *et al.*, (2000) High levels of platelet inhibition with abciximab despite heightened platelet activation and aggregation during thrombolysis for acute myocardial infarction: results from TIMI (thrombolysis in myocardial infarction) 14. *Circulation*, 101(23): 2690–5.
[46] Merlini, P.A., *et al.*, (1995) Thrombin generation and activity during thrombolysis and concomitant heparin therapy in patients with acute myocardial infarction. *J Am Coll Cardiol*, 25(1): 203–9.
[47] ISIS-2 (Second International Study of Infarct Survival) Collaborative Group, (1988) Randomised trial of intravenous streptokinase, oral aspirin, both, or neither among 17,187 cases of suspected acute myocardial infarction: ISIS-2. *Lancet*, 2(8607): 349–60.
[48] Roux, S., Christeller, S., Ludin, E., (1992) Effects of aspirin on coronary reocclusion and recurrent ischemia after thrombolysis: a meta-analysis. *J Am Coll Cardiol*, 19(3): p. 671–7.
[49] Lewis, H.D., Jr., *et al.*, (1983) Protective effects of aspirin against acute myocardial infarction and death in men with unstable angina. Results of a Veterans Administration Cooperative Study. *N Eng J Med*, 309(7): 396–403.
[50] Cairns, J.A., *et al.*, (1985) Aspirin, sulfinpyrazone, or both in unstable angina. Results of a Canadian multicenter trial. *N Eng J Med*, 313(22): 1369–75.
[51] The RISC Group, (1990) Risk of myocardial infarction and death during treatment with low dose aspirin and intravenous heparin in men with unstable coronary artery disease. *Lancet*, 336(8719): 827–30.
[52] Theroux, P., *et al.*, (1988) Aspirin, heparin, or both to treat acute unstable angina. *N Eng J Med*, 319(17): 1105–11.
[53] Yusuf, S., *et al.*, (2001) Effects of clopidogrel in addition to aspirin in patients with acute coronary syndromes without ST-segment elevation. *N Eng J Med*, 345(7): 494–502.
[54] Braunwald, E., *et al.*, (2002) ACC/AHA 2002 guideline update for the management of patients with unstable angina and non-ST-segment elevation myocardial infarction–summary article: a report of the American College of Cardiology/American Heart Association task force on practice guidelines (Committee on the Management of Patients With Unstable Angina). *J Am Coll Cardiol*, 40(7): 1366–74.
[55] Spencer, F.A., *et al.*, (2002) Impact of aspirin on presentation and hospital outcomes in patients with acute coronary syndromes (The Global Registry of Acute Coronary Events [GRACE]). *Am J Cardiol*, 90(10): 1056–61.
[56] Garcia-Dorado, D., *et al.*, (1995) Previous aspirin use may attenuate the severity of the manifestation of acute ischemic syndromes. *Circulation*, 92(7): 1743–8.
[57] Alexander, J.H., *et al.*, (1999) Prior aspirin use predicts worse outcomes in patients with non-ST-elevation acute coronary syndromes. PURSUIT Investigators. Platelet IIb/IIIa in Unstable angina: Receptor Suppression Using Integrilin Therapy. *Am J Cardiol*, 83(8): 1147–51.
[58] Santopinto, J., *et al.*, (2001) Prior aspirin users with acute non-ST-elevation coronary syndromes are at increased risk of cardiac events and benefit from enoxaparin. *Am Heart J*, 141(4): 566–72.
[59] Antman, E.M., *et al.*, (2000) The TIMI risk score for unstable angina/non-ST elevation MI: A method for prognostication and therapeutic decision making. *JAMA*, 284(7): 835–42.
[60] Borzak, S., *et al.*, (1998) Effects of prior aspirin and anti-ischemic therapy on outcome of patients with unstable angina. TIMI 7 Investigators. Thrombin Inhibition in Myocardial Ischemia. *Am J Cardiol*, 81(6): 678–81.
[61] International Stroke Trial Collaborative Group, (1997) The International Stroke Trial (IST): a randomised trial of aspirin, subcutaneous heparin, both, or neither among 19435 patients with acute ischaemic stroke. *Lancet*, 349(9065): 1569–81.
[62] CAST (Chinese Acute Stroke Trial) Collaborative Group, (1997) CAST: randomised placebo-controlled trial of early aspirin use in 20,000 patients with acute ischaemic stroke. *Lancet*, 349(9066): 1641–9.
[63] Antiplatelet Trialists' Collaboration, (1994) Collaborative overview of randomised trials of antiplatelet therapy—III: Reduction in venous thrombosis and pulmonary embolism by antiplatelet prophylaxis among surgical and medical patients. *Br Med J*, 308(6923): 235–46.

[64] Powers, P.J., *et al.*, (1989) A randomized trial of less intense postoperative warfarin or aspirin therapy in the prevention of venous thromboembolism after surgery for fractured hip. *Arch Intern Med*, 149(4): 771–4.
[65] Gent, M., *et al.*, (1996) Low-molecular-weight heparinoid orgaran is more effective than aspirin in the prevention of venous thromboembolism after surgery for hip fracture. *Circulation*, 93(1): 80–4.
[66] Gum, P.A., *et al.*, (2003) A prospective, blinded determination of the natural history of aspirin resistance among stable patients with cardiovascular disease. *J Am Coll Cardiol*, 41(6): 961–5.
[67] Chen, W.H., *et al.*, (2004) Aspirin resistance is associated with a high incidence of myonecrosis after non-urgent percutaneous coronary intervention despite clopidogrel pretreatment. *J Am Coll Cardiol*, 43(6): 1122–6.
[68] Eikelboom, J.W., *et al.*, (2002) Aspirin-resistant thromboxane biosynthesis and the risk of myocardial infarction, stroke, or cardiovascular death in patients at high risk for cardiovascular events. *Circulation*, 105(14): 1650–5.
[69] Helgason, C.M., *et al.*, (1993) Aspirin response and failure in cerebral infarction. *Stroke*, 24(3): 345–50.
[70] Helgason, C.M., *et al.*, (1994) Development of aspirin resistance in persons with previous ischemic stroke. *Stroke*, 25(12): 2331–6.
[71] Weksler, B.B., *et al.*, (1985) Effects of low dose aspirin on platelet function in patients with recent cerebral ischemia. *Stroke*, 16(1): 5–9.
[72] Berglund, U., Wallentin, L., (1991) Persistent inhibition of platelet function during long-term treatment with 75 mg acetylsalicylic acid daily in men with unstable coronary artery disease. *Eur Heart J*, 12(3): 428–33.
[73] Yilmaz, M.B., *et al.*, (2005) Late saphenous vein graft occlusion in patients with coronary bypass: possible role of aspirin resistance. *Thromb Res*, 115(1–2): 25–9.
[74] Roth, G.J., Calverley, D.C., (1994) Aspirin, platelets, and thrombosis: theory and practice. *Blood*, 83(4): 885–98.
[75] Hirsh, J., *et al.*, (1995) Aspirin and other platelet-active drugs. The relationship among dose, effectiveness, and side effects. *Chest*, 108(4 Suppl): 247S-57S.
[76] Patrono, C., *et al.*, (1998) Platelet-active drugs: the relationships among dose, effectiveness, and side effects. *Chest*, 114(5 Suppl): 470S-88S.
[77] Catella-Lawson, F., *et al.*, (2001) Cyclooxygenase inhibitors and the antiplatelet effects of aspirin. *N Eng J Med*, 345(25): 1809–17.
[78] MacDonald, T.M., Wei, L., (2003) Effect of ibuprofen on cardioprotective effect of aspirin. *Lancet*, 361(9357): 573–4.
[79] Curtis, J.P., *et al.*, (2003) Aspirin, ibuprofen, and mortality after myocardial infarction: retrospective cohort study. *Brit Med J*, 327(7427): 1322–3.
[80] Garcia Rodriguez, L.A., *et al.*, (2004) Nonsteroidal antiinflammatory drugs and the risk of myocardial infarction in the general population. *Circulation*, 109(24): 3000–6.
[81] Guazzi, M.D., *et al.*, (1998) Antihypertensive efficacy of angiotensin converting enzyme inhibition and aspirin counteraction. *Clin Pharmacol Ther*, 63(1): 79–86.
[82] Davie, A.P., McMurray, J.J., (2002) Effect of aspirin on vasodilation to bradykinin and substance P in patients with heart failure treated with ACE inhibitor. *Br J Clin Pharmacol*, 53(1): 37–42.
[83] Dubey, K., Balani, D.K. and Pillai, K.K., (2003) Potential adverse interaction between aspirin and lisinopril in hypertensive rats. Hum Exp Toxicol, 22(3): 143–7.
[84] Nguyen, K.N., Aursnes, I., Kjekshus, J., (1997) Interaction between enalapril and aspirin on mortality after acute myocardial infarction: subgroup analysis of the Cooperative New Scandinavian Enalapril Survival Study II (CONSENSUS II). *Am J Cardiol*, 79(2): 115–19.
[85] Peterson, J.G., *et al.*, (2000) Evaluation of the effects of aspirin combined with angiotensin-converting enzyme inhibitors in patients with coronary artery disease. *Am J Med*, 109(5): 371–7.
[86] Leor, J., *et al.*, (1999) Aspirin and mortality in patients treated with angiotensin-converting enzyme inhibitors: a cohort study of 11,575 patients with coronary artery disease. *J Am Coll Cardiol*, 33(7): 1920–5.

[87] Latini, R., *et al.*, (2000) Aspirin does not interact with ACE inhibitors when both are given early after acute myocardial infarction: results of the GISSI-3 Trial. Heart Dis, 2(3): 185–90.

[88] Krumholz, H.M., *et al.*, (2001) Aspirin and angiotensin-converting enzyme inhibitors among elderly survivors of hospitalization for an acute myocardial infarction. *Arch Intern Med*, 161(4): 538–44.

[89] Teo, K.K., *et al.*, (2002) Effects of long-term treatment with angiotensin-converting-enzyme inhibitors in the presence or absence of aspirin: a systematic review. *Lancet*, 360(9339): 1037–43.

[90] Barnathan, E.S., *et al.*, (1987) Aspirin and dipyridamole in the prevention of acute coronary thrombosis complicating coronary angioplasty. *Circulation*, 76(1): 125–34.

[91] White, C., *et al.*, (1987) Antiplatelet agents are effective in reducing the immediate complications of PTCA: results of the ticlopidine multicenter trial [abstract]. *Circulation*, 76: IV–400.

[92] Knudtson, M.L., *et al.*, (1990) Effect of short-term prostacyclin administration on restenosis after percutaneous transluminal coronary angioplasty. *J Am Coll Cardiol*, 15(3): 691–7.

[93] Taylor, R.R., *et al.*, (1991) Effects of low-dose aspirin on restenosis after coronary angioplasty. *Am J Cardiol*, 68(9): 874–8.

[94] Valles, J., *et al.*, (1991) Erythrocytes metabolically enhance collagen-induced platelet responsiveness via increased thromboxane production, adenosine diphosphate release, and recruitment. *Blood*, 78(1): 154–62.

[95] Santos, M.T., *et al.*, (1991) Enhancement of platelet reactivity and modulation of eicosanoid production by intact erythrocytes. A new approach to platelet activation and recruitment. *J Clin Invest*, 87(2): 571–80.

[96] Kawasaki, T., *et al.*, (2000) Increased platelet sensitivity to collagen in individuals resistant to low-dose aspirin. *Stroke*, 31(3): 591–5.

[97] Larsson, P.T., Wallen, N.H., Hjemdahl, P., (1994) Norepinephrine-induced human platelet activation in vivo is only partly counteracted by aspirin. *Circulation*, 89(5): 1951–7.

[98] Hurlen, M., Seljeflot, I., Arnesen, H., (2000) Increased platelet aggregability during exercise in patients with previous myocardial infarction. Lack of inhibition by aspirin. *Thromb Res*, 99(5): 487–94.

[99] Cipollone, F., *et al.*, (1997) Differential suppression of thromboxane biosynthesis by indobufen and aspirin in patients with unstable angina. *Circulation*, 96(4): 1109–16.

[100] Cambria-Kiely, J.A., Gandhi, P.J., (2002) Aspirin resistance and genetic polymorphisms. *J Thromb Thrombolysis*, 14(1): 51–8.

[101] Caughey, G.E., *et al.*, (2001) Roles of cyclooxygenase (COX)-1 and COX-2 in prostanoid production by human endothelial cells: selective up-regulation of prostacyclin synthesis by COX-2. J Immunol, 167(5): 2831–8.

[102] Macchi, L., *et al.*, (2003) Resistance in vitro to low-dose aspirin is associated with platelet PlA1 (GP IIIa) polymorphism but not with C807T(GP Ia/IIa) and C-5T Kozak (GP Ibalpha) polymorphisms. *J Am Coll Cardiol*, 42(6): 1115–19.

[103] Andersen, K., *et al.*, (2002) Aspirin non-responsiveness as measured by PFA-100 in patients with coronary artery disease. *Thromb Res*, 108(1): 37–42.

[104] Patrono, C., *et al.*, (2004) Platelet-active drugs: the relationships among dose, effectiveness, and side effects: the Seventh ACCP Conference on Antithrombotic and Thrombolytic Therapy. *Chest*, 126(3 Suppl): 234S–64S.

3 Thienopyridines – Ticlopidine and Clopidogrel

3.1 INTRODUCTION

The central role of platelets in the pathophysiology of arterial vascular disease has focused attention on the development of effective platelet inhibitor modalities to mitigate the clinical consequences of atherothrombotic disease. Aspirin inhibits platelet cyclooxygenase and the conversion of AA to the potent platelet agonist thromboxane A(2) and has been the gold standard of therapy. Its beneficial effects have been well documented in cerebral, coronary and peripheral arterial disease, with an approximately 25% reduction in MI, stroke and vascular death. However, the known limitations and incomplete platelet inhibition with aspirin have prompted the search for more 'optimal' antiplatelet agents.

The platelet ADP receptor antagonists were developed to further improve the clinical results of antiplatelet therapy with aspirin. Ticlopidine provides an additional 10% relative risk reduction over aspirin alone in stroke prevention and coronary stent placement. However, ticlopidine is accompanied by occasional life-threatening adverse hematological events. The action of clopidogrel is similar to that of ticlopidine, and it is comparably effective with a much more favorable side-effect profile. This chapter will serve to review the pharmacology, the utility across the spectrum of CVD and the evolving limitations of these versatile antiplatelet agents.

3.2 PHARMACOLOGY

ADP AND THROMBOSIS

ADP plays a key role in hemostasis and thrombosis. Several lines of evidence support the role of ADP in both physiologic and pathologic thrombus formation. ADP is contained at high concentrations in the platelet dense granules and is released when platelets are stimulated by other agents, such as thrombin or collagen, thus reinforcing platelet aggregation [1]. As a consequence, inhibitors of ADP-induced platelet aggregation are effective antithrombotic drugs [2]. Furthermore, defects of ADP receptors or an absence of ADP in platelet granules have been associated with bleeding diatheses [1, 3, 4].

Despite its early identification in 1961 as the first known aggregating agent, the molecular basis of ADP-induced platelet activation is only beginning to be understood [5]. ADP released from damaged vessels and red blood cells induces platelet aggregation through activation of the integrin GPIIb-IIIa and subsequent binding of fibrinogen [4]. This occurs through at least two biochemical events resulting from ADP stimulation, a phospholipase C-mediated rise in

Management Strategies in Antithrombotic Therapy Arman T. Askari, Adrian W. Messerli and A. Michael Lincoff

intracellular calcium and a $G_{\alpha i2}$-mediated inhibition of adenylyl cyclase [6]. ADP secreted from platelets on activation also acts in a paracrine fashion, providing positive feedback that potentiates the actions of many platelet activators [4, 7].

ADP RECEPTORS

The platelet response to ADP is mediated by a family of membrane-bound nucleotide receptors called P2 receptors (Figure 3.1). These are further subdivided into P2X ligand-gated 'ionotropic' receptors [8] and P2Y G-protein-linked 'metabotropic' receptors [9–11]. P2X1 induces transmembrane calcium flux in response to ADP but does not play a major role in platelet aggregation and is unaffected by the thienopyridines [8, 12].

The P2Y metabotropic family of ADP receptors has been shown to be essential in mediating ADP-associated platelet aggregation [10]. Seven subtypes of the P2Y receptor have been identified and cloned [13]. Of these, the P2Y1 and P2Y12 receptors are integrally involved in ADP-induced platelet activation and aggregation [10, 11, 14–18]. The P2Y1 receptor mediates the ADP-induced platelet shape change and calcium mobilization essential for platelet aggregation [10, 14, 19]. The P2Y12 receptor, coupled to the inhibition of adenylyl cyclase, is necessary for the full aggregation potential of platelets [5]. Importantly, the activation of platelets through this pathway is independent of that induced by thromboxane

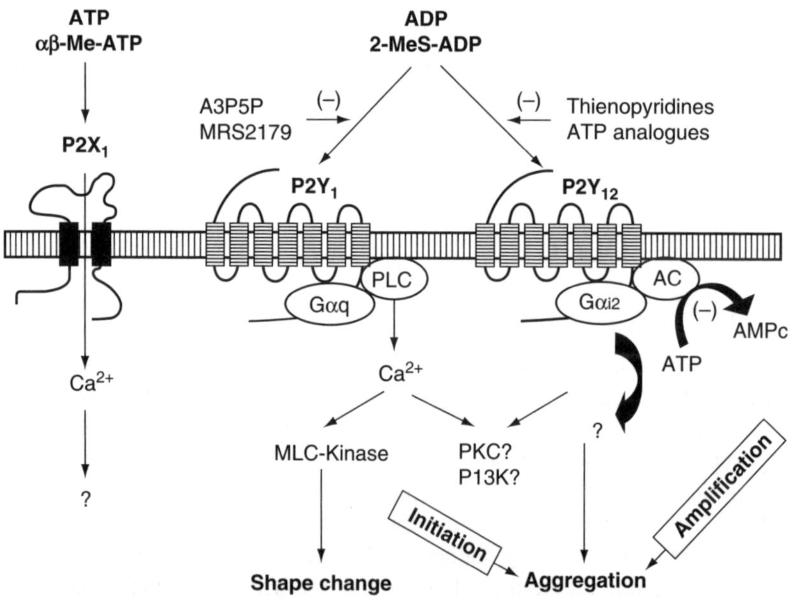

Figure 3.1 Three-receptor model of the ADP-induced platelet aggregation. Two ADP receptors are involved in ADP-induced platelet aggregation; the P2Y1 receptor responsible for intracellular Ca2+ mobilization, shape change, and initiation of aggregation and P2Y12, coupled to adenylyl cyclase inhibition, enhance P2Y1-mediated platelet activation and secretion. P2Y12 is the molecular target of the ADP-specific antiplatelet drug thienopyridines. Both receptors are required for normal platelet aggregation in response to ADP. P2X1 is a receptor responsible for a rapid influx of calcium into the cytosol, but its role in the process of ADP-induced aggregation remains unknown. Adapted from Herbert and Savi [16].

A2. Thus, the utility of medications that target ADP-induced platelet aggregation alone or in addition to agents that inhibit thromboxane-induced platelet activation (i.e. aspirin) is evident [19, 20].

MECHANISM OF ACTION

Anti-thrombotic effects

Ticlopidine and its more recently developed analogue, clopidogrel, are thienopyridine derivatives that inhibit ADP-induced platelet aggregation. Clopidogrel differs structurally from ticlopidine by the addition of a carboxymethyl side group (Figure 3.2), the presence of which provides enhanced pharmacological activity and a better safety profile. The inhibitory effects of ticlopidine and clopidogrel are abolished by increasing the concentration of potential agonists such as collagen and thrombin. This suggests that the thienopyridines also function by inhibiting the ADP-mediated amplification of the platelet response to other agonists [21, 22].

In order to impart their antiplatelet effects, both ticlopidine and clopidogrel require hepatic metabolism to active metabolites [23, 24]. Through these metabolites, clopidogrel and ticlopidine irreversibly inhibit the P2Y12 receptor at its ADP binding site [11, 25]. The irreversible modification of this ADP receptor site could be explained by the formation of a disulfide bridge between the reactive thiol group of the active metabolite of clopidogrel and one or more cysteine residues of the platelet P2Y12 receptor [25]. This permanent alteration of the ADP binding site is consistent with the observation of a cumulative effect on platelet inhibition with repeated thienopyridine dosing and a protracted recovery of platelet function following cessation of thienopyridine administration [26, 27].

Additional beneficial effects of clopidogrel in CVD

Evidence from recent clinical trials and mechanistic studies underlines the importance of an inflammatory etiology in acute IHD. Growing evidence indicates that platelets act as prominent players in the inflammatory component of atherothrombotic diseases. Upon activation, platelets release a series of cytokines and growth factors and express the CD40 ligand, which interacts with the CD40 receptor on other major cell types involved in atherosclerosis/atherothrombosis [28]. In healthy volunteers, CD40L expression in platelets

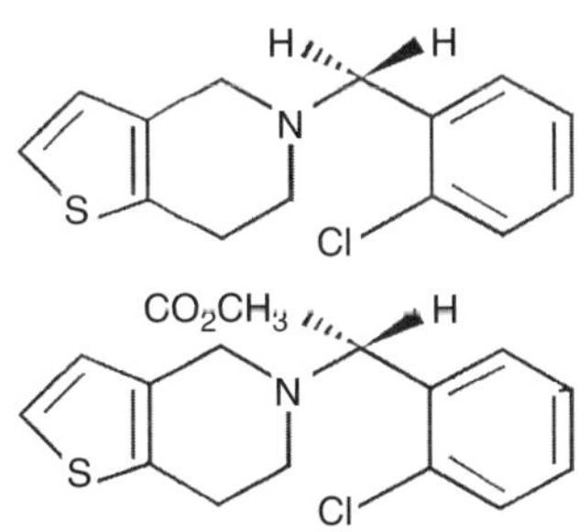

Figure 3.2 Chemical structures of ticlopidine (top) and clopidogrel (bottom)

is not significantly inhibited by acetylsalicylic acid (ASA) alone, but is inhibited after treatment with the ADP-receptor antagonist clopidogrel or with clopidogrel plus ASA. In addition, clopidogrel has been shown to attenuate platelet secretion, aggregation, and formation of platelet–monocyte and platelet–neutrophil conjugates in patients with ACS [29]. Furthermore, clopidogrel pretreatment reduces platelet inflammatory marker (CD40 ligand and P-selectin) expression in patients undergoing PCI [30]. These effects may all contribute to the clinical benefits of this drug across the spectrum of CVD.

The importance of C-reactive protein (CRP) in predicting and contributing to an individual's risk of cardiovascular events and the benefits of treatments in atherothrombotic diseases is well established [31]. The effect of clopidogrel on serum CRP has been studied in various populations of patients with atherothrombotic diseases including those with cerebrovascular [32] and cardiovascular [33–35] disease. One study demonstrated that clopidogrel significantly attenuated the rise of CRP by 65% following PCI [35]. However, the precise contribution of this anti-inflammatory effect to the beneficial effects of clopidogrel in patients with atherothrombotic diseases remains to be more optimally defined.

PHARMACOKINETICS AND PHARMACODYNAMICS

Ticlopidine

Ticlopidine is well absorbed after oral administration, with peak plasma concentrations occurring 1–3 h after administration of a single 250 mg oral dose [36]. Administration after meals results in a 20% increase in the area under the curve (AUC) of ticlopidine [37]. Plasma levels of ticlopidine increase approximately threefold on repeated twice-daily dosing over two to three weeks because of drug accumulation. Ticlopidine hydrochloride binds reversibly (98%) to plasma proteins, mainly to serum albumin and lipoproteins [37].

Inhibition of platelet aggregation is both dose- and time-related, with its onset of activity being 24–48 h, its maximal activity occurring after 3–5 days, and its activity still being present 72 h after a final dose [37]. The apparent elimination half-life of ticlopidine is 24–36 h after a single oral dose and 4–5 days after 14–21 days of repeated dosing [37]. As noted, a delay in maximal antithrombotic effect is seen with ticlopidine administration. Therefore, ticlopidine therapy is not useful when a rapid antiplatelet effect is required.

Ticlopidine is metabolized extensively by the liver and only one of its metabolites, the 2-keto derivative, is a more potent inhibitor of ADP-induced platelet aggregation than the parent compound [23]. Following an oral dose of radioactive ticlopidine administered in solution, 60% of the radioactivity is recovered in the urine and 23% in the feces. Approximately 1/3 of the dose excreted in the feces is intact ticlopidine hydrochloride, possibly excreted in the bile. Clearance of ticlopidine decreases with age. Steady-state trough values in elderly patients (mean age 70 years) are about twice those in younger volunteer populations [38].

Clopidogrel

Clopidogrel is rapidly absorbed after oral administration of repeated doses of 75 mg clopidogrel, with peak plasma levels of the main circulating metabolite, SR 26334, occurring approximately 1 h after dosing. The pharmacokinetics of SR 26334 are linear (plasma concentrations increased in proportion to dose) in the dose range of 50–150 mg of clopidogrel. Clopidogrel and SR 26334 bind reversibly *in vitro* to human plasma proteins (98% and 94%, respectively).

Dose-dependent inhibition of platelet aggregation can be seen after single oral doses of clopidogrel and remains relatively stable up to 48 h [39]. Maximum inhibition by 40–50% is observed 2–5 h after a single 400 mg dose. On repeated daily dosing of 50–100 mg clopidogrel in healthy volunteers, ADP-induced platelet aggregation was inhibited 25–30% by the second day of treatment and reached a steady state of 50–60% inhibition after 4–7 days [40]. No appreciable differences in the maximum inhibitory effects of therapy with 50, 75, and 100 mg clopidogrel were noted, suggesting that a dose of 50 mg daily may be at or close to the top of the dose–response curve. These features are consistent with the observation that a loading dose (300 mg) of clopidogrel results in a much more rapid onset of platelet inhibition than is achieved with the 75 mg dose [41]. However, the optimal timing and dosing regimen of clopidogrel in the acute setting remain poorly defined and doses up to 600 mg have been assessed in patients with CAD [42] and in those prior to PCI [43, 44]. Platelet aggregation and bleeding time gradually return to baseline values after treatment is discontinued, generally in about five days.

The plasma elimination half-life of SR 26334, the active platelet inhibitor, is approximately 8 h. However, the interindividual variability in this metabolic activation is still being assessed, and whether liver impairment decreases the ability of clopidogrel to inhibit platelet function remains poorly understood. The cytochrome P450 isozymes CYP3A4 and 3A5 metabolize clopidogrel faster than other human P450 isozymes and are felt to be predominantly responsible for the activation of clopidogrel *in vivo*.

3.3 CLINICAL USES OF THE THIENOPYRIDINES

The utility of the thienopyridines ticlopidine and clopidogrel has been assessed across the spectrum of CVD. Where they have made the greatest impact has been as an adjunctive medication to the percutaneous management of atherothrombotic diseases. In fact, when coupled to aspirin, ticlopidine revolutionized the post-PCI therapeutic regimen and markedly improved the beneficial effects of intracoronary stenting [45].

The thienopyridines have also been beneficial in several other arenas, including management of patients with acute coronary syndromes [46] as well as those with established atherothrombotic diseases [47], and as an alternative for those with hypersensitivity to aspirin. Furthermore, when utilized as part of a dual antiplatelet regimen, these agents have improved outcomes for patients with acute coronary syndromes or those who have experienced 'aspirin failures' [48–53]. Of the currently available thienopyridines, clopidogrel is the agent of choice as a result of the unfavorable side-effect profile of ticlopidine which includes aplastic anemia [54] and thrombotic thrombocytopenic purpura (TTP) [55].

TICLOPIDINE

Ticlopidine offers a substantial benefit to patients who have experienced TIAs or stroke, and in those with peripheral arterial disease (PAD) or IHD (Tables 3.1 and 3.2). Although the biggest impact of ticlopidine has been within the realm of interventional cardiology, ticlopidine has demonstrated benefit in non-invasive arenas, where its use has been associated

Table 3.1 Selected trials of ticlopidine in patients with cardiovascular disease

Trial	Population	Trial type	*N*	Comparative arm	Primary endpoint	Outcome control (%)	Outcome ticlopidine (%)	*p*-value	Comment
Balsano *et al.* [56]	ACS	Open-label RCT	652	'Conventional therapy'	Vascular Death/MI	13.6	7.3	0.009	Ticlopidine (500 mg/day) was more effective in reducing adverse events in patients with ACS than conventional therapy
Scrutinio *et al.* [57]	MI	RCT	1,470	Aspirin 160 mg/day	D/MI/Stroke/ Angina/Vascular D within 6 months	8.0	8.0	NS	Randomization took place a mean of 13 days after treatment for acute MI. No difference was found between the ticlopidine (500 mg/day) and aspirin groups in the rate of the primary combined endpoint of death, recurrent MI, stroke, and angina
Schomig *et al.* [59]	Intracoronary stenting	RCT	517	IV UH, phenpro-couman, aspirin (100 mg bid)	D/MI/CABG/PCI 30 days	6.2	1.6	0.01	Ticlopidine (250 mg bid) plus aspirin (100 mg bid) therapy post-PCI (stents) reduces the incidence of both cardiac events and hemorrhagic and vascular complications

Hall *et al.* [58]	Intracoronary stenting	RCT	226	Aspirin 325 mg/day	D/MI/CABG/PCI VC at 30 days	3.9	0.8	0.1	Treatment group consisted of aspirin (325 mg/day) followed by ticlopidine (250 mg bid) for 1 month
FANTASTIC [61]	Intracoronary stenting	RCT	485	Aspirin + IV UH then OAC	Bleeding or PV complications	21	13.5	0.03	Ticlopidine (500 mg in catheter lab then 250 mg bid × 6 weeks) + aspirin (100–325 mg/day) associated with less MACE in electively stented patients (2.4% vs 9.9% with anticoagulation)
MATTIS [60]	Intracoronary stenting	RCT	350	Aspirin + OAC (INR 2.5–3)	D/MI/ revascularization at 30 days	11	5.6	0.07	Ticlopidine (500 mg/d) + aspirin (250 mg/d) decreased adverse events after stenting. Significant decrease in bleeding and vascular complications with antiplatelet therapy after PCI

Table 3.1 (*Continued*)

Trial	Population	Trial type	*N*	Comparative arm	Primary endpoint	Outcome control (%)	Outcome ticlopidine (%)	*p*-value	Comment
STARS [45]	Intracoronary stenting	RCT	1653	Aspirin 325 mg/day	D/MI/UR/CABG	3.6	0.5	<0.001	This trial revolutionized the peri-procedural antithrombotic regimen following stenting
				Aspirin + warfarin		2.7		0.007	Aspirin 325 mg/day plus ticlopidine 250 mg bid significantly decreased adverse events
Goods *et al.* [146]	Intracoronary stenting	OT	384	Aspirin 325 mg before PCI then bid for 30 days then daily	Stent thrombosis	6.5	0.9	0.02	Ticlopidine (250 mg bid) + aspirin (325 mg bid × 30 days then daily) decreased rate of stent thrombosis compared with aspirin alone. This regimen also decreased deaths (0.3% vs 4.4%) and Q-wave MI (0% vs 6.5%)
Steinhubl *et al.* [62]	Intracoronary stenting	OT	175	NA	Procedure-related MI	NA	NA	NA	Ticlopidine pretreatment of ≥3 days was associated with a significant reduction in the risk of non-Q-wave MI (unadjusted odds

									ratio 0.18, 95% CI = 0.04–0.78, p-value = 0.01) compared with pretreatment of <3 days
Berger *et al.* [63]	Intracoronary stenting	OT	827	NA	Adverse cardiac events at 14 days	NA	1.3%	NA	In patients receiving intracoronary stents, the discontinuation of ticlopidine therapy 14 days after stent placement is associated with a very low frequency of stent thrombosis and other adverse events
Limet *et al.* [74]	Coronary bypass	RCT	173	Placebo	Graft occlusion at 360 days	26.1	15.9	<0.01	The incidence of occlusion is significantly reduced by ticlopidine (250 mg bid) therapy

bid = twice daily; D = death; MACE = major adverse cardiac events; NA = not applicable; NS = non-significant; OAC = oral anticoagulation; OT = observational trial; UR = urgent revascularization

Table 3.2 Selected trials of ticlopidine in patients with extra-cardiac atherothrombotic disease

Trial	Population	Trial type	*N*	Comparative arm	Primary endpoint	Outcome control (%)	Outcome ticlopidine (%)	*p*-value	Comment
CATS [66]	Recent thromboembolic stroke	RCT	1,072	Placebo	Stroke/MI and vascular D	15.3	10.8	0.006	Ticlopidine (250 mg bid) beneficial in both men and women over a mean of 24 months of follow up. Toxicity of ticlopidine: neutropenia (1%) and skin rash and diarrhea (2%)
TASS [67]	Recent TIA or minor stroke	RCT	3,069	Aspirin 1300 mg/d	D/stroke	19.0	17.0	0.048	Over a mean of 3 years, ticlopidine (500 mg/day) somewhat more effective than aspirin in preventing strokes, albeit at increased risk: diarrhea (20%), skin rash (14%), severe neutropenia ($<1\%$)
TISS [65]	Recent TIA or minor stroke	RCT	1,632	Indobufen 200 mg/d	D/stroke/MI at 1 year	5.8	2.9	0.004	Ticlopidine (250 mg/day) reduced adverse events compared with indobufen with a similar side-effect profile
STIMS [71]	Intermittent claudication	RCT	687	Placebo	MI/stroke/TIA	29.0	25.0	<0.05	34% RRR in coronary and cerebrovascular events with

									ticlopidine RRR of mortality was 29% with ticlopidine at a median of 5.6 years of follow up. Reversible leucopenia noted in ~1%
Arcan *et al.* [73]	Chronic intermittent claudication	RCT	169	Placebo	Stroke/TIA /peripheral ischemia requiring surgery at 6 months	10.5	2.4	0.03	Ticlopidine (250 mg bid) is beneficial for the treatment of the symptoms and the prevention of vascular complications in patients with intermittent claudication
Blanchard *et al.* [72]	Intermittent claudication	RCT	615	Placebo	D/MI/stroke and CV intervention	6.4	1	0.002	Ticlopidine (250 mg bid) for 24 weeks decreased the rate of CV events in the patient population
Becquemin *et al.* [75]	LE SV Bypass	RCT	243	Placebo	Graft patency at 2 years	63	82	0.002	Ticlopidine (250 mg bid) significantly improved the long-term patency of saphenous-vein bypass grafts in the legs

bid=twice daily; D=death; LE=lower extremity; PV=peripheral vascular; SV=saphenous vein with a decreased risk of further stroke, MI or vascular death, in patients with extra-cardiac (recent stroke, TIAs or intermittent claudication) atherothrombotic diseases. Ticlopidine has been shown to be superior to placebo and to aspirin in these circumstances (Table 3.2). However, given the associated risks of severe neutropenia and TTP and the availability of an effective alternative, clopidogrel, use of ticlopidine has become marginalized.

Cardiovascular disease

A paucity of data exists with respect to the utility of ticlopidine in the management of patients presenting across the spectrum of the acute ischemic syndromes (Table 3.1). Compared to conventional treatment, the addition of ticlopidine was associated with a 46% relative risk reduction of adverse events in patients presenting with unstable angina in one small study [56]. Although no randomized trial has compared ticlopidine to placebo or aspirin as an adjunct to fibrinolytic therapy in patients with STEMI, one trial revealed that the use of ticlopidine, beginning an average of 13 days after fibrinolysis for a STEMI, resulted in similar rates of adverse events compared with aspirin [57]. Approximately 93–94% of the patients in that trial received aspirin during the acute phase of treatment.

Where ticlopidine has imparted the greatest benefit has been within the realm of interventional cardiology, historically, as an integral member of a dual antiplatelet regimen following intracoronary stent implantation (Table 3.1). Several small trials revealed the utility and safety of ticlopidine combined with aspirin compared with aspirin alone [58] or aspirin followed by oral anticoagulation [59–61] after successful intracoronary stent placement. Warfarin-based regimens were severely limited, however, by incomplete suppression of stent thrombosis events, high rates of hemorrhagic complications and prolonged hospitalizations for initiation of therapy. Since the mid-1990s, however, a combination of aspirin and thienopyridine (initially ticlopidine) has been demonstrated to provide superior efficacy and safety following stenting compared with aspirin and coumadin. The seminal study that revolutionized the periprocedural antithrombotic regimen compared the safety and efficacy of aspirin alone, aspirin plus warfarin, and aspirin plus ticlopidine for 30 days following successful stent implantation in 1653 patients [45]. Dual antiplatelet therapy with aspirin plus ticlopidine was associated with a statistically significant reduction in the thirty-day endpoint of death, revascularization of the target lesion, angiographically evident thrombosis or MI (0.5% vs 2.7% aspirin + warfarin; 3.6% aspirin alone, p-value <0.001). Hemorrhagic complications occurred in 1.8% who received aspirin alone, 6.2% who received aspirin plus warfarin, and 5.5% who received aspirin plus ticlopidine. Issues regarding the length of pretreatment with ticlopidine prior to PCI [62] and the minimally effective duration of dual antiplatelet therapy with ticlopidine after PCI [63] have been addressed by small studies (Table 3.1). However, the frequency and risk of rheologic derangements (neutropenia, TTP) with ticlopidine and the availability of an efficacious alternative ADP-receptor antagonist, clopidogrel, have made these more of an exercise in academics. Nevertheless, there remain potential clinical situations where ticlopidine may need to be utilized, such as in patients with hypersensitivity to clopidogrel and aspirin.

Cerebrovascular disease

Stroke is the third leading cause of mortality in the United States. As the leading cause of neurological deficits worldwide, stroke is associated with tremendous costs both to society and to the individuals and families that stroke impacts. Antiplatelet agents have demonstrated efficacy in preventing recurrent atherothrombotic strokes and are the principal pharmacologic modality employed [64].

The efficacy of ticlopidine in patients with symptomatic cerebrovascular disease has been evaluated in three large clinical trials (Table 3.2) [65–67]. In the first trial, among 1072 patients with TIA or stroke, ticlopidine (500 mg/d) compared with placebo or untreated control reduced the risk of stroke, MI, or vascular death by 30.2% (10.8% vs 15.3%, p-value = 0.006) after a mean of two years [66]. The beneficial effects of ticlopidine persisted when compared with aspirin (1300 mg/day) [67]. In another trial of 3069 patients following a recent TIA or minor stroke, ticlopidine was associated with a reduction in the risk of death or recurrent stroke after three years of follow up (17% vs 19% with aspirin, p-value = 0.048). Despite these encouraging data as well as data that ticlopidine maintains its therapeutic edge in patients with cerebrovascular disease compared with an alternative antiplatelet agent [65], the toxicity associated with ticlopidine has precluded its widespread use.

Peripheral arterial disease

It is increasingly becoming recognized that the presence of PAD imparts a significant risk of future adverse cardiovascular events [68–70]. That ticlopidine would be able to decrease the risk of future CV events in patients with symptomatic PAD has been assessed in two moderately sized clinical studies (Table 3.2) [71, 72]. In the Swedish Ticlopidine Multicenter Study of 687 patients, a significant 34% reduction in coronary and cerebrovascular events was observed with ticlopidine (250 mg twice daily) over a mean of 5.6 years (25.0% vs 29.0% with placebo; 95% CI, 0.45 to 0.96) [71]. The short-term benefit of ticlopidine has also been demonstrated with respect to decreasing future CV [72] and peripheral vascular [73] events. Furthermore, consistent with its beneficial effects in coronary saphenous vein graft patency [74], ticlopidine significantly improved the long-term patency of peripheral saphenous vein bypass grafts [75]. Despite these results, potential adverse effects associated with ticlopidine, in particular neutropenia and TTP, have limited its use.

Limitations of ticlopidine

Despite the beneficial effects described above, ticlopidine is associated with a number of serious and potentially life-threatening limitations that have precluded its widespread use for the management of atherothrombotic disorders. The most feared complications reside within the field of hematology, and include life-threatening neutropenia and TTP. Neutropenia (absolute neutrophil count <450 cells/mm^3) occurs in approximately 1% of patients treated with ticlopidine, typically within the first three months after the initiation of therapy; however, it is infrequently seen within the first two to three weeks [65–67]. Another serious and often fatal side effect of ticlopidine therapy, TTP, occurs in significantly more patients receiving ticlopidine than in the general population [76]. Most of the cases have been shown to occur between 4 and 12 weeks after the initiation of therapy [77], although one study demonstrated a persistent risk of TTP even within the first two weeks after the initiation of therapy [76]. Therefore, even with short-term use of ticlopidine a significant risk of hematologic toxicity remains.

Other side effects that have hindered ticlopidine use have included the gastro-intestinal (GI) effects of the medication. Usually occurring within the first two to three weeks of therapy, various GI toxicities ranging from diarrhea (up to 20% of patients) [65–67, 71] prompting drug discontinuation to cholestatic jaundice [78] have been reported with ticlopidine use. Given that ticlopidine's GI effects are dose-related, the use of an adequate loading dose is unlikely to occur. Thus, coupled with the availability of an alternative thienopyridine, clopidogrel, these factors have contributed to ticlopidine's very limited role in atherothrombotic diseases.

CLOPIDOGREL

The search for an alternative antiplatelet agent that would address the limitations of aspirin (Chapter 2) and ticlopidine without compromising efficacy in patients with CV disease is actively ongoing. Clopidogrel is a thienopyridine that addresses some of the limitations of both agents. While proven to be effective in the prevention of secondary episodes in patients with IHD when used as the sole antiplatelet agent [47], clopidogrel has demonstrated an additive effect when combined with aspirin in patients undergoing PCI [79] as well as in those presenting with ACS [46]. Given the beneficial effects and the improved safety profile compared with ticlopidine, clopidogrel should be the additional or alternative oral antiplatelet therapy of choice.

Although clopidogrel reduces the risk of CV episodes after coronary events and stenting, a substantial number of incidents continue to occur. Although incompletely understood, 'clopidogrel resistance' has been suggested to contribute to these adverse events [80–83]. In addition, the incidence of TTP occurring early after the initiation of clopidogrel therapy has been documented [55] and, in one trial, at a similar rate as that seen with aspirin [47]. Nevertheless, clopidogrel currently holds a strong position as an alternative to as well as in combination with aspirin for the treatment of atherothrombotic diseases (Tables 3.3 and 3.4).

Cardiovascular disease

Secondary prevention of CV events

Clopidogrel was approved by the FDA in 1998 based in part on the results of the Clopidogrel Versus Aspirin in Patients at Risk of Ischemic Events (CAPRIE) tria1 [47]. CAPRIE randomized 19,185 patients with atherosclerotic vascular disease manifested as a recent ischemic stroke (onset >1 week and <6 months before randomization), recent MI (onset ~35 days before randomization), or symptomatic PAD to clopidogrel (75 mg once daily) or aspirin (325 mg once daily) and assessed the effects on the composite outcome of ischemic stroke, MI or vascular death. In an intention-to-treat analysis, treatment with clopidogrel modestly but significantly reduced the annual rate of atherothrombotic events compared with aspirin (5.32% vs 5.83%, p-value = 0.043) [47]. Long-term administration of clopidogrel to patients with atherosclerotic vascular disease was shown to be more effective than aspirin in reducing future CV events with an overall safety profile at least as good as that of medium-dose aspirin.

The efficacy of clopidogrel in the CAPRIE trial was heterogeneous depending on presenting enrollment criteria. Whereas the majority of benefit was seen in patients with PAD (clopidogrel 3.71% vs ASA 4.86%; p-value <0.003), a non-significant increased

Table 3.3 Selected clinical trials of clopidogrel in patients with atherothrombotic disease

Trial	Population	Trial type	*N*	Comparative arm	Primary endpoint	Outcome control (%)	Outcome clopidogrel (%)	*p*-value	Comment
CAPRIE [47]	Established AVD	RCT	19,185	Aspirin 325 mg daily	Ischemic stroke, MI, vascular D	5.83	5.32	0.043	Long-term (mean 1.91 years) administration of clopidogrel to patients with atherosclerotic vascular disease is more effective than aspirin in reducing the combined risk of ischemic stroke, MI, or vascular D with a safety profile at least as good as aspirin
CURE [46]	ACS	RCT	12,562	Placebo	D/MI/Stroke	11.4	9.3	<0.001	Demonstrated the benefit of clopidogrel (300 mg upon randomization then 75 mg daily) in patients with ACS. Note that a minority of patients underwent 'early invasive' therapy. Bleeding events increased with clopidogrel
CLARITY – TIMI 28 [93]	STEMI – within 12 h of symptom onset	RCT	3,491	Placebo	Efficacy: D/MI/occluded IRA at angiography	21.7	15.0	<0.001	Clopidogrel given as loading dose of 300 mg followed by 75 mg daily. No increase in bleeding complications seen with clopidogrel
					Clinical: D/MI/UR at 30 d	14.1	11.6	0.03	No increase in CABG-related bleeding (7.5% vs 7.2% with placebo, *p*-value = 1.0), even in those undergoing CABG within 5 days after discontinuation of clopidogrel (9.1% vs 7.9% with placebo, *p*-value = 1.0)

Table 3.3 (*Continued*)

Trial	Population	Trial type	N	Comparative arm	Primary endpoint	Outcome control (%)	Outcome clopidogrel (%)	p-value	Comment
COMMIT [94]	AMI – within 24 h	RCT	45,852	Placebo	D/MI/Stroke at hospital discharge	10.1	9.3	$2p = 0.002$	Clopidogrel 75 mg daily (mean 16 days). Excluded patients undergoing primary PCI or those at high risk of bleeding. 67% presented within 12 h. 49% received fibrinolytics. No increased risk of bleeding seen with clopidogrel. All patients received aspirin (162 mg daily).
PCI-CURE [106]	PCI in ACS	Sub-study of CURE	2,658	Placebo	CVD/MI/UTVR	6.4	4.5	0.03	Patients were pretreated with aspirin and study drug for a median of 6 days before PCI during the initial hospital admission, and for a median of 10 days overall. After PCI, most patients (>80%) received open-label thienopyridine for about 4 weeks, after which study drug was restarted for a mean of 8 months.
CREDO [79]	Elective PCI	RCT	2,116	Placebo	D/MI/UTVR at 28 days	8.3	6.8	NS	Patients were randomized to receive a 300 mg clopidogrel loading dose or placebo 3–24 h before PCI. All patients received clopidogrel, 75 mg/day, through day 28. From day 29 to 12 months, the loading-dose group received clopidogrel, 75 mg/day, and the control group received placebo. Both groups received aspirin throughout the study.

					D/MI/Stroke at 1 year	11.5	8.5	0.02	
ISAR-REACT [44]	Elective PCI	OBS Trial	2,159	Placebo	D/MI/UTVR at 30 days	4	4	0.82	Abciximab is not associated with a measurable benefit at 30 days in low-to-intermediate risk patients who undergo elective PCI after pretreatment with a high (600 mg $\geq$2 h before PCI) loading dose of clopidogrel.
ARMYDA-2 [107]	Elective PCI	RCT	255	Clopidogrel 600 mg vs 300 mg 4–8 h prior to PCI	D/MI/UTVR at 30 days	12	4	0.041	Benefit of high loading dose entirely due to decreased peri-procedural MI. High loading dose unassociated with increased bleeding complications
Diener *et al.* [109]	Recent ischemic stroke or TIA	RCT	7,599	Clopidogrel alone	Stroke/MI/VD/re-hospitalization for acute ischemia at 18 months	16.7	15.7	NS	Adding aspirin to clopidogrel in these patients does not improve outcomes but does increase the risk of bleeding

AMI = acute myocardial infarction; AVD = atherosclerotic vascular disease; CVD = cardiovascular death; D = death; NS = not significant; OBS = observational; UR = urgent revascularization; UTVR = urgent target vessel revascularization

Table 3.4 Selected trials comparing ticlopidine with clopidogrel in patients undergoing coronary stenting

Trial	Population	Trial type	*N*	Treatment groups	Primary endpoint	Outcome ticlopidine (%)	Outcome clopidogrel (%)	*p*-value	Comment
CLASSICS [105]	Elective stenting	RCT	1020	1) Ticlopidine 250 mg bid + aspirin 325 mg daily 2) Clopidogrel 300 mg f/b 75 mg daily + aspirin 325 mg daily 3) Clopidogrel 75 mg + aspirin 325 mg daily	B, neutropenia, TCP, D/C drug due to non-cardiac complications at 28 days	9.1	4.6	0.005	MACE (D/MI/TLR) at 28 days: 0.9% with ticlopidine, 1.5% clopidogrel, 1.2% loading dose clopidogrel *p*-value = NS
Taniuchi *et al.* [104]	Elective stenting	RCT	1016	1) Ticlopidine 500 mg load after stent then 250 mg bid + aspirin 325 mg daily 2) Clopidogrel 300 mg load after stent then 75 mg daily + aspirin 325 mg daily	Failure to complete 2 weeks of therapy	3.64	1.62	0.043	30 days SAT: 1.92% ticlopidine and 2.02% clopidogrel. MACE: ticlopidine, 4.6% clopidogrel, 3.85%

Juergens *et al.* [147]	Elective stenting	RCT	307	1) Ticlopidine 500 mg load after stent then 250 mg bid + aspirin 300 mg 24 h before stent then 100 mg daily 2) Clopidogrel 150 mg load then 75 mg daily + aspirin 300 mg 24 h before stent then 100 mg daily	Failure to complete 2 weeks of therapy	3.3	0.6	.121	SAT: 0.7% with ticlopidine, 1.9% with clopidogrel (*p*-value = 0.623). MACE occurred in 1.9% in each group at 30 days
Muller *et al.* [102]	Unselected patients	RCT	700	1) Ticlopidine 500mg load after stent then 250 mg bid + aspirin 100 mg daily 2) Clopidogrel 75 mg after stent + aspirin 100 mg daily	CVD/MI/TVR/TSO at 30 days	1.7	3.1	0.24	D/stroke/severe PV or hemorrhagic complications decreased with clopidogrel
Mueller *et al.* [103]	Unselected patients	RCT	700	1) Ticlopidine 500 mg load after stent then 250 mg bid + aspirin 100 mg daily 2) Clopidogrel 75 mg after stent + aspirin 100 mg daily	CVD at 28 months	2.3	7.4	0.003	In this long-term follow-up of a prior trial, ticlopidine was associated with a significantly lower mortality than clopidogrel

Trial	Population	Trial type	N	Treatment groups	Primary endpoint	Outcome ticlopidine (%)	Outcome clopidogrel (%)	p-value	Comment
L'Allier *et al.* [148]	Elective stenting	Registry	2372	1) Ticlopidine 500 mg load after stent then 250 mg bid + aspirin 325 mg daily	30-day Mortality	1.46	0.31	NS	Improved clinical outcomes without an increase in bleeding complications suggested by this study
				2) Clopidogrel 300 mg load then 75 mg daily + aspirin 325 mg daily	30-day D/MI/TVR	9.1	6.2	0.05	
Berger *et al.* [149]	Unselected patients	Registry	1327	1) Ticlopidine 500 mg load immediately before stent then 250 mg bid + aspirin ≥325 mg daily for 14 days 2) Clopidogrel 300 mg load immediately before stent then 75 mg daily + aspirin ≥325 mg daily for 14 days	D/MI/SAT and need for CABG or Re-PCI at 30 days	1.6	0.8	NS	Clopidogrel was as effective as ticlopidine at preventing stent thrombosis within 30 days of PCI
Moussa *et al.* [150]	Unselected patients	Registry	1689	1) Ticlopidine 500 mg load then 250 mg bid + aspirin 325 mg daily for 2 weeks	SAT at 30 days	1.5	1.4	1.00	Clopidogrel demonstrated an improved safety profile
				2) Clopidogrel 300 mg load then 75 mg daily + aspirin 325 mg daily for 4 weeks	MACE at 30 days	3.1	2.4	0.85	
Dangas *et al.* [101]	Unselected patients	Registry	827	1) Ticlopidine 500 mg before and 250 mg bid after stenting for 2–4 weeks + aspirin 325 mg daily	SAT at 30 days	0.2	1.3	0.10	These results suggest that aspirin + clopidogrel may have marginally higher subacute stent thrombosis than aspirin + ticlopidine

				2) Clopidogrel: 300 mg 1–5 h before,150 mg bid for 1–3 days or 75 mg daily 1–3 days before stenting then 75 mg daily after stenting for 4 weeks + aspirin 325 mg daily	D/MI/TLR at 30 days	0.5	2.0	0.09	
Mishkel *et al.* [151]	Elective or bail-out stenting	Registry	875	1) Ticlopidine 250 mg bid + aspirin 325 mg daily	D/MI/TVR at 30 days	1.4	2.1	0.57	Clopidogrel + aspirin was an effective alternative to ticlopidine + aspirin
				2) Clopidogrel 75 mg + aspirin 325 mg daily	SAT at 30 days	0.3	0.2	0.99	
Calver [152]	Unselected patients	Registry	361	1) Ticlopidine 500 mg + aspirin 300 mg on day of procedure then ticlopidine 250 mg bid + aspirin 150 mg daily for 1 month	MACE at 30 days	5.3	2.3	NS	Suggested clopidogrel + aspirin a safe alternative to ticlopidine + aspirin in vessels ≤3.0 mm.
				2) Clopidogrel 300 mg + aspirin 300 mg on day of procedure then Clopidogrel 75 mg + aspirin 150 mg for 1 month	SAT	1.6	0	NS	

B = bleeding; bid = twice daily; CVD = cardiovascular death; D = death; D/C = discontinue; f/b = followed by; MACE = major adverse cardiac event; NS = not significant; PV = peripheral vascular; SAT = subacute stent thrombosis; TCP = thrombocytopenia; TLR = target lesion revascularization; TSO = thrombotic stent occlusion; TVR = target vessel revascularization risk of CV events was observed in those enrolled with a prior MI (5.03% vs 4.84%, respectively) [47]. It is unclear whether this heterogeneity was real or a spurious finding of statistical chance. More recent substudy analyses of the CAPRIE data have suggested enhanced efficacy of clopidogrel compared with aspirin in specific subgroups of patients. Given the increased cumulative rate of graft closure and recurrent ischemic events in patients following CABG surgery, the efficacy of clopidogrel compared to aspirin was assessed in this population [84]. The use of clopidogrel was associated with significant reduction in the combined annual event rates of all-cause mortality, vascular death, myocardial infarction, stroke and rehospitalization in the 1480 patients with a history of cardiac surgery [84]. The greater benefit of clopidogrel over that of aspirin was also recently demonstrated in patients with diabetes, a subgroup of patients at increased risk of recurrent events across the spectrum of atherothrombotic diseases [85].

Acute coronary syndromes

The need for an antithrombotic regimen that provides a seamless beneficial effect on both the short- and long-term outcomes in patients presenting with ACS is evident by the lack of an existing therapeutic strategy that can address the specific needs of these patients when they initially present, when they undergo an early invasive strategy and after they have received definitive therapy. Although a small but significant benefit of clopidogrel monotherapy has been demonstrated over aspirin alone, the markedly enhanced efficacy of combining a thienopyridine with aspirin on reducing stent thrombosis provided the backdrop for investigating the utility of clopidogrel for the management of ACS. Given its beneficial effects with limited toxicity, clopidogrel's role in ACS was assessed in the Clopidogrel in Unstable Angina to Prevent Recurrent Events (CURE) trial [46]. In this trial of 12,562 patients presenting within 24 h of symptom onset, clopidogrel (300 mg immediately, followed by 75 mg once daily) in addition to aspirin was associated with a significant, 20% reduction compared with aspirin alone in the relative risk of the composite endpoint, death from cardiovascular causes, non-fatal MI, or stroke (RRR compared to placebo 0.80; 95% CI, 0.72 to 0.90; p-value <0.001). The percentages of patients with in-hospital refractory or severe ischemia, heart failure, and revascularization procedures were also significantly lower with clopidogrel.

That the addition of clopidogrel to standard care may provide an avenue for the seamless transition between the pharmacologic and percutaneous management of patients with ACS was suggested by the CURE trial. Clopidogrel was shown to be effective in these patients regardless of treatment strategy received, invasive or conservative, and regardless of baseline risk profile [46, 86]. This is in contrast to the data regarding the use of GP IIb/IIIa inhibitors, which demonstrate that the beneficial effects of these agents is primarily limited to those patients with the highest baseline risk [87, 88]. Furthermore, given the widespread use of GP IIb/IIIa inhibitors in these patients, data have suggested that the addition of thienopyridines to GP IIb/IIIa inhibitors in patients with ACS provides additional platelet inhibition [89] and may be safe and effective [90–92]. Coupled with the consistent benefit of clopidogrel amongst trials regardless of patient population and setting [79, 93, 94], these data have strongly positioned clopidogrel as an integral component of the armamentarium available for these patients.

The benefit of clopidogrel in patients with ACS is not without risk. The complication of clopidogrel use of greatest concern remains the increased risk of bleeding. In the CURE trial there were significantly more patients with major bleeding in the clopidogrel group than in the placebo group (3.7% vs 2.7%; RR, 1.38; p-value = 0.001) [46]. A significant increase in transfusion requirements and minor bleeding episodes was also demonstrated in this trial. Although there was no increase in CABG-related hemorrhagic events in this trial, clopidogrel was held for median of 5 days in patients slated to undergo surgical revascularization. Although the data addressing the increase in peri-CABG hemorrhagic events with pre-operative clopidogrel use are conflicting [95, 96], the growing understanding is that clopidogrel as an adjunctive therapy for patients with ACS improves outcomes when utilized in these patients [97].

STEMI

The central paradigm in the management of acute STEMI remains rapid and complete restoration of antegrade coronary perfusion. The benefits of primary PCI have established it as the reperfusion modality of choice. However, given the lack of widespread, readily available catheterization laboratories, fibrinolysis remains an important alternative to primary PCI. Although fibrinolysis is effective in improving outcomes in STEMI, failure to achieve reperfusion and/or reocclusion of the infarct-related artery occur in substantial proportions of patients [98]. This has prompted the development of enhanced reperfusion strategies that simultaneously target multiple pathways of thrombogenesis and, in particular, the platelet [99, 100]. Despite its favorable role in ACS and peri-PCI the effect of clopidogrel in addition to aspirin and fibrinolytics on outcomes in patients had not been studied. However, the completion of two large randomized trials assessing the effects of clopidogrel in addition to either fibrinolytics [93, 94] or primary PCI [94] has improved our understanding of the benefits of clopidogrel in this setting (Table 3.3).

The Clopidogrel as Adjunctive Reperfusion TherapY (CLARITY) trial sought to assess the effects of clopidogrel, in addition to standard-dose fibrinolytics and aspirin, in the management of STEMI [93]. In this trial, 3491 patients presenting within 12 h after the onset of a STEMI were randomized to receive clopidogrel (300 mg loading dose, followed by 75 mg daily) or placebo. Patients received a fibrinolytic agent, aspirin, and, when appropriate, weight-based UH and were scheduled to undergo angiography 48 to 192 h after the start of study medication. The primary efficacy endpoint, a composite of an occluded infarct-related artery on angiography or death or recurrent MI before angiography, was significantly reduced with clopidogrel therapy (15% vs 21.7%; RRR, 36%; p-value <0.001) [93]. Clopidogrel therapy was also associated with a reduced risk of cardiovascular death, recurrent MI, or recurrent ischemia leading to the need for urgent revascularization by 20% (from 14.1% to 11.6%, p-value = 0.03). Importantly, clopidogrel was not associated with an increase in hemorrhagic events among the population as a whole or among the 136 patients who underwent CABG during the hospitalization. Enthusiasm for clopidogrel in this setting, however, must be tempered by the fact that this trial assessed its effects in a relatively young (<75 years of age) and low-risk (30-day mortality in both groups <5%) population.

The Clopidogrel Metoprolol Myocardial Infarction (COMMIT) trial addressed some of the limitations of CLARITY and broadened the scope of utility of clopidogrel in this setting [94]. COMMIT randomized 45,852 patients with an MI (either ST change or left bundle branch block) within 24 h of symptom onset to treatment with clopidogrel (75 mg daily) or placebo for the duration of hospital stay (mean 16 days). The primary endpoint, a composite of death, reinfarction or stroke at hospital discharge, was significantly reduced with clopidogrel (9.3% vs 10.1%, $2p = 0.002$). The benefit in the primary endpoint occurred regardless of gender, age (26% older than 70), time to presentation (67% within 12 h) and reperfusion strategy received (49% fibrinolysis), and was not associated with an increase in hemorrhagic complications.

Taken together, these trials may stimulate a change in the management of patients with STEMI. They both demonstrated a significant benefit with the addition of clopidogrel to fibrinolytics and aspirin that appeared to be safe. Although primary PCI remains the reperfusion modality of choice, these data provide an improved pharmacologic reperfusion protocol that will also benefit those in whom PCI is not readily available. In addition, the safe use of clopidogrel in this setting may bridge the medical and interventional management of these patients.

PCI

Given the limitations of ticlopidine described above, the development of clopidogrel, with its similar mechanism of action, more rapid platelet inhibition and improved safety profile, was a welcome addition to the peri-interventional armamentarium. The safety and efficacy of clopidogrel compared to ticlopidine as an adjunct to PCI with stent (bare metal) implantation has been evaluated in several randomized trials and registries across a broad spectrum of patients (Table 3.4). Whereas the majority of the data suggest a similar efficacy of clopidogrel and ticlopidine in this patient population, one registry [101] and the short- [102] and long-term [103] assessment of outcomes from a randomized trial suggested increased adverse events with clopidogrel. However, the two largest randomized controlled trials revealed improved tolerability and a trend towards improved outcomes with clopidogrel [104, 105]. Although these data fostered clopidogrel's role as the ADP-receptor antagonist of choice in patients undergoing PCI with stent (bare metal) implantation, issues regarding the need for and timing and strength of a loading dose, optimal duration of therapy, safety of long-term therapy and need for additional antiplatelet agents have only recently been addressed (Table 3.3) [44, 79, 106]. Issues regarding drug eluting stents will be addressed in the clinical consideration section of this chapter.

The Clopidogrel for the Reduction of Events During Observation (CREDO) trial attempted to shed light on several of the previously unanswered issues of clopidogrel use in the setting of PCI [79]. The purpose of this trial was to determine the benefit of initiating clopidogrel with a pre-procedure loading dose (300 mg 3–24 h before PCI) and to evaluate the benefit of long-term (12-month) treatment with clopidogrel after PCI, both in addition to aspirin therapy. Clopidogrel pretreatment did not significantly reduce the combined risk of death, MI, or urgent target vessel revascularization at 28 days among the 2116 patients enrolled in this trial. However, in a pre-specified subgroup analysis, patients who received clopidogrel at least 6 h before PCI experienced a relative risk reduction of 38.6% (95% CI, −1.6% to 62.9%; p-value = 0.051) for this endpoint compared with no reduction with treatment less than 6 h before PCI. Long-term clopidogrel use (75 mg daily) resulted in a significant relative reduction in the combined risk of death, MI, or stroke (26.9%, p-value = 0.02) with an insignificant increase in the risk of major bleeding at 1 year (8.8% vs 6.7% with placebo; p-value = 0.07).

Although questions remained regarding the utility of clopidogrel pretreatment, the subgroup analysis of the CREDO trial suggested that pretreatment given greater than 6 h before elective stenting may be necessary to improve short-term outcomes. This idea was recently addressed in a randomized controlled trial comparing high (600 mg) versus standard (300 mg) loading doses of clopidogrel given 4–8 h before elective PCI [107]. Not only was pretreatment with a high loading dose associated with improved 30-day clinical outcomes, it was as safe as the standard dose loading regimen (Table 3.3). Combined with a recent trial suggesting that a 600 mg loading dose of clopidogrel given at least 2 h prior to PCI may obviate the need for adjunctive glycoprotein IIb/IIIa inhibition with abciximab in low- to intermediate-risk patients [44], these data support the high loading dose of clopidogrel and should influence current practice patterns.

Taken in totality, clopidogrel is an effective and well-tolerated alternative to ticlopidine in the peri-procedural pharmacologic armamentarium. The data delineated above has vastly improved the current understanding of clopidogrel's utility in this setting. However, several questions remain, among them: (i) How long before PCI should a patient be on clopidogrel? (ii) Does clopidogrel in addition to aspirin obviate the need for glycoprotein IIb/IIIa inhibitors during higher-risk PCI with stenting? and (iii) In what patient populations does clopidogrel impart the most benefit?

Cerebrovascular disease

The importance of antiplatelet therapy in the management of patients with cerebrovascular disease is supported by the avoidance of 36 events per 1000 patients with a previous stroke or TIA treated with these agents for two years [64]. The utility of clopidogrel for the secondary prevention of cerebrovascular disease has largely been extrapolated from data which demonstrated the benefits of ticlopidine in this setting. The CAPRIE trial also suggested the beneficial effects of clopidogrel in this setting with the demonstration of a significant, albeit small, decrease in the combined endpoint of ischemic stroke, MI or vascular death in 19,185 patients with atherosclerotic vascular disease [47]. Clopidogrel was associated with a trend towards a decreased annual recurrent event rate (7.15% vs 7.71% with aspirin, p-value = 0.26) in the 6413 patients who composed the stroke subgroup. In addition, in a recent meta-analysis combining the results of all studies comparing thienopyridines and aspirin, thienopyridines seem to be modestly more, or at least equally, effective in the secondary prevention of ischemic stroke or other major vascular events [108]. Arising out of this paucity of data, clopidogrel has assumed the role of an alternative agent to aspirin in patients with cerebrovascular disease.

Whether clopidogrel in addition to aspirin would afford improved outcomes compared with clopidogrel alone has been assessed [109]. In this trial of high-risk patients with recent ischemic stroke or TIA and at least one additional vascular risk factor already receiving clopidogrel 75 mg/day, 7599 patients were randomized receive aspirin (75 mg/day) or placebo. The combination of aspirin plus clopidogrel resulted in marginal improvement over clopidogrel alone. However, this was at the expense of increased life-threatening or major bleeding. Therefore, current recommendations suggest the use of either aspirin or clopidogrel for the secondary prevention of ischemic cerebrovascular events. Whether current outcomes can be improved with alternative antiplatelet strategies is actively being assessed in several clinical trials [110].

PAD

Patients with PAD are at increased risk of generalized atherothrombotic events [111, 112]. Epidemiologic data shows a high rate of co-prevalence of PAD and atherosclerosis in other vascular beds [113]. Aggressive risk-factor modification and antiplatelet therapy has become the cornerstone of treatment to prevent ischemic events associated with PAD. Although a paucity of data exists evaluating the clinical benefit of clopidogrel in patients with PAD, the beneficial effects of clopidogrel in patients with symptomatic atherothrombotic disease in other vascular territories allows for extrapolation to patients with PAD. In the CAPRIE trial, clopidogrel was associated with a relative risk reduction of 23.8% in the average annual event rate within the 6452 patients that comprised the PAD subgroup (compared with aspirin, p-value = 0.0028) [47]. Furthermore, evaluation of the CAPRIE data suggested that the true benefit of clopidogrel over aspirin might be much greater in patients with PAD [47]. Based on these results, clopidogrel was approved in 1997 by the FDA for the reduction of ischemic events in patients with PAD.

CLINICAL CONSIDERATIONS

Clopidogrel resistance

Similar to the situation seen with aspirin, a significant proportion of patients receiving clopidogrel exhibit a failure of clopidogrel to adequately inhibit platelet aggregation [80, 114, 115] and, more importantly, experience recurrent thrombotic events [81, 82, 116]. Whether this is the result of true 'resistance' to the antiplatelet effects of clopidogrel or simply a treatment failure of a multifactorial disease process remains a topic of debate. The question remains does pharmacologic resistance to the antiplatelet effects of clopidogrel result in treatment failures in patients with atherothrombotic disease?

The extent of the platelet aggregation response *in vitro* to ADP has been used to define 'clopidogrel resistance' in the large majority of studies that have been published so far [80–82, 115]. Using less than or equal to 10% inhibition of platelet aggregation relative to baseline values by 5 μmol/L ADP, clopidogrel resistance has been identified in up to 31% of patients. However, using this definition may over-estimate the true incidence of non-response to clopidogrel, owing to the presence of an additional ADP receptor, P2Y1, that is responsible for the initial wave of platelet aggregation (see section Mechanism of action). Development of a test that could measure the effects of ADP antagonism directly on the P2Y12 receptor would more accurately identify clopidogrel non-responders [117, 118].

Equally important to the understanding of clopidogrel resistance is the potential mechanism to account for its occurrence. Because clopidogrel is a prodrug, it requires metabolism into its active metabolite by hepatic cytochrome P450 (CYP) 3A4 in order to impart its anti-aggregating effects. As a result, the plasma levels of the active metabolite may vary widely among individuals, resulting in a widely variable inhibition of ADP-induced platelet aggregation, which has been correlated with inter-individual differences in CYP3A4 metabolism [119]. Other potential mechanisms, either extrinsic (inappropriate dosing or underdosing of clopidogrel, drug–drug interactions, variable absorption of the prodrug or variable clearance of the active metabolite) or intrinsic (polymorphisms of the P2Y12 receptor, increase in number of receptors, increased release of ADP or upregulation of other platelet activation pathways) may be involved in the phenomenon of clopidogrel resistance but remain, as yet, incompletely identified.

Until recently, there has been a dearth of information demonstrating the clinical relevance of this laboratory entity. To determine whether variability in response to clopidogrel affects clinical outcomes, the antiplatelet effect of clopidogrel was prospectively studied in 60 consecutive patients treated with primary PCI with stenting for acute STEMI [82]. Patients with clopidogrel resistance (ADP-induced platelet aggregation at day 6, 103 ±8% of baseline) were significantly more likely to sustain recurrent cardiovascular events (p-value = 0.007).

Despite these data, the routine assessment of individual responses to clopidogrel can not be advocated owing to (i) a lack of data in larger, randomized trials, (ii) a lack of a standardized, reproducible test to assess clopidogrel-induced inhibition of platelet aggregation and (iii) a paucity of therapies identified to overcome clopidogrel resistance.

Optimal duration of clopidogrel in the drug-eluting stent era

The development of coronary stents revolutionized the field of interventional cardiology. However, the use of intracoronary stents was accompanied by an Achilles' heel, restenosis, in a significant proportion of cases depending on clinical risk factors, lesion characteristics, and technical aspects of the intervention [120]. Recently, several randomized clinical trials have once again pushed the frontier of interventional cardiology further with the demonstration that restenosis rates could be substantially decreased with the use of drug-eluting stents. Despite no clear warning in the clinical trials (Table 3.5), after-market case reports of a potentially devastating complication, subacute thrombosis (SAT), became increasingly frequent, prompting the FDA to publish a Web notification of the reported events [121, 122]. Furthermore, several case reports of late SAT have, disturbingly, surfaced [123–126]. Nevertheless, it remains unclear whether SAT rates are actually elevated with drug-eluting stents above those experienced with conventional bare metal stents.

Although the risk factors for and mechanisms involved in early and late SAT are incompletely defined, enhanced platelet aggregation induced by the local delivery of these anti-proliferative medications has been implicated as an integral component [127, 128]. That said, the utility of dual antiplatelet therapies, primarily with clopidogrel and aspirin, for longer durations, in general, than previously assessed with bare metal stents is understandable (Table 3.5). The optimal duration of dual antiplatelet therapy in patients receiving drug-eluting stents (DES) has not been formally addressed. However, current practice patterns have arisen from extrapolation of data demonstrating the benefit of use for one year following DES implantation. Furthermore, that late SAT has been shown to occur in a temporally related fashion with cessation of antiplatelet therapy has prompted the continuation of these regimens for increasing lengths of time. Nevertheless, the optimal duration of antiplatelet therapy with clopidogrel combined with aspirin remains a moving target.

Clopidogrel–atorvastatin interaction

Clopidogrel and atorvastatin are frequently co-administered to patients across the spectrum of CV disease. Atorvastatin is extensively metabolized by the hepatic CYP 3A4 isoenzyme, and has been shown to inhibit the metabolism of clopidogrel into its active metabolite by more than 90% [129]. Several additional studies of the interaction between atorvastatin and clopidogrel have been performed with conflicting results. Whereas three *ex vivo* studies of

Table 3.5 Duration of dual antiplatelet therapy in trials of drug-eluting stents

Trial	Stent type	Lesion type	Trial type	*N*	Antiplatelet regimen	Duration of antiplatelet therapy	SAT rate with DES (%)	SAT rate with BMS (%)	*p*-value	Comment
Colombo *et al.* [153]	Paclitaxel – SR or Paclitaxel – MR vs control stent	Single, lesions in native vessel	RCT	536	Clopidogrel 300 mg 24 h before catheterization or at least 4 h before stent placement then 75 mg daily + Aspirin 75 mg 24 h before catheterization or at least 4 h before stent placement, then aspirin 75 mg daily	Clopidogrel – 6 months aspirin – indefinitely	0.7% between 6 and 12 months	0	NS	MACE at 12 months 10.9% (TAXUS-SR), 22% (Control), 9.9% (TAXUS MR) 21.4% (control)
Stone *et al.* [154]	Paclitaxel – SR vs BMS	Single, lesions in native vessel	RCT	1314	Clopidogrel 300 mg before and 75 mg after procedure + aspirin 325 mg before and after procedure	Clopidogrel – 6 months Aspirin – indefinitely	0.6	0.8	0.75	Aspirin was continued indefinitely at an intermediate dose which was higher than the other DES trials
Park *et al.* [155]	Low-dose or high-dose paclitaxel vs BMS	Single, lesions in native vessel	RCT	177	Ticlopidine before and after stent, OR clopidogrel before and after stent OR clopidogrel or ticlopidine before and cilostazol after stent + aspirin	Aspirin + ticlopidine or clopidogrel for 1 month and 6 months. Aspirin + cilostazol in 37 patients	0 10.8	0	NS	Cilostazol + aspirin was associated with increased MACE

Gershlick *et al.* [156]	Paclitaxel – escalating doses vs BMS	Single, lesions in native vessel	RCT	190	Clopidogrel + aspirin	Clopidogrel + aspirin for 3 months	2.7	2.6	NS	SAT occurred in the group receiving a paclitaxel eluting stent with the highest dose density
Lansky *et al.* [157]	Non-polymer based paclitaxel coated stent vs BMS	Single, lesions in native vessel	RCT	1043	Clopidogrel 300 mg 24 h before or immediately after stent then 75 mg daily + aspirin 325 mg 24 h before and after stent	Clopidogrel – 3 months Aspirin – 1 year	–	–	–	ACHIEVE paclitaxel-coated stent failed to meet the primary end point of TV failure
Morice *et al.* [158]	Sirolimus-eluting vs BMS	Single, lesions in native vessel	RCT	238	Clopidogrel 300 mg 48 h before stent then 75 mg daily OR Ticlopidine 250 mg bid one day before then daily after stent + aspirin 100 mg per day, was begun 12 h before the procedure and continued indefinitely	Clopidogrel or ticlopidine – 8 weeks Aspirin – indefinitely	–	–	–	MACE 5.8% (sirolimus) 28.8% (BMS)
Moses *et al.* [159]	Sirolimus-eluting vs BMS	Single, lesions in native vessel	RCT	1058	Clopidogrel 300–375 mg 24 h before and 75 mg daily after procedure + aspirin 325 mg 24 h before and daily after procedure	Clopidogrel – 3 months Aspirin – indefinitely	0.4	0.8	NS	SAT: 1, 1–30 days after stent in each group; 4, 31–270 days after stent – one in the sirolimus-stent group and three in the standard- stent group

Table 3.5 (*Continued*)

Trial	Stent type	Lesion type	Trial type	*N*	Antiplatelet regimen	Duration of antiplatelet therapy	SAT rate with DES (%)	SAT rate with BMS (%)	*p*-value	Comment
Schofer *et al.* [160]	Sirolimus-eluting vs BMS	Long lesions, small coronary arteries	RCT	352	Clopidogrel 300 mg immediately before or after stent or 75 mg daily for 3 days before and daily after stent OR Ticlopidine 250 mg bid 24 h before and daily after stent + Aspirin 100 mg 12 h before and daily after stent	Clopidogrel – 2 months Ticlopidine – 2 months Aspirin – indefinitely	1.1	0	0.25	SAT occurred at 5 and 10 days after the procedure
Schampaert *et al.* [161]	Sirolimus-eluting vs BMS	Long lesions, small coronary arteries	RCT	100	Clopidogrel 300mg immediately before or after stent or 75 mg daily after stent + aspirin 81–325 mg ~12 h before and daily after stent	Clopidogrel – 2 months Aspirin – indefinitely	2	2	NS	SAT occurred on day 8 in the DES patient and day 57 in the BMS patient

bid = twice daily; BMS = bare metal stent; DES = drug-eluting stent; MACE = major adverse cardiac events; MR = medium release; NS = not significant; SR = slow release; SAT = subacute thrombosis; TV = target vessel platelet function have suggested a negative effect of atorvastatin on clopidogrel's ability to inhibit platelet aggregation [130–132], four *ex vivo* studies assessing the effects of combined atorvastatin and clopidogrel administration in various sub-populations of patients have not [133–136]. More importantly, atorvastatin has not been shown to mitigate the beneficial effects of clopidogrel in patients undergoing PCI with stenting [137] or in those presenting with ACS [138]. Unfortunately, the dose–response attenuation of clopidogrel's antiplatelet activity by atorvastatin at doses shown to provide the optimal clinical benefit, 80 mg daily [139, 140], has not been adequately assessed. Thus, the debate will, undoubtedly, continue.

Clopidogrel and the risk of CABG-related bleeding

Approximately one in five patients presenting with an ACS will ultimately undergo CABG [141]. The relationship between clopidogrel use and the incidence of CABG-related hemorrhagic complications continues to evolve. An increased risk of hemorrhagic complications has been demonstrated when CABG is performed within 5 days of clopidogrel administration [46, 142–144]. These data have limited the widespread acceptance of early clopidogrel use, including pretreatment for PCI, in these patients and, especially, those presenting with ACS. Furthermore, the potential increased risk of bleeding associated with clopidogrel use preoperatively has prompted the development of clinical prediction rules that may assist in identifying patients with ACS who are likely to require CABG during the index hospitalization [145]. Ultimately, the purpose of these models is to optimize therapy with clopidogrel for those least likely to require CABG.

Recent data has emerged that contradicts the increased incidence of bleeding seen with clopidogrel use pre-CABG [93, 94, 96, 97]. In patients with STEMI an increased risk of CABG-related bleeding was not observed with the use of clopidogrel (7.5% vs 7.2% with placebo, p-value $= 1.0$) even when given within 5 days of surgery (9.1% vs 7.9% with placebo, p-value $= 1.0$) [93]. A similar lack of a relationship between clopidogrel use and CABG-related bleeding was also seen in the COMMIT trial [94]. Coupled with data illustrating that the benefits outweigh the risks in patients with ACS who proceed to CABG during the initial hospitalization [97], these data may serve to alter current clinical practice. However, more data supporting the lack of an increased bleeding risk peri-operatively may be required before this change occurs.

3.4 CONCLUSIONS

With its enhanced pharmacokinetic, pharmacodynamic and safety profile, clopidogrel has been catapulted into the position of antiplatelet agent of choice in combination with or in lieu of aspirin. However, that clopidogrel may have a chink in its antiplatelet armor has been suggested by the presence of 'non-responders' and its implicated treatment failures in these patients. This has fostered the ever-continuing quest for the optimal antiplatelet agent that possesses a totally effective and safe profile across the spectrum of atherothrombotic diseases. Given that this agent does not exist and is unlikely to do so in the near future, clopidogrel's stronghold in the management of atherothrombotic diseases is likely to persist.

REFERENCES

[1] Rao, A.K., (1990) Congenital disorders of platelet function. *Hematol Oncol Clin North Am*, 4(1):65–86.

[2] Yusuf, S., *et al.*, (2003) Early and late effects of clopidogrel in patients with acute coronary syndromes. *Circulation*, 107(7):966–72.

[3] Cattaneo, M., Gachet, C., (1999) ADP receptors and clinical bleeding disorders. *Arterioscler Thromb Vasc Biol*, 19(10):281–5.

[4] Hollopeter, G., *et al.*, (2001) Identification of the platelet ADP receptor targeted by antithrombotic drugs. Nature, 409(6817):202–7.

[5] Gachet, C., (2001) Identification, characterization, and inhibition of the platelet ADP receptors. Int J Hematol, 74(4):375–81.

[6] Gachet, C., (2000) Platelet activation by ADP: the role of ADP antagonists. Ann Med, 32 Suppl 1:15–20.

[7] Martinson, E.A., *et al.*, (1998) Secreted ADP plays a central role in thrombin-induced phospholipase D activation in human platelets. *Thromb Haemost*, 80(6):976–81.

[8] Vial, C., *et al.*, (1997) Presence of P2X1 purinoceptors in human platelets and megakaryoblastic cell lines. *Thromb Haemost*, 78(6):1500–4.

[9] Daniel, J.L., *et al.*, (1998) Molecular basis for ADP-induced platelet activation. I. Evidence for three distinct ADP receptors on human platelets. *J Biol Chem*, 273(4):2024–9.

[10] Jin, J., Daniel, J.L., Kunapuli, S.P., (1998) Molecular basis for ADP-induced platelet activation. II. The P2Y1 receptor mediates ADP-induced intracellular calcium mobilization and shape change in platelets. *J Biol Chem*, 273(4):2030–4.

[11] Savi, P., *et al.*, (2001) P2y(12), a new platelet ADP receptor, target of clopidogrel. *Biochem Biophys Res Commun*, 283(2):379–83.

[12] Savi, P., *et al.*, (1997) Characterization of P2x1 purinoreceptors on rat platelets: effect of clopidogrel. *Br J Haematol*, 98(4):880–6.

[13] Ziganshin, A.U., Ziganshina, L.E., Burnstock, G., (2002) P2 receptors: theoretical background for the use in clinical practice. *Bull Exp Biol Med*, 134(4):313–17.

[14] Hechler, B., *et al.*, (1998) The P2Y1 receptor is necessary for adenosine 5'-diphosphate-induced platelet aggregation. *Blood*, 92(1):152–9.

[15] Leon, C., *et al.*, (2003) Differential involvement of the P2Y1 and P2Y12 receptors in platelet procoagulant activity. *Arterioscler Thromb Vasc Biol*, 23(10):1941–7.

[16] Herbert, J.M., Savi, P., (2003) P2Y12, a new platelet ADP receptor, target of clopidogrel. *Semin Vasc Med*, 3(2):113–22.

[17] Fox, S.C., Behan, M.W., Heptinstall, S., (2004) Inhibition of ADP-induced intracellular Ca2+ responses and platelet aggregation by the P2Y12 receptor antagonists AR-C69931MX and clopidogrel is enhanced by prostaglandin E1. *Cell Calcium*, 35(1):39–46.

[18] Matsuno, H., *et al.*, (2005) P2Y12 receptors play a significant role in the development of platelet microaggregation in patients with diabetes. *J Clin Endocrinol Metab*, 90(2):920–7.

[19] Mangin, P., *et al.*, (2004) The P2Y1 receptor plays an essential role in the platelet shape change induced by collagen when TxA2 formation is prevented. *J Thromb Haemost*, 2(6):969–77.

[20] Jagroop, I.A., *et al.*, (2004) The effect of clopidogrel, aspirin and both antiplatelet drugs on platelet function in patients with peripheral arterial disease. *Platelets*, 15(2):117–25.

[21] Mills, D.C., *et al.*, (1992) Clopidogrel inhibits the binding of ADP analogues to the receptor mediating inhibition of platelet adenylate cyclase. *Arterioscler Thromb*, 12(4):430–6.

[22] Heptinstall, S., *et al.*, (1995) Effects of ticlopidine administered to healthy volunteers on platelet function in whole blood. *Thromb Haemost*, 74(5):1310–15.

[23] Kam, P.C., Nethery, C.M., (2003) The thienopyridine derivatives (platelet adenosine diphosphate receptor antagonists), pharmacology and clinical developments. *Anaesthesia*, 58(1): 28–35.

[24] Savi, P., *et al.*, (2000) Identification and biological activity of the active metabolite of clopidogrel. *Thromb Haemost*, 84(5):891–6.

[25] Ding, Z., *et al.*, (2003) Inactivation of the human P2Y12 receptor by thiol reagents requires interaction with both extracellular cysteine residues, Cys17 and Cys270. *Blood*, 101(10):3908–14.

[26] Boneu, B., Destelle, G., (1996) Platelet anti-aggregating activity and tolerance of clopidogrel in atherosclerotic patients. *Thromb Haemost*, 76(6):939–43.
[27] Di Minno, G., *et al.*, (1985) Functionally thrombasthenic state in normal platelets following the administration of ticlopidine. *J Clin Invest*, 75(2):328–38.
[28] Vishnevetsky, D., Kiyanista, V.A., Gandhi, P.J., (2004) CD40 ligand: a novel target in the fight against cardiovascular disease. *Ann Pharmacother*, 38(9):1500–8.
[29] Xiao, Z., Theroux, P., (2004) Clopidogrel inhibits platelet-leukocyte interactions and thrombin receptor agonist peptide-induced platelet activation in patients with an acute coronary syndrome. *J Am Coll Cardiol*, 43(11):1982–8.
[30] Quinn, M.J., *et al.*, (2004) Effect of clopidogrel pretreatment on inflammatory marker expression in patients undergoing percutaneous coronary intervention. *Am J Cardiol*, 93(6):679–84.
[31] Koenig, W., (2005) Predicting risk and treatment benefit in atherosclerosis: the role of C-reactive protein. *Int J Cardiol*, 98(2):199–206.
[32] Cha, J.K., *et al.*, (2002) Changes in platelet P-selectin and in plasma C-reactive protein in acute atherosclerotic ischemic stroke treated with a loading dose of clopidogrel. *J Thromb Thrombolysis*, 14(2):145–50.
[33] Chew, D.P., *et al.*, (2001) Effect of clopidogrel added to aspirin before percutaneous coronary intervention on the risk associated with C-reactive protein. *Am J Cardiol*, 88(6):672–4.
[34] Woodward, M., *et al.*, (2004) A randomized comparison of the effects of aspirin and clopidogrel on thrombotic risk factors and C-reactive protein following myocardial infarction: the CADET trial. *J Thromb Haemost*, 2(11):1934–40.
[35] Vivekananthan, D.P., *et al.*, (2004) Effect of clopidogrel pretreatment on periprocedural rise in C-reactive protein after percutaneous coronary intervention. *Am J Cardiol*, 94(3):358–60.
[36] Saltiel, E., Ward, A., (1987) Ticlopidine. A review of its pharmacodynamic and pharmacokinetic properties, and therapeutic efficacy in platelet-dependent disease states. *Drugs*, 34(2):222–62.
[37] Desager, J.P., (1994) Clinical pharmacokinetics of ticlopidine. *Clin Pharmacokinet*, 26(5): 347–55.
[38] Shah, J., *et al.*, (1991) Single and multiple dose pharmacokinetics of ticlopidine in young and elderly subjects. *Br J Clin Pharmacol*, 32(6):761–4.
[39] Coukell, A.J., Markham, A., (1997) Clopidogrel. *Drugs*, 54(5):745–50; discussion 751.
[40] Caplain, H., *et al.*, (1999) Pharmacokinetics of clopidogrel. *Semin Thromb Hemost*, 25 Suppl 2:25–8.
[41] Savcic, M., *et al.*, (1999) Clopidogrel loading dose regimens: kinetic profile of pharmacodynamic response in healthy subjects. *Semin Thromb Hemost*, 25 Suppl 2:15–19.
[42] Kastrati, A., *et al.*, (2004) Loading with 600 mg clopidogrel in patients with coronary artery disease with and without chronic clopidogrel therapy. *Circulation*, 110(14):1916–19.
[43] Kandzari, D.E., *et al.*, (2004) Influence of treatment duration with a 600-mg dose of clopidogrel before percutaneous coronary revascularization. *J Am Coll Cardiol*, 44(11):2133–6.
[44] Kastrati, A., *et al.*, (2004) A clinical trial of abciximab in elective percutaneous coronary intervention after pretreatment with clopidogrel. *N Eng J Med*, 350(3):232–8.
[45] Leon, M.B., *et al.*, (1998) A clinical trial comparing three antithrombotic-drug regimens after coronary-artery stenting. Stent Anticoagulation Restenosis Study Investigators. *N Eng J Med*, 339(23):1665–71.
[46] Yusuf, S., *et al.*, (2001) Effects of clopidogrel in addition to aspirin in patients with acute coronary syndromes without ST-segment elevation. *N Eng J Med*, 345(7):494–502.
[47] CAPRIE Steering Committee. (1996) A randomised, blinded, trial of clopidogrel versus aspirin in patients at risk of ischaemic events (CAPRIE). *Lancet*, 348(9038):1329–39.
[48] Moshfegh, K., *et al.*, (2000) Antiplatelet effects of clopidogrel compared with aspirin after myocardial infarction: enhanced inhibitory effects of combination therapy. *J Am Coll Cardiol*, 36(3):699–705.
[49] Bhatt, D.L., *et al.*, (2001) Dual antiplatelet therapy with clopidogrel and aspirin after carotid artery stenting. *J Invasive Cardiol*, 13(12):767–71.
[50] Nappi, J., Talbert, R., (2002) Dual antiplatelet therapy for prevention of recurrent ischemic events. *Am J Health Syst Pharm*, 59(18):1723–35.
[51] Payne, D.A., *et al.*, (2002) Combined therapy with clopidogrel and aspirin significantly increases the bleeding time through a synergistic antiplatelet action. *J Vasc Surg*, 35(6):1204–9.

[52] Bhatt, D.L., Topol, E.J., (2004) Clopidogrel added to aspirin versus aspirin alone in secondary prevention and high-risk primary prevention: rationale and design of the Clopidogrel for High Atherothrombotic Risk and Ischemic Stabilization, Management, and Avoidance (CHARISMA) trial. *Am Heart J*, 148(2):263–8.

[53] Zhao, L., *et al.*, (2005) Effects of aspirin, clopidogrel and dipyridamole administered singly and in combination on platelet and leucocyte function in normal volunteers and patients with prior ischaemic stroke. *Thromb Haemost*, 93(3):527–34.

[54] Yeh, S.P., *et al.*, (1998) Ticlopidine-associated aplastic anemia. A case report and review of literature. *Ann Hematol*, 76(2):87–90.

[55] Bennett, C.L., *et al.*, (2000) Thrombotic thrombocytopenic purpura associated with clopidogrel. *N Eng J Med*, 342(24):1773–7.

[56] Balsano, F., *et al.*, (1990) Antiplatelet treatment with ticlopidine in unstable angina. A controlled multicenter clinical trial. The Studio della Ticlopidina nell'Angina Instabile Group. *Circulation*, 82(1):17–26.

[57] Scrutinio, D., *et al.*, (2001) Ticlopidine versus aspirin after myocardial infarction (STAMI) trial. *J Am Coll Cardiol*, 37(5):1259–65.

[58] Hall, P., *et al.*, (1996) A randomized comparison of combined ticlopidine and aspirin therapy versus aspirin therapy alone after successful intravascular ultrasound-guided stent implantation. *Circulation*, 93(2):215–22.

[59] Schomig, A., *et al.*, (1996) A randomized comparison of antiplatelet and anticoagulant therapy after the placement of coronary-artery stents. *N Eng J Med*, 334(17):1084–9.

[60] Urban, P., *et al.*, (1998) Randomized evaluation of anticoagulation versus antiplatelet therapy after coronary stent implantation in high-risk patients: the multicenter aspirin and ticlopidine trial after intracoronary stenting (MATTIS). *Circulation*, 98(20):2126–32.

[61] Bertrand, M.E., *et al.*, (1998) Randomized multicenter comparison of conventional anticoagulation versus antiplatelet therapy in unplanned and elective coronary stenting. The full anticoagulation versus aspirin and ticlopidine (fantastic) study. *Circulation*, 98(16):1597–603.

[62] Steinhubl, S.R., *et al.*, (1998) The duration of pretreatment with ticlopidine prior to stenting is associated with the risk of procedure-related non-Q-wave myocardial infarctions. *J Am Coll Cardiol*, 32(5):1366–70.

[63] Berger, P.B., *et al.*, (1999) Safety and efficacy of ticlopidine for only 2 weeks after successful intracoronary stent placement. *Circulation*, 99(2):248–53.

[64] Collaborative meta-analysis of randomised trials of antiplatelet therapy for prevention of death, myocardial infarction, and stroke in high risk patients. (2002) *Br Med J*, 324(7329):71–86.

[65] Bergamasco, B., *et al.*, (1997) A randomized trial comparing ticlopidine hydrochloride with indobufen for the prevention of stroke in high-risk patients (TISS Study). Ticlopidine Indobufen Stroke Study. *Funct Neurol*, 12(1):33–43.

[66] Gent, M., *et al.*, (1989) The Canadian American Ticlopidine Study (CATS) in thromboembolic stroke. *Lancet*, 1(8649):1215–20.

[67] Hass, W.K., *et al.*, (1989) A randomized trial comparing ticlopidine hydrochloride with aspirin for the prevention of stroke in high-risk patients. Ticlopidine Aspirin Stroke Study Group. *N Eng J Med*, 321(8):501–7.

[68] Narins, C.R., *et al.*, (2004) Relationship between intermittent claudication, inflammation, thrombosis, and recurrent cardiac events among survivors of myocardial infarction. *Arch Intern Med*, 164(4):440–6.

[69] Nikolsky, E., *et al.*, (2004) Impact of symptomatic peripheral arterial disease on 1-year mortality in patients undergoing percutaneous coronary interventions. *J Endovasc Ther*, 11(1):60–70.

[70] Violi, F., *et al.*, (1996) Relation between risk factors and cardiovascular complications in patients with peripheral vascular disease. Results from the A.D.E.P. study. *Atherosclerosis*, 120(1–2): 25–35.

[71] Janzon, L., *et al.*, (1990) Prevention of myocardial infarction and stroke in patients with intermittent claudication; effects of ticlopidine. Results from STIMS, the Swedish Ticlopidine Multicentre Study. *J Intern Med*, 227(5):301–8.

[72] Blanchard, J., Carreras, L.O., Kindermans, M., (1994) Results of EMATAP: a double-blind placebo-controlled multicentre trial of ticlopidine in patients with peripheral arterial disease. *Nouv Rev Fr Hematol*, 35(6):523–8.

[73] Arcan, J.C., *et al.*, (1988) Multicenter double-blind study of ticlopidine in the treatment of intermittent claudication and the prevention of its complications. *Angiology*, 39(9):802–11.
[74] Limet, R., *et al.*, (1987) Prevention of aorta-coronary bypass graft occlusion. Beneficial effect of ticlopidine on early and late patency rates of venous coronary bypass grafts: a double-blind study. *J Thorac Cardiovasc Surg*, 94(5):773–83.
[75] Becquemin, J.P., (1997) Effect of ticlopidine on the long-term patency of saphenous-vein bypass grafts in the legs. Etude de la Ticlopidine apres Pontage Femoro-Poplite and the Association Universitaire de Recherche en Chirurgie. *N Eng J Med*, 337(24):1726–31.
[76] Steinhubl, S.R., *et al.*, (1999) Incidence and clinical course of thrombotic thrombocytopenic purpura due to ticlopidine following coronary stenting. EPISTENT Investigators. Evaluation of Platelet IIb/IIIa Inhibitor for Stenting. *JAMA*, 281(9):806–10.
[77] Bennett, C.L., *et al.*, (1999) Thrombotic thrombocytopenic purpura associated with ticlopidine in the setting of coronary artery stents and stroke prevention. *Arch Intern Med*, 159(21):2524–8.
[78] Yim, H.B., Lieu, P.K., Choo, P.W., (1997) Ticlopidine induced cholestatic jaundice. *Singapore Med J*, 38(3):132–3.
[79] Steinhubl, S.R., *et al.*, (2002) Early and sustained dual oral antiplatelet therapy following percutaneous coronary intervention: a randomized controlled trial. *JAMA*, 288(19): 2411–20.
[80] Gurbel, P.A., *et al.*, (2003) Clopidogrel for coronary stenting: response variability, drug resistance, and the effect of pretreatment platelet reactivity. *Circulation*, 107(23):2908–13.
[81] Muller, I., *et al.*, (2003) Prevalence of clopidogrel non-responders among patients with stable angina pectoris scheduled for elective coronary stent placement. *Thromb Haemost*, 89(5): 783–7.
[82] Matetzky, S., *et al.*, (2004) Clopidogrel resistance is associated with increased risk of recurrent atherothrombotic events in patients with acute myocardial infarction. *Circulation*, 109(25):3171–5.
[83] Serebruany, V.L., *et al.*, (2005) Variability in platelet responsiveness to clopidogrel among 544 individuals. *J Am Coll Cardiol*, 45(2):246–51.
[84] Bhatt, D.L., *et al.*, (2001) Superiority of clopidogrel versus aspirin in patients with prior cardiac surgery. *Circulation*, 103(3):363–8.
[85] Bhatt, D.L., *et al.*, (2002) Amplified benefit of clopidogrel versus aspirin in patients with diabetes mellitus. *Am J Cardiol*, 90(6):625–8.
[86] Mehta, S.R., Yusuf, S., (2003) Short- and long-term oral antiplatelet therapy in acute coronary syndromes and percutaneous coronary intervention. *J Am Coll Cardiol*, 41(4 Suppl S): 79S-88S.
[87] Cannon, C.P., *et al.*, (2001) Comparison of early invasive and conservative strategies in patients with unstable coronary syndromes treated with the glycoprotein IIb/IIIa inhibitor tirofiban. *N Eng J Med*, 344(25):1879–87.
[88] Heeschen, C., *et al.*, (1999) Troponin concentrations for stratification of patients with acute coronary syndromes in relation to therapeutic efficacy of tirofiban. PRISM Study Investigators. Platelet Receptor Inhibition in Ischemic Syndrome Management. *Lancet*, 354(9192): 1757–62.
[89] Dalby, M., *et al.*, (2004) Eptifibatide provides additional platelet inhibition in non-ST-elevation myocardial infarction patients already treated with aspirin and clopidogrel. Results of the platelet activity extinction in non-Q-wave myocardial infarction with aspirin, clopidogrel, and eptifibatide (PEACE) study. *J Am Coll Cardiol*, 43(2):162–8.
[90] Novel dosing regimen of eptifibatide in planned coronary stent implantation (ESPRIT): a randomised, placebo-controlled trial, (2000) *Lancet*, 356(9247):2037–44.
[91] Kapadia, S.R., *et al.*, (2001) Initial experience of platelet glycoprotein IIb/IIIa inhibition with abciximab during carotid stenting: a safe and effective adjunctive therapy. *Stroke*, 32(10):2328–32.
[92] Chan, A.W., *et al.*, (2003) Triple antiplatelet therapy during percutaneous coronary intervention is associated with improved outcomes including one-year survival: results from the Do Tirofiban and ReoProGive Similar Efficacy Outcome Trial (TARGET). *J Am Coll Cardiol*, 42(7):1188–95.

[93] Sabatine, M.S., *et al.*, (2005) Addition of clopidogrel to aspirin and fibrinolytic therapy for myocardial infarction with ST-segment elevation. *N Eng J Med*, 352.

[94] Chen, Z., (2005) Clopidogrel Metoprolol Myocardial Infarction (COMMIT) trial, in *American College of Cardiology Scientific Sessions*. Orlando, Fl.

[95] Yende, S., Wunderink, R.G., (2001) Effect of clopidogrel on bleeding after coronary artery bypass surgery. *Crit Care Med*, 29(12):2271–5.

[96] Karabulut, H., *et al.*, (2004) Clopidogrel does not increase bleeding and allogenic blood transfusion in coronary artery surgery. *Eur J Cardiothorac Surg*, 25(3):419–23.

[97] Fox, K.A., *et al.*, (2004) Benefits and risks of the combination of clopidogrel and aspirin in patients undergoing surgical revascularization for non-ST-elevation acute coronary syndrome: the Clopidogrel in Unstable angina to prevent Recurrent ischemic Events (CURE) Trial. *Circulation*, 110(10):1202–8.

[98] Hudson, M.P., *et al.*, (2001) Early reinfarction after fibrinolysis: experience from the global utilization of streptokinase and tissue plasminogen activator (alteplase) for occluded coronary arteries (GUSTO I) and global use of strategies to open occluded coronary arteries (GUSTO III) trials. *Circulation*, 104(11):1229–35.

[99] The GUSTO V Investigators, (2001) Reperfusion therapy for acute myocardial infarction with fibrinolytic therapy or combination reduced fibrinolytic therapy and platelet glycoprotein IIb/IIIa inhibition: the GUSTO V randomized trial. *Lancet*, 357:1905–1914.

[100] Efficacy and safety of tenecteplase in combination with enoxaparin, abciximab, or unfractionated heparin: the ASSENT-3 randomised trial in acute myocardial infarction, (2001) *Lancet*, 358(9282):605–13.

[101] Dangas, G., *et al.*, (2001) Combination therapy with aspirin plus clopidogrel versus aspirin plus ticlopidine for prevention of subacute thrombosis after successful native coronary stenting. *Am J Cardiol*, 87(4):470–2, A7.

[102] Muller, C., *et al.*, (2000) A randomized comparison of clopidogrel and aspirin versus ticlopidine and aspirin after the placement of coronary-artery stents. *Circulation*, 101(6): 590–3.

[103] Mueller, C., *et al.*, (2003) A randomized comparison of clopidogrel and aspirin versus ticlopidine and aspirin after the placement of coronary artery stents. *J Am Coll Cardiol*, 41(6): 969–73.

[104] Taniuchi, M., Kurz, H.I., Lasala, J.M., (2001) Randomized comparison of ticlopidine and clopidogrel after intracoronary stent implantation in a broad patient population. *Circulation*, 104(5):539–43.

[105] Bertrand, M.E., *et al.*, (2000) Double-blind study of the safety of clopidogrel with and without a loading dose in combination with aspirin compared with ticlopidine in combination with aspirin after coronary stenting: the clopidogrel aspirin stent international cooperative study (CLASSICS). *Circulation*, 102(6):624–9.

[106] Mehta, S.R., *et al.*, (2001) Effects of pretreatment with clopidogrel and aspirin followed by long-term therapy in patients undergoing percutaneous coronary intervention: the PCI-CURE study. *Lancet*, 358(9281):527–33.

[107] Patti, G., *et al.*, (2005) Randomized Trial of High Loading Dose of Clopidogrel for Reduction of Periprocedural Myocardial Infarction in Patients Undergoing Coronary Intervention. Results From the ARMYDA-2 (Antiplatelet therapy for Reduction of MYocardial Damage during Angioplasty) Study. *Circulation*, 111: 2099–106.

[108] Hankey, G.J., Sudlow, C.L., Dunbabin, D.W., (2000) Thienopyridines or aspirin to prevent stroke and other serious vascular events in patients at high risk of vascular disease? A systematic review of the evidence from randomized trials. *Stroke*, 31(7):1779–84.

[109] Diener, H.C., *et al.*, (2004) Aspirin and clopidogrel compared with clopidogrel alone after recent ischaemic stroke or transient ischaemic attack in high-risk patients (MATCH): randomised, double-blind, placebo-controlled trial. *Lancet*, 364(9431):331–7.

[110] Hankey, G.J., (2004) Ongoing and planned trials of antiplatelet therapy in the acute and long-term management of patients with ischaemic brain syndromes: setting a new standard of care. *Cerebrovasc Dis*, 17 Suppl 3:11–16.

[111] Criqui, M.H., Denenberg, J.O., (1998) The generalized nature of atherosclerosis: how peripheral arterial disease may predict adverse events from coronary artery disease. *Vasc Med*, 3(3):241–5.

[112] Newman, A.B., *et al.*, (1999) Ankle-arm index as a predictor of cardiovascular disease and mortality in the Cardiovascular Health Study. The Cardiovascular Health Study Group. *Arterioscler Thromb Vasc Biol*, 19(3):538–45.

[113] Criqui, M.H., (2001) Peripheral arterial disease—epidemiological aspects. *Vasc Med*, 6(3 Suppl):3–7.

[114] Jaremo, P., *et al.*, (2002) Individual variations of platelet inhibition after loading doses of clopidogrel. *J Intern Med*, 252(3):233–8.

[115] Mobley, J.E., *et al.*, (2004) Frequency of nonresponse antiplatelet activity of clopidogrel during pretreatment for cardiac catheterization. *Am J Cardiol*, 93(4):456–8.

[116] Soffer, D., *et al.*, (2003) Impact of angina class on inhibition of platelet aggregation following clopidogrel loading in patients undergoing coronary intervention: do we need more aggressive dosing regimens in unstable angina? *Catheter Cardiovasc Interv*, 59(1):21–5.

[117] Geiger, J., *et al.*, (1999) Specific impairment of human platelet P2Y(AC) ADP receptor-mediated signaling by the antiplatelet drug clopidogrel. *Arterioscler Thromb Vasc Biol*, 19(8):2007–11.

[118] Aleil, B., *et al.*, (2005) Flow cytometric analysis of intraplatelet VASP phosphorylation for the detection of clopidogrel resistance in patients with ischemic cardiovascular diseases. *J Thromb Haemost*, 3(1):85–92.

[119] Lau, W.C., *et al.*, (2004) Contribution of hepatic cytochrome P450 3A4 metabolic activity to the phenomenon of clopidogrel resistance. *Circulation*, 109(2):166–71.

[120] Lowe, H.C., Oesterle, S.N., Khachigian, L.M., (2002) Coronary in-stent restenosis: current status and future strategies. *J Am Coll Cardiol*, 39(2):183–93.

[121] Regar, E., *et al.*, (2004) Incidence of thrombotic stent occlusion during the first three months after sirolimus-eluting stent implantation in 500 consecutive patients. *Am J Cardiol*, 93(10):1271–5.

[122] Muni, N.I., Gross, T.P., (2004) Problems with drug-eluting coronary stents—the FDA perspective. *N Eng J Med*, 351(16):1593–5.

[123] Virmani, R., *et al.*, (2004) Localized hypersensitivity and late coronary thrombosis secondary to a sirolimus-eluting stent: should we be cautious? *Circulation*, 109(6):701–5.

[124] McFadden, E.P., *et al.*, (2004) Late thrombosis in drug-eluting coronary stents after discontinuation of antiplatelet therapy. *Lancet*, 364(9444):1519–21.

[125] Lee, C.H., *et al.*, (2004) Late thrombotic occlusion of paclitaxel eluting stent more than one year after stent implantation. *Heart*, 90(12):1482.

[126] Kerner, A., *et al.*, (2003) Late stent thrombosis after implantation of a sirolimus-eluting stent. *Catheter Cardiovasc Interv*, 60(4):505–8.

[127] Babinska, A., *et al.*, (1998) Enhancement of human platelet aggregation and secretion induced by rapamycin. *Nephrol Dial Transplant*, 13(12):3153–9.

[128] Jeremias, A., *et al.*, (2004) Stent thrombosis after successful sirolimus-eluting stent implantation. *Circulation*, 109(16):1930–2.

[129] Clarke, T.A., Waskell, L.A., (2003) The metabolism of clopidogrel is catalyzed by human cytochrome P450 3A and is inhibited by atorvastatin. *Drug Metab Dispos*, 31(1):53–9.

[130] Lau, W.C., *et al.*, (2003) Atorvastatin reduces the ability of clopidogrel to inhibit platelet aggregation: a new drug-drug interaction. *Circulation*, 107(1):32–7.

[131] Neubauer, H., *et al.*, (2003) Lipophilic statins interfere with the inhibitory effects of clopidogrel on platelet function—a flow cytometry study. *Eur Heart J*, 24(19):1744–9.

[132] Piorkowski, M., *et al.*, (2004) ADP induced platelet degranulation in healthy individuals is reduced by clopidogrel after pretreatment with atorvastatin. *Thromb Haemost*, 92(3): 614–20.

[133] Muller, I., *et al.*, (2003) Effects of statins on platelet inhibition by a high loading dose of clopidogrel. *Circulation*, 108(18):2195–7.

[134] Gorchakova, O., *et al.*, (2004) Antiplatelet effects of a 600 mg loading dose of clopidogrel are not attenuated in patients receiving atorvastatin or simvastatin for at least 4 weeks prior to coronary artery stenting. *Eur Heart J*, 25(21):1898–902.

[135] Mitsios, J.V., *et al.*, (2004) Atorvastatin does not affect the antiplatelet potency of clopidogrel when it is administered concomitantly for 5 weeks in patients with acute coronary syndromes. *Circulation*, 109(11):1335–8.

[136] Serebruany, V.L., *et al.*, (2004) Absence of interaction between atorvastatin or other statins and clopidogrel: results from the interaction study. *Arch Intern Med*, 164(18):2051–7.

[137] Saw, J., *et al.*, (2003) Lack of adverse clopidogrel-atorvastatin clinical interaction from secondary analysis of a randomized, placebo-controlled clopidogrel trial. *Circulation*, 108(8):921–4.
[138] Wienbergen, H., *et al.*, (2003) Comparison of clinical benefits of clopidogrel therapy in patients with acute coronary syndromes taking atorvastatin versus other statin therapies. *Am J Cardiol*, 92(3):285–8.
[139] Cannon, C.P., *et al.*, (2004) Intensive versus moderate lipid lowering with statins after acute coronary syndromes. *N Eng J Med*, 350(15):1495–504.
[140] LaRosa, J.C., *et al.*, (2005) Intensive Lipid Lowering with Atorvastatin in Patients with Stable Coronary Disease. *N Eng J Med*, 352(14):1425–35.
[141] Ferguson, J.J., *et al.*, (2004) Enoxaparin vs unfractionated heparin in high-risk patients with non-ST-segment elevation acute coronary syndromes managed with an intended early invasive strategy: primary results of the SYNERGY randomized trial. *JAMA*, 292(1): 45–54.
[142] Englberger, L., *et al.*, (2004) Impact of clopidogrel in coronary artery bypass grafting. *Eur J Cardiothorac Surg*, 26(1):96–101.
[143] Chen, L., *et al.*, (2004) Clopidogrel and bleeding in patients undergoing elective coronary artery bypass grafting. *J Thorac Cardiovasc Surg*, 128(3):425–31.
[144] Kapetanakis, E.I., *et al.*, (2005) Clopidogrel administration prior to coronary artery bypass grafting surgery: the cardiologist's panacea or the surgeon's headache? *Eur Heart J*, 26(6):576–83.
[145] Sadanandan, S., *et al.*, (2004) A risk score to estimate the likelihood of coronary artery bypass surgery during the index hospitalization among patients with unstable angina and non-ST-segment elevation myocardial infarction. *J Am Coll Cardiol*, 44(4):799–803.
[146] Goods, C.M., *et al.*, (1996) Comparison of aspirin alone versus aspirin plus ticlopidine after coronary artery stenting. *Am J Cardiol*, 78(9):1042–4.
[147] Juergens, C.P., *et al.*, (2004) A randomized comparison of clopidogrel and aspirin versus ticlopidine and aspirin after coronary stent implantation. *Am Heart J*, 147(4):E15.
[148] L'Allier, P.L., *et al.*, (2003) Clopidogrel is associated with better in-hospital and 30-day outcomes than ticlopidine after coronary stenting. *Can J Cardiol*, 19(9):1041–6.
[149] Berger, P.B., *et al.*, (1999) Clopidogrel versus ticlopidine after intracoronary stent placement. *J Am Coll Cardiol*, 34(7):1891–4.
[150] Moussa, I., *et al.*, (1999) Effectiveness of clopidogrel and aspirin versus ticlopidine and aspirin in preventing stent thrombosis after coronary stent implantation. *Circulation*, 99(18): 2364–6.
[151] Mishkel, G.J., *et al.*, (1999) Clopidogrel as adjunctive antiplatelet therapy during coronary stenting. *J Am Coll Cardiol*, 34(7):1884–90.
[152] Calver, A.L., *et al.*, (2000) Clopidogrel for prevention of major cardiac events after coronary stent implantation: 30-day and 6-month results in patients with smaller stents. *Am Heart J*, 140(3):483–91.
[153] Colombo, A., *et al.*, (2003) Randomized study to assess the effectiveness of slow- and moderate-release polymer-based paclitaxel-eluting stents for coronary artery lesions. *Circulation*, 108(7):788–94.
[154] Stone, G.W., *et al.*, (2004) A polymer-based, paclitaxel-eluting stent in patients with coronary artery disease. *N Eng J Med*, 350(3):221–31.
[155] Park, S.J., *et al.*, (2003) A paclitaxel-eluting stent for the prevention of coronary restenosis. *N Eng J Med*, 348(16):1537–45.
[156] Gershlick, A., *et al.*, (2004) Inhibition of restenosis with a paclitaxel-eluting, polymer-free coronary stent: the European evaLUation of pacliTaxel Eluting Stent (ELUTES) trial. *Circulation*, 109(4):487–93.
[157] Lansky, A.J., *et al.*, (2004) Non-polymer-based paclitaxel-coated coronary stents for the treatment of patients with de novo coronary lesions: angiographic follow-up of the DELIVER clinical trial. *Circulation*, 109(16):1948–54.
[158] Morice, M.C., *et al.*, (2002) A randomized comparison of a sirolimus-eluting stent with a standard stent for coronary revascularization. *N Eng J Med*, 346(23):1773–80.
[159] Moses, J.W., *et al.*, (2003) Sirolimus-eluting stents versus standard stents in patients with stenosis in a native coronary artery. *N Eng J Med*, 349(14):1315–23.

[160] Schofer, J., *et al.*, (2003) Sirolimus-eluting stents for treatment of patients with long atherosclerotic lesions in small coronary arteries: double-blind, randomised controlled trial (E-SIRIUS). *Lancet*, 362(9390):1093–9.

[161] Schampaert, E., *et al.*, (2004) The Canadian study of the sirolimus-eluting stent in the treatment of patients with long de novo lesions in small native coronary arteries (C-SIRIUS). *J Am Coll Cardiol*, 43(6):1110–15.

4 Platelet Glycoprotein IIb/IIIa Inhibitors

4.1 INTRODUCTION

Platelet activity plays a major role in the pathogenesis of the acute ischemic syndromes and the complications of PCI. Rupture of the atherosclerotic plaque is the initiating event, exposing thrombogenic lipids and other subendothelial components, resulting in platelet adhesion, activation and aggregation, thrombin generation and fibrin deposition, with formation of occlusive thrombus. Aggregating platelets form the core of the growing thrombotic mass, with upstream and/or downstream propagation. Pathologic or angioscopic examinations have revealed the presence of characteristic platelet-rich ('white') thrombus at the site of plaque rupture, with proximal and distal extension of fibrin- and erythrocyte-rich ('red') clot [1, 2]. Thrombus that becomes occlusive or subocclusive or embolizes the coronary vessel may lead to UA or MI. The central role of platelet activity in the development of ischemic complications in these settings is highlighted by several studies demonstrating unequivocal clinical benefit derived from aspirin therapy in patients with UA [3–6] or undergoing percutaneous coronary revascularization [7, 8].

Platelet deposition along a rupture or eroded arterial plaque occurs almost immediately after arterial injury, mediated by platelet interaction with adhesive proteins in the subendothelium such as vWF, collagen, fibrinonectin or thrombospondin. The resulting monolayer of platelets on the luminal surface is not obstructive. Subsequently, however, platelet activation is initiated by a number of redundant pathways, including soluble agonists such as thrombin and ADP or adhesive proteins such as collagen or fibrinogen. Release of the contents of platelet storage granules, including serotonin, thromboxane A2 and epinephrine, amplifies the platelet activation response. Although platelet activation by these various pathways can trigger inflammatory, mitogenic and vasoactive responses in the vascular wall, aggregation of platelets to form a thrombostatic mass requires participation of the GP IIb/IIIa receptor protein on the platelet surface.

GP IIb/IIIa is a member of a family of adhesion molecules known as integrins, found on virtually all cell surfaces, which consist of a non-covalent dimeric association of alpha and beta subunits. Although a variety of different integrins are present on platelets, the GP IIb/IIIa integrin (alpha-IIb, beta-3) is by far the most abundant, with approximately 50–80,000 copies per platelet. On the unstimulated platelet, GP IIb/IIIa is in its inactive configuration and is not competent for ligand binding. Upon stimulation of the platelet by the various agonists, GP IIb/IIIa undergoes a conformation change and avidly binds circulating adhesion molecules, most prominently fibrinogen or vWF. Upon binding to GP IIb/IIIa, the bivalent fibrinogen or vWF molecules mediate platelet aggregation by bridging to activated GP IIb/IIIa receptors on the surfaces of adjacent platelets. The platelet plug propagates as platelets entering the

Management Strategies in Antithrombotic Therapy Arman T. Askari, Adrian W. Messerli and A. Michael Lincoff

injured vascular bed become activated, express the competent GP IIb/IIIa receptor, and become incorporated into the thrombotic mass through crosslinking fibrinogen or vWF.

4.2 GP IIB/IIIA RECEPTOR INHIBITORS

Given the multiplicity of pathways by which platelets are activated, it is not surprising that antiplatelet agents such as aspirin or clopidogrel, each acting on only one pathway, are themselves relatively weak platelet inhibitors [9]. Because the GP IIb/IIIa receptor is required for recruitment of platelets, regardless of the pathways by which they are activated, it has been termed the ‘final common pathway’ of platelet aggregation and is a logical target for pharmacologic inhibition of platelet thrombosis. An inherited autosomal recessive disorder known as Glanzmann’s Thrombasthenia exists in which GP IIb/IIIa receptors are functionally deficient; the hallmark of this disease is failure of platelets to aggregate in response to all known agonists. The clinical hemorrhagic syndrome of Glanzmann’s Thrombasthenia is characterized by spontaneous mucocutaneous bleeding and easy bruising, but spontaneous organ or central nervous system hemorrhage rarely occurs. The relatively mild nature of the bleeding complications associated with this disorder, in contrast to those associated with inherited deficiencies of other components of the hemostatic system, suggested that pharmacologic blockade of the GP IIb/IIIa receptor might be well tolerated for at least brief periods of time. Pharmacologic compounds have been developed that block this receptor, prevent binding of circulating adhesion molecules and potently inhibit platelet aggregation. Antithrombotic effects are observed both in animal models and clinically with doses that achieve levels of GP IIb/IIIa receptor blockade >50%, with nearly complete abrogation of aggregability at >80% receptor occupancy. Four intravenous GP IIb/IIIa antagonists have undergone large-scale Phase III and Phase IV trial evaluation in the setting of percutaneous coronary revascularization (Table 4.1), and three have been approved for clinical use by the FDA. Several orally available agents have also been evaluated, although results with these compounds were unfavorable and none has been approved for clinical use. The oral GP IIb/IIIa inhibitors will not be discussed in this chapter.

Abciximab, the first agent of the class of GP IIb/IIIa antagonists, is a human–murine chimeric monoclonal Fab antibody fragment, which binds with high affinity and a slow dissociation rate to the GP IIb/IIIa receptor [10, 11]. Abciximab is derived from a murine antibody (7E3) produced by immunization of mice with human platelets. To limit the risk of thrombocytopenia due to cross-linking of platelets or clearance of 7E3-coated platelets by binding of the Fc region to the reticuloendothelial system, 7E3 was cleaved into Fab fragments. To reduce the risk of immunogenicity to murine protein, genetic reconstruction was used to produce the chimeric c7E3 Fab antibody fragment currently in clinical use (abciximab), consisting of human constant regions and murine variable regions of the IgG antibody. In preclinical canine and primate animal models, abciximab was shown to markedly diminish thrombus formation and platelet-mediated cyclic flow reductions in injured and stenosed coronary arteries and to facilitate t-PA-induced fibrinolysis and abolish reocclusion. In humans, abciximab binds with high affinity to both activated and unactivated platelet GP IIb/IIIa, and free drug is cleared rapidly from the plasma (half life ~25 min) [12]. Clearance of abciximab is not related to renal function, and likely occurs through catabolic activity of cells in the reticuloendothelial system. Although binding is reversible, dissociation of the agent from the platelet receptor is slow, and normalization of platelet aggregation does

Table 4.1 IV GP IIb/IIIa receptor antagonists

	Abciximab	Eptifibatide	Tirofiban	Lamifiban
Brand name	ReoPro	Integrilin	Aggrastat	—
Structure	antibody Fab fragment	cyclic heptapeptide	non-peptide	non-peptide
Molecular weight (kDa)	47.6	0.832	0.495	0.468
Plasma half-life	10–30 min	~2.5 h	~2h	~2h
Excretion	unknown	~50% renal	39–69% renal	90% renal
Approved indications*	PCI Refractory UA when PCI is planned within 24 h	ACS (UA and non-Q-wave MI) PCI	ACS (UA and non-Q-wave MI)	Not approved
Approved dose	0.25 mg/kg bolus, 0.125 μg/kg per min (max 10 mg/min) infusion × 12 h	*For ACS*: 180 μg/kg bolus, 2.0 μg/kg per min infusion × 72–96 h *For PCI*: Two180 μg/kg boluses 10 min apart, 2.0 μg/kg per min infusion × 18–24 h	*For ACS*: 0.4 μg/kg per min × 30 min, then 0.1 μg/kg per min × 48–108 h or × 12–24 h post PCI	Not approved

kDa = kilodalton

*Approved indications according to the FDA

not occur until 24–36 h following discontinuation of abciximab infusion [11, 13]. By flow cytometry, decreasing but measurable levels of platelet-bound abciximab are present for as long as 15 days, beyond the normal circulating platelet lifespan, indicating redistribution of abciximab to new platelets entering the circulation [14]. Binding of abciximab is not specific for the platelet GP IIb/IIIa receptor; this agent has equal affinity for the vitronectin receptor (alpha-v, beta-3), which appears to play a role in cell adhesion, migration and proliferation, and Mac-1 (alpha-M, beta-3), which is involved in leukocyte activation.

Eptifibatide is a synthetic disulfide-linked cyclic heptapeptide designed around the arginine-glycine-aspartic acid (RGD) amino acid sequence, a binding site for ligands to GP IIb/IIIa. In eptifibatide, specificity of binding to GP IIb/IIIa is increased by substitution of lysine for arginine, forming the KGD amino acid sequence found in the snake venom disintegrin. Blockade of the receptor by eptifibatide is rapidly reversible and dependent upon circulating drug concentrations, with a plasma half-life in humans of 1.5–2.5 h [15]. Eptifibatide is cleared from the body via excretion of the unchanged molecule through the kidneys; dose reductions are recommended in patients with renal insufficiency.

Tirofiban is a tyrosine-derivative non-peptide mimetic inhibitor of GP IIb/IIIa, which also selectively and competitively binds to the GP IIb/IIIa receptor in a rapidly reversible fashion [16]. Tirofiban is cleared by renal and biliary excretion and has a short (~1.6 h) plasma half-life. As with eptifibatide, elimination half-life is prolonged and dosage reductions are recommended in patients with renal insufficiency.

Lamifiban has been studied in two major trials of patients in the setting of unstable angina, but this agent was never approved for clinical use. Lamifiban is a synthetic non-peptide inhibitor, which binds specifically to GP IIb/IIIa with reversible pharmacodynamics. Plasma half-life of lamifiban has been estimated at 40 min.

4.3 GP IIB/IIIA INHIBITORS DURING PERCUTANEOUS CORONARY REVASCULARIZATION

Proof of concept that GP IIb/IIIa inhibition would diminish ischemic complications of percutaneous coronary revascularization was provided by the first large-scale study of this class of agents, the EPIC trial. EPIC evaluated two dosing strategies of abciximab versus placebo among patients considered to be at high risk for coronary intervention on the basis of acute ischemic syndromes or clinical and angiographic characteristics 27. Nearly 2100 patients were randomized to placebo, abciximab 0.25 mg/kg bolus only, or abciximab 0.25 mg/kg bolus followed by a 10 mcg/min infusion for 12 hours. The composite endpoint of death, myocardial infarction, or urgent revascularization was reduced from 12.8% among patients receiving placebo to 11.4% among patients randomized to the abciximab bolus (10% relative risk reduction, $p = 0.43$) and to 8.3% among patients randomized to the abciximab bolus and 12 hour infusion (35% relative risk reduction, $p = 0.008$).

Hemorrhagic complications were significantly increased by abciximab in the EPIC trial, however, raising concerns regarding the potential clinical utility of this form of therapy. Compared with placebo, the bolus and infusion of abciximab resulted in a doubling in the rates of major bleeding (7 versus 14%, $p = 0.001$) and red blood cell transfusions (7 versus 15%, $p < 0.001$) 27. Conjunctive heparin therapy appeared to have played a key role in the pathogenesis of bleeding among these patients 28. Heparin dosages in EPIC were not weight-adjusted, and a relationship was observed between the risk of bleeding and lighter body weight, total heparin dose, and the intensity of anticoagulation as measured by peak activated clotting time (ACT). Moreover, femoral artery vascular access sheaths had been left in place for the 12-hour abciximab infusion, requiring ongoing heparin during that period. A subsequent pilot study suggested that bleeding associated with abciximab might be attenuated by using lower, weight-adjusted doses of heparin as well as by early removal of the vascular sheath (during infusion of abciximab) to eliminate the need for post-procedural heparin therapy 29.

Subsequent trials of GP IIb/IIIa blockade during PCI generally utilized low-dose weight-adjusted heparin regimens (60–70 U/kg bolus, adjusted as necessary to maintain ACT >200–225 seconds). The treatment effect of abciximab appeared to be amplified (up to a 56% risk reduction) in the EPILOG trial 30:the composite endpoint event rate was 11.7% in the placebo group, 5.2% in the abciximab with low-dose heparin group (56% relative risk reduction, $p < 0.0001$), and 5.4% in the abciximab with standard-dose heparin group (54% relative reduction, $p < 0.0001$). Similar clinical efficacy was observed among patients receiving abciximab compared with placebo during stenting in the EPISTENT trial 31; the primary efficacy composite endpoint occurred in 10.8% of patients in the stent plus placebo arm versus 5.3% of patients in the stent plus abciximab arm (51% relative risk reduction, $p < 0.001$). In neither of these trials was an increase in rates of major bleeding or transfusions observed with abciximab.

With eptifibatide, the IMPACT II trial suggested that this agent diminished periprocedural ischemic events, although the magnitude of treatment effect was less marked than in the abciximab trials and did not reach statistical significance 32. The composite endpoint in IMPACT II occurred in 11.4% of patients in the placebo group, 9.2% of patients in the eptifibatide 135 mcg/kg bolus, 0.50 mg/kg/min infusion group (19% relative risk reduction, $p = 0.063$), and 9.9% of patients in the eptifibatide 135 mcg/kg bolus, 0.75 mcg/kg/min group (16% relative risk reduction, $p = 0.22$). The higher double-bolus dose of eptifibatide (discussed above) led to a substantially greater treatment effect in the ESPRIT trial 33, where the composite endpoint was reduced from 10.5% to 6.8% (35% risk reduction, $p = 0.0034$).

In the RESTORE trial 34, the efficacy of tirofiban (10 mcg/kg bolus, 0.15 mcg/kg/min infusion for 24 hours) during high-risk balloon angioplasty was also less than had been anticipated based upon the results of the EPIC trial. The 30-day composite of death, myocardial infarction, or urgent revascularization occurred in 10.5% of patients in the placebo group vs 8.0% of those in the tirofiban group (24% relative risk reduction, $p = 0.052$). When directly compared with abciximab among patients undergoing stenting in the TARGET trial 35, tirofiban was found to provide inferior protection from acute ischemic events. The 30-day composite endpoint occurred in 7.6% of patients receiving tirofiban, compared with 6.0% of patients randomized to abciximab (hazard ratio for tirofiban 1.26, 95% confidence interval 1.01–1.57, $p = 0.038$). Whether this observed difference in outcome reflects true differences in efficacy between the two agents or inadequate dosing of tirofiban remains unknown.

During the GP IIb/IIIa inhibitor trials that followed EPIC, wherein heparin doses were limited and vascular sheaths removed early, bleeding rates were diminished in all treatment groups and appreciable increases in major hemorrhagic risk were no longer associated with GP IIb/IIIa therapy. Minor bleeding events (defined as gastrointestinal or genitourinary bleeding or hemoglobin drop of 3–5 gm/dL) tended to occur more frequently in these trials among patients receiving GP IIb/IIIa agents as compared with placebo, however, even with reduced-dose heparin regimens. In the two recent major stent trials, for example, rates of minor bleeding were 1.7% versus 2.9% in the placebo and abciximab groups of EPISTENT and 1.7% versus 2.8% in the placebo and eptifibatide groups of ESPRIT.

The treatment effect in reducing ischemic events which was achieved early (by 30 days) with GP IIb/IIIa blockade in these PCI trials was maintained without attenuation over the long term (6 month or longer follow-up). Moreover, therapy with abciximab in the EPIC trial was associated with a 26% reduction in the need for target vessel revascularization procedures (elective or urgent) at 6 months, a finding which led to speculation that this agent may reduce restenosis following coronary angioplasty. Routine angiographic follow up was not performed in EPIC; thus, the influence of abciximab on angiographic restenosis could not be confirmed. A significant reduction in the need for late target vessel revascularization procedures by abciximab was not observed at 6 months or 1 year in the subsequent EPILOG trial, however, nor have any of the other interventional trials with GP IIb/IIIa blockade during balloon angioplasty or stenting demonstrated a significant decrease in "clinical restenosis."

Moreover, the influence 12-hr or 24-hr infusions of abciximab on in-stent restenosis was assessed among 225 patients in the mechanistic ERASER study utilizing intravascular ultrasound (IVUS) measurements of in-stent neointimal tissue volume 36. No effect of either abciximab regimen on neointimal hyperplasia following stenting was observed by IVUS, a finding confirmed by quantitative coronary angiography. The only intriguing exception to the apparent lack of effect of GP IIb/IIIa blockade on restenosis has been suggested in 3 trials of abciximab which found ~50% reductions in rates of target vessel revascularization among patients with diabetes mellitus 37–39. Nonetheless, two other prospective trials among diabetic patients failed to confirm a reduction with abciximab of revascularization rates, angiographic restenosis, or in-stent intimal hyperplasia by IVUS 40, 41.

A compelling result of these interventional trials was the finding of a long-term mortality benefit following abciximab therapy. In EPISTENT, the mortality rate was reduced by 60% among patients randomized to abciximab compared with placebo during stenting (2.4 vs 1.0%, $p = 0.037$). Further support for the veracity of this finding of a mortality reduction by abciximab during PCI was obtained by pooling the long-term findings of the different abciximab interventional trials 42. Among all studies using the bolus and 12-hour infusion regimen of abciximab, mortality rates compared with placebo were significantly diminished by 25–30% for as long as 3 years (Figure 2). The mechanism of mortality reduction with abciximab in these studies remains to be defined. Although the occurrence of a periprocedural myocardial infarction or urgent revascularization clearly increased the risk of subsequent death over the ensuing year, 70–75% of the observed mortality by 1 year occurred in patients who had not suffered an ischemic event within the early period after their index intervention 42. Thus, abciximab did not appear to exert its mortality benefit exclusively through prevention of early ischemic complications. A significant reduction in long-term mortality by the small molecule GP IIb/IIIa inhibitors has not yet been clearly demonstrated. No effects of eptifibatide or tirofiban on long-term death rates were observed in the IMPACT II or RESTORE trials, although there was a trend toward mortality reduction at one year with the high-dose eptifibatide regimen in the ESPRIT trial (2.0 vs 1.4%, $p = 0.28$) 43. One year mortality rates were not significantly different in the tirofiban and abciximab treatment arms in the comparative TARGET trial (1.92% vs 1.74%, respectively), although TARGET was not statistically powered to assess for equivalence with regard to this infrequent mortality endpoint.

GP IIB/IIIA INHIBITORS DURING PCI WITH UNDERLYING ASPIRIN AND HEPARIN THERAPY

The clinical efficacy of GP IIb/IIIa inhibition was first tested in the setting of PCI. By the early 1990s, balloon angioplasty could be performed with high rates of technical success, but ischemic complications of abrupt vessel closure or peri-procedural MI continued to occur despite adjunctive antithrombotic therapy with aspirin and heparin. Event rates for a composite endpoint of death, MI (defined as new electrocardiographic Q-waves or CK-MB elevations more than three times control), or emergency repeat revascularization typically ranged from 10–15% during the 30 days after PCI. Attempts to prevent ischemic complications by intensification of dosing or prolongation of post-procedural infusions of heparin were not successful. Intracoronary stents, while effective in reducing long-term (over 6 months) restenosis due to vascular remodeling and recoil, did not diminish the risk of peri-procedural complications. The pathogenesis of these ischemic events appears predominantly related to thrombosis at the site of plaque injury during coronary intervention (induced by balloons, stents or atherectomy devices), resulting in thrombotic obstruction at the epicardial injury site and/or microvascular obstruction due to distal embolization of platelet aggregates, platelet–leukocyte aggregates, thrombotic plaque material and platelet- or leukocyte-derived vasoactive substances. The most frequent ischemic event in this setting is MI, predominantly non-Q-wave infarction. Although the clinical importance of such peri-procedural non-Q-wave infarctions following percutaneous coronary revascularization was initially controversial, most studies that examined the impact of peri-procedural enzyme release over an adequate follow-up period demonstrated that patients who experience MI during or after coronary intervention are at greater risk of late cardiac death than those who do not [17–21]. While an increased risk of late events has been observed in these studies even among patients with 'small' CK-MB elevations (>1 to 1.5 times control) [19, 20], the extent of mortality risk appears to be proportional to the degree of enzyme elevation.

A series of Phase II studies attempted to identify doses of the various GP IIb/IIIa inhibitors which produced and maintained >80% blockade of GP IIb/IIIa receptors and similar degrees of inhibition of platelet aggregation. For abciximab, a bolus dose of 0.25 mg/kg followed by an infusion of 0.125 mcg/kg/min (maximum 10 mcg/min) results in immediate inhibition to this target level in most patients, although substantial inter-individual variability is observed over the period of infusion. For eptifibatide, early dose-finding studies suggested that a bolus dose of 135 mcg/kg followed by infusions of 0.50 or 0.75 mcg/kg/min would achieve target levels of platelet inhibition, and these doses was used in the initial Phase III trial of eptifibatide (IMPACT II). The disappointing treatment effect of eptifibatide observed in that trial was subsequently attributed to the discovery that eptifibatide's inhibition of platelet aggregation during dose-finding studies had likely been artifactually augmented by the use of citrate (a calcium chelating agent) as an *in vitro* anticoagulant for blood samples. Doses employed in the IMPACT II trial actually resulted in blockade of only 30–50% of GP IIb/IIIa receptors [22] in samples anticoagulated with agents that do not chelate calcium. Further dosing studies [23] and pharmacodynamic modeling demonstrated that a double bolus of 180 mcg/kg given 10 min apart with a 2.0 mcg/kg per min infusion of eptifibatide uniformly produced and maintained >80% blockade of GP IIb/IIIa receptors. This high-dose eptifibatide regimen was tested with better results among patients in the setting of coronary stenting in the later ESPRIT trial. The experience with dose selection of tirofiban may have been similar to that with eptifibatide. Although an influence of calcium-chelating anticoagulants on pharmacodynamics has not been conclusively demonstrated with this agent, the 10 mcg/kg bolus and 0.15 mcg/kg per min infusion of tirofiban used in the RESTORE and TARGET trials results in significantly less early inhibition of platelet aggregation than abciximab or (high-dose) eptifibatide [24,25]. A higher dose of tirofiban (25 mcg/kg bolus, 0.15 mg/kg per min infusion) is under evaluation, and preliminary data in small numbers of patients suggest the efficacy and safety of this regimen [26].

The role of GP IIb/IIIa inhibitors administered as peri-procedural intravenous therapy in the setting of PCI was then tested in a number of large-scale, randomized controlled trials enrolling in total over 26,000 patients (Table 4.2). Six of these trials were placebo-controlled evaluations during elective or urgent PCI (Figure 4.1): EPIC of abciximab among patients considered to be at high risk during balloon angioplasty, EPILOG of abciximab in a broad spectrum of patients undergoing elective or urgent balloon angioplasty, EPISTENT of abciximab among patients during stent implantation, IMPACT II of lower-dose eptifibatide in a broad patient population undergoing balloon angioplasty, ESPRIT of a high-dose, double-bolus eptifibatide regimen during elective or urgent stenting, and RESTORE of tirofiban during balloon angioplasty for unstable ischemic syndromes. TARGET is the only large-scale trial comparing two GP IIb/IIIa inhibitors to be carried out thus far, testing the relative efficacy of abciximab and tirofiban during PCI. Five trials have tested abciximab versus placebo or 'conventional care' among patients with acute MI undergoing primary reperfusion, and will be discussed in a later section. Most recently, the ISAR-REACT trial evaluated the incremental effect of abciximab versus placebo among lower-risk patients who had been pretreated with high-dose clopidogrel at least 2 h before undergoing coronary stenting.

GP IIB/IIIA INHIBITORS DURING PCI WITH NEWER ANTITHROMBOTIC REGIMENS

The consistent finding among the over 15,000 patients enrolled in the previously described trials of GP IIb/IIIa blockade during PCI was that of reduction in the risk of important acute ischemic events by as much as 50–60%, a treatment effect that was maintained without attenuation thereafter and was associated with a long-term mortality benefit. Improved outcome with this therapy was apparent in every subgroup of patients tested and was independent of the modality of percutaneous coronary revascularization (balloon angioplasty, stenting or atherectomy). Underlying antithrombotic therapy in those studies consisted of aspirin, heparin, and, in patients receiving stents, post-procedural thienopyridine platelet inhibitors (ticlopidine or clopidogrel). These studies therefore unequivocally demonstrated the efficacy of GP IIb/IIIa blockade when added to traditional antithrombotic regimens. A growing body of evidence, however, indicates that high loading doses of clopidogrel (300–600 mg) given two or more hours prior to an interventional procedure may reduce acute ischemic events relative to initial administration of clopidogrel at the time of PCI (Chapter 3). The recent ISAR-REACT trial suggested that GP IIb/IIIa blockade may not provide important clinical benefit among low-risk patients undergoing coronary stenting after such a pre-treatment regimen [44]. In this study, 2159 patients were pretreated with clopidogrel 600 mg at least 2 h prior to PCI, then randomized to low-dose heparin (70 U/kg) with abciximab or to high-dose heparin (140 U/kg) alone. No differences were observed in ischemic endpoints between the treatment groups (30-day composite endpoint event rate of 4.0% vs 4.2% in the control and abciximab groups, respectively, p-value = NS). In the absence of confirmatory data from other trials, however, the exclusion of patients with high-risk characteristics from

Table 4.2 GP IIb/IIIa interventional trials – patient populations

Trial	Agent tested	*N*	Enrollment Period	Entry criteria
EPIC	abciximab	2099	11/91 to 11/92	*High risk PTCA or DCA* Acute MI – within 12 h (direct or rescue PTCA) Recent MI – within prior 7 days UA – within 24 h of chest pain (rest or post-infarction angina with ischemic ECG changes) Clinical–morphologic criteria (ACC/AHA lesion score B2 or C, ACC/AHA score B1 with DM or with female of age >65 years)
EPILOG	abciximab	2792	2/95 to 12/95	*Urgent or elective PTCA, DCA, TEC, or laser* Excluding UA or acute MI (EPIC criteria) within prior 24 h, elective stents, rotational atherectomy
EPISTENT	abciximab	2399	7/96 to 9/97	*Coronary intervention suitable for PTCA or elective stent* Excluding acute MI within 24 h, rotational atherectomy
IMPACT II	eptifibatide	4010	11/93 to 11/94	*All clinical indications, all approved interventions*
ESPRIT	eptifibatide	2064	6/99 to 2/00	*Elective stent for which GP IIb/IIIa inhibitor would not be routinely used* Excluding acute MI within 24 h or unstable ischemia with ongoing chest pain or prior thienopyridine use
RESTORE	tirofiban	2139	1/95 to 12/95	*High risk PTCA or DCA* Acute MI – within 72 h (Q-wave or non-Q-wave) UA – within 72 h (chest pain at rest or on minimal effort with ECG changes, hemodynamic changes, or angiographic thrombus)
RAPPORT	abciximab	483	11/95 to 2/97	*Primary PTCA for acute ST elevation MI* – within 12 h
ISAR-2	abciximab	401	N/A	*Primary stent for acute ST elevation MI* – within 48 h
ADMIRAL	abciximab	300	7/97 to 12/98	*Primary PCI for acute ST elevation MI* – within 12 h
CADILLAC	abciximab	2681	11/97 to 9/99	*Primary PCI for acute ST elevation MI* – within 12 h
ACE	abciximab	400	1/01 to 8/02	*Primary PCI for acute STEMI* – within 24 h
TARGET	abciximab vs tirofiban	4809	12/99 to 8/00	*Coronary intervention suitable for stent* Excluding acute MI or cardiogenic shock

DCA = directional coronary atherectomy; DM = diabetes mellitus; ECG = electrocardiographic; N/A = not available; PTCA = coronary balloon angioplasty; TEC = transluminal extraction catheter atherectomy

Trial / Treatment	Control % (n)	GP IIb/IIIa % (n)	p-value
EPIC			
Abciximab B	12.8% (696)	11.4% (695)	0.430
Abciximab B+I	12.8% (696)	8.3% (708)	0.008
EPILOG			
Abciximab LDH	11.7% (939)	5.2% (935)	<0.001
Abciximab SDH	11.7% (939)	5.4% (918)	<0.001
EPISTENT			
Abciximab + Stent	10.8% (809)	5.3% (794)	<0.001
Abciximab + PTCA*	10.8% (809)	6.9% (796)	0.007
IMPACT II			
Eptifibatide 135/0.5	11.4% (1328)	9.2% (1349)	0.063
Eptifibatide 135/0.75	11.4% (1328)	9.9% (1333)	0.220
ESPRIT			
Eptifibatide 180/2.0/180	10.5% (1024)	6.8% (1040)	0.003
RESTORE			
Tirofiban	10.5% (1070)	8.0% (1071)	0.052

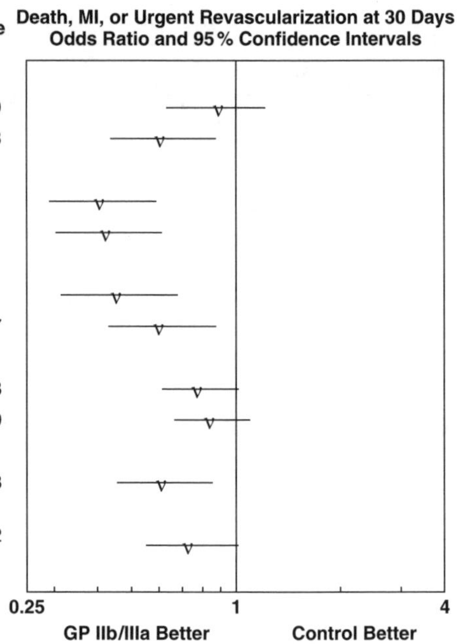

Figure 4.1 Composite 30-day endpoint (death, myocardial infarction, or urgent repeat revascularization) event rates and odds ratios for the 6 trials of GP IIb/IIIa inhibition during elective or urgent percutaneous interventional (TARGET excluded, as it was an active control trial). *EPISTENT trial groups compared with reference group of Placebo + Stent; thus, the "placebo control" for the Abciximab + PTCA group underwent stenting rather than PTCA. B = bolus, B+I=bolus plus infusion; LDH = low-dose, weight-adjusted heparin; SDH = standard-dose, weight-adjusted heparin, 135/0.5, 135/0.75, and 180/2.0/180 = eptifibatide doses

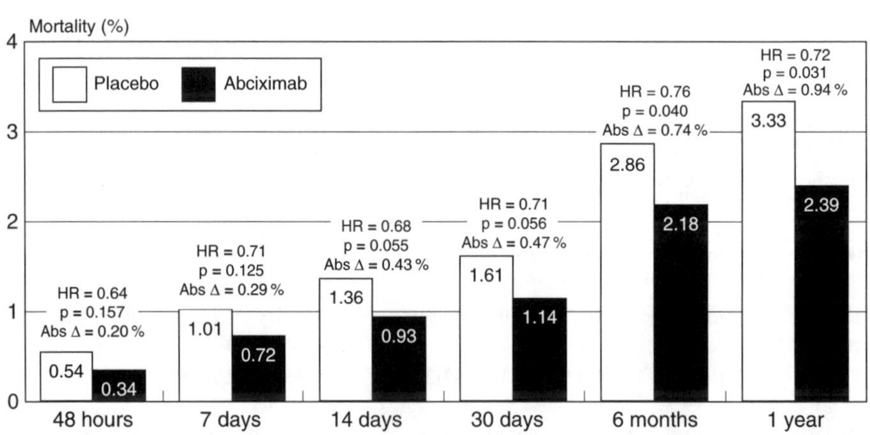

Figure 4.2 Pooled results of mortality reduction over time by abciximab relative to control for all interventional trials using the bolus and 12-hour infusion regimen of abciximab during percutaneous coronary intervention. Abs Δ = absolute % reduction in mortality; HR = hazard ratio. Data from Anderson *et al.* [42]

ISAR-REACT (recent MI, UA, bypass graft interventions, chronic occlusion, angiographic thrombus, LV ejection fraction <30%, hemodynamic instability or insulin-dependent diabetes mellitus) and the inadequate statistical power to assess equivalence or non-inferiority of the two treatment strategies limit the applicability of these trial findings to broad clinical practice. Moreover, a requirement to administer clopidogrel at least 2 h prior to PCI may be associated with logistic difficulties and catheterization laboratory delays when procedures are performed on an *ad hoc* basis (immediately after definition of coronary anatomy by diagnostic catheterization) and may substantially increase the risk of peri-operative bleeding if patients subsequently require emergent or urgent CAPG surgery.

Additional evidence supporting a selective rather than universal role for GP IIb/IIIa blockade during PCI was derived from the REPLACE-2 trial (Chapter 7) [45, 46]. In that study of over 6000 patients undergoing elective or urgent PCI, monotherapy with the direct thrombin inhibitor bivalirudin was compared with the combination of low-dose heparin (65 U/kg) plus GP IIb/IIIa blockade (abciximab or eptifibatide). Clopidogrel was given to all patients, nearly half of whom had been pretreated more than 2 h before PCI. GP IIb/IIIa inhibitors could be used on a 'provisional' basis in the event of procedural complications among patients receiving bivalirudin and were administered to 7.2% of patients in that treatment arm. The 30-day composite ischemic event rates were 7.1% vs 7.6% in the heparin plus GP IIb/IIIa blockade vs bivalirudin arms, respectively, meeting formal statistical criteria for non-inferiority of the bivalirudin regimen. Bleeding was reduced by 41% (4.1% vs 2.4%, p-value <0.001) with bivalirudin treatment. No difference in 1-year mortality was observed between the two antithrombotic strategies. Patients with acute MI or those with UA requiring ongoing therapy with heparin or GP IIb/IIIa blockade were excluded from enrollment in the REPLACE-2 trial, however, thus limiting extrapolation of these findings to patients with severe acute coronary syndromes. Given the sizeable body of evidence demonstrating the distinctive efficacy of GP IIb/IIIa blockade in patients with unstable ischemic syndromes, GP IIb/IIIa inhibitors should not be withheld in this setting unless subsequent trials show similar clinical benefit achieved with bivalirudin.

4.4 GP IIB/IIIA INHIBITORS IN THE MANAGEMENT OF NON-ST-ELEVATION ACS

Antithrombotic therapies in patients with ACS are not only targeted at limiting the arterial thrombotic response to revascularization but would also be expected to prevent propagation and embolization of a clot formed at the site of plaque rupture, and to shift the balance of the endogenous hemostatic system towards spontaneous fibrinolysis. Thus, GP IIb/IIIa blockade has been investigated as a medical therapy in this setting, independent of whether coronary revascularization is performed. Evidence from the first of the GP IIb/IIIa interventional trials, EPIC, suggested that particular benefit from these platelet antagonists might be derived among patients with ACS. Although the treatment effect of abciximab in that trial was present in all subgroups, the composite endpoint was decreased by 71% among those with UA; the most serious endpoints of death or MI were reduced by 94% (11.1% in the placebo group vs 0.6% in the abciximab bolus and infusion group; p-value <0.001) [47]. Over 3-year follow-up in EPIC, mortality was significantly reduced by abciximab from 12.7% to 5.1% (p-value = 0.01) among the 555 highest risk patients enrolled with UA or acute MI [21].

The intravenous GP IIb/IIIa inhibitors have therefore been evaluated in six large-scale, placebo-controlled trials (Table 4.3) among a total of over 31,000 patients with acute ischemic syndromes without ST-segment elevation, including PURSUIT (eptifibatide) [48], PRISM [49] and PRISM PLUS [50] (tirofiban), PARAGON-A and PARAGON-B (lamifiban) [51], and GUSTO-IV (abciximab) [52]. In each of these trials, patients were randomized to receive the GP IIb/IIIa antagonist or placebo initiated at the time of hospital presentation and continued for 24–96 h, superimposed upon aspirin, heparin (except in PRISM, where tirofiban was used without heparin) and other standard medical therapies. The study protocols varied substantially in their approaches to coronary revascularization, but in no trial was percutaneous intervention or bypass surgery mandated. In PARAGON-A and GUSTO-IV, revascularization was prohibited during the first 48 and 60 h of study drug therapy, respectively. Angiography and revascularization were discouraged for the first 48 h in PRISM and PRISM PLUS, but then encouraged during the study drug infusion of PRISM PLUS between 48 and 96 h. In PURSUIT and PARAGON-B, utilization of revascularization was according to physician preference.

The results of the 6 ACS trials are summarized in Figure 4.3. As with the interventional trials, ischemic event rates were generally reduced by glycoprotein IIb/IIIa blockade among patients with unstable ischemic syndromes. The largest trial was PURSUIT, in which treatment with eptifibatide among almost 11,000 patients was associated with a 10% reduction the incidence of death or MI at 30 days (15.7% vs 14.2%, p-value = 0.04). The other four trials of reversible small molecule inhibitors, ranging in size from 1500 to 5225 patients, similarly demonstrated reductions in the risk of death or MI ranging from 8% to 27%. Most recently, the GUSTO-IV trial failed to show any efficacy of abciximab administered for 24 or 48 h in a population of patients managed medically for unstable ischemic syndromes; reasons for the lack of benefit of abciximab in this setting are unknown, but may be related to inadequate platelet inhibition during prolonged infusion or the infrequent use of coronary revascularization in that trial.

The treatment effect of GP IIb/IIIa blockade in the setting of unstable ischemic syndromes appears to be greatest among those who undergo early percutaneous coronary revascularization, with clear evidence of stabilization during the period prior to intervention as well as suppression of post-procedural ischemic events. The interaction between GP IIb/IIIa blockade and coronary revascularization was not tested in a randomized fashion in the large acute ischemic syndrome trials. Nevertheless, in three of these studies, PURSUIT, PRISM PLUS, and PARAGON B, important information regarding the effect of these agents as pre-procedural and post-procedural therapy was derived from the substantial number of patients who underwent early coronary intervention while on study drug (GP IIb/IIIa inhibitor or matching placebo) infusion. In PURSUIT, 1228 patients were treated with coronary balloon angioplasty within the first 72 h after randomization [48]. Eptifibatide was associated with a significant reduction in the risk of MI prior to the revascularization procedure (5.5% vs 1.8%, p-value <0.001), as well as an important reduction in the composite endpoint of death or MI by 30 days (16.8% vs 11.8%, 30% relative risk reduction, p-value = 0.01). In PRISM PLUS, catheterization and percutaneous revascularization were encouraged, but to be deferred for 48 h, and 475 patients underwent coronary angioplasty while receiving study drug [50]. During the first 48 h (before intervention), death or MI rates were reduced from 2.6% to 0.9% by tirofiban in the overall 1570 patient trial cohort (p-value = 0.01); among the 475 patients undergoing intervention, 30-day rates of death or MI were 10.2% and 5.9% in the placebo and tirofiban groups, respectively (42% relative risk reduction, p-value = 0.12).

Table 4.3 GP IIb/IIIa acute ischemic syndrome trials – patient populations

Trial	Agent tested	*N*	Enrollment period	Angiography and revascularization	PCI during study (%)	CABG during study (%)
PURSUIT	eptifibatide	10,948	11/95 to 1/97	Physician's discretion	24	14
PRISM PLUS	tirofiban	1,915	11/94 to 9/96	Deferred for first 48 h, then performed during study drug infusion	31	23
PRISM	tirofiban	3,232	3/94 to 10/96	Discouraged	21	17
PARAGON A	lamifiban	2,282	8/95 to 5/96	Discouraged	13	11
PARAGON B	lamifiban	5,225	2/98 to 6/99	Physician's discretion	28	15
GUSTO IV	abciximab	7,800	7/98 to 4/00	Discouraged	19	11

Trial / Treatment	Control % (n)	GP IIb/IIIa % (n)	p-value
PURSUIT Eptifibatide	15.7% (4739)	14.2% (4722)	0.04
PRISM PLUS Tirofiban	11.9% (797)	8.7% (793)	0.03
PRISM Tirofiban	7.1% (1616)	5.8% (1616)	0.11
PARAGON A Lamifiban	11.7% (758)	10.6% (755)	0.71
PARAGON B Lamifiban	11.5% (2597)	10.6% (2628)	0.34
GUSTO IV Abciximab	8.0% (2598)	8.6% (5202)	0.36

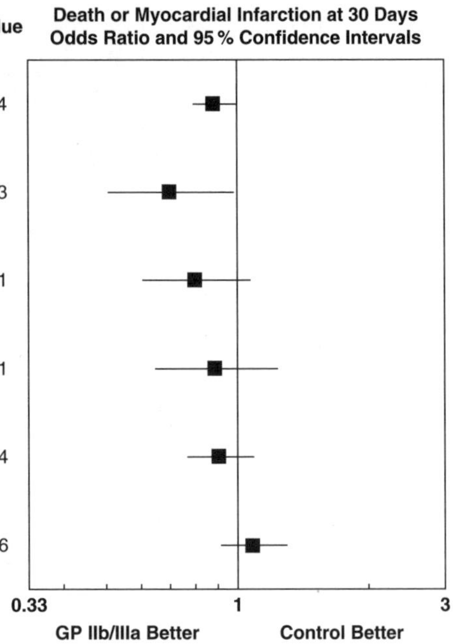

Figure 4.3 Composite 30-day endpoint (death or myocardial infarction) event rates and odds ratios for the 6 trials of GP IIb/IIIa inhibition among patients with non-ST-segment elevation acute coronary syndromes

Revascularization Strategy	Control %	GP IIb/IIIa %	N	p-value
Medically managed	9.7%	9.3%	20,054	0.27
PCI after discontinuation of study drug	12.3%	10.9%	4088	0.17
PCI on study drug	13.6%	10.5%	2249	0.02

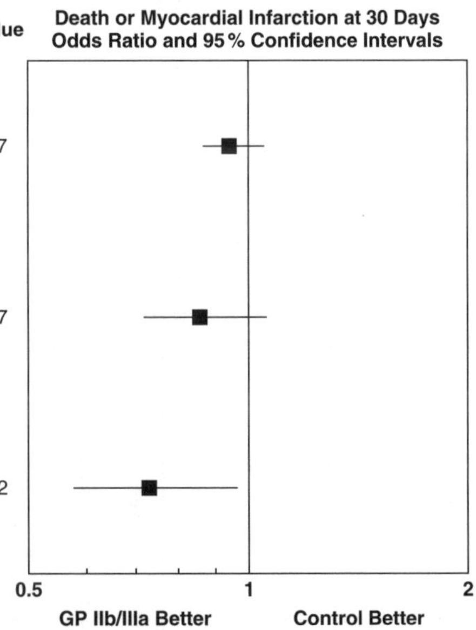

Figure 4.4 Pooled results of the trials of GP Iib/IIIa inhibition during non-ST segment elevation acute coronary syndromes, demonstrating treatment effect on 30-day death or myocardial infarction according to revascularization strategy. Data from Roffi *et al.* [54]

Among the 678 patients undergoing PCI while on study drug in PARAGON B, the composite endpoint of death or MI was reduced from 0.85% to 0.31% prior to PCI and from 12.8% to 8.9% following PCI [53]. In contrast, the clinical benefit of GP IIb/IIIa inhibition among patients who are not ultimately revascularized is less clear. In a pooled analysis of these ACS trials, no significant reductions in the risk of death or MI by 30 days with GP IIb/IIIa blockade were observed among patients managed without revascularization or in whom revascularization was performed after the study drug infusion had been discontinued [54] (Figure 4.4). These findings suggest that although GP IIb/IIIa inhibitors may stabilize patients with ACS during the medical phase of management, revascularization under the protection of these agents is required to sustain a durable improvement in clinical outcome.

4.5 GP IIB/IIIA INHIBITORS IN THE MANAGEMENT OF ACUTE STEMI

The presence of ST-segment elevations on the electrocardiogram of a patient with acute ischemic chest pain predicts a more than 80% likelihood of complete coronary occlusion and resultant MI. Immediate reperfusion therapy by pharmacologic fibrinolysis or primary percutaneous coronary revascularization has become the mainstay of early management in this setting, and has been demonstrated to limit infarct size and reduce mortality. Contemporary reperfusion strategies remain subject to a number of limitations, however, including diminished efficacy with time delays between symptom onset and treatment, arterial reocclusion or incomplete microvascular and tissue level reperfusion, an apparent 'ceiling' of patency and the risk of intracranial hemorrhage with fibrinolytic therapy, and logistic difficulties and the need for rapid access to specialized expertise with primary intervention. Given the unequivocal efficacy of aspirin in improving mortality and reducing recurrent ischemia and infarction among patients with acute ST-segment elevation MI, the potential role of platelet inhibition with GP IIb/IIIa inhibitors has been investigated. Based upon evidence of the platelet disaggregatory properties of abciximab, it had even been suggested that coronary reperfusion might be achieved by potent GP IIb/IIIa inhibition alone without administration of exogenous plasminogen activators or percutaneous coronary revascularization. In fact, phase II studies demonstrated rates of complete coronary patency 45–90 min after receiving abciximab or eptifibatide ranging from 18% to 32% [55–58], comparable to patency rates achieved with SK. Thus, GP IIb/IIIa antagonists appear to have modest 'fibrinolytic' properties, but their optimal role in these patients seems to be as adjuncts to traditional reperfusion therapies.

GP IIB/IIIA INHIBITORS AS AN ADJUNCT TO PRIMARY PERCUTANEOUS CORONARY REVASCULARIZATION

The efficacy of GP IIb/IIIa blockade during elective PCI might logically be expected to extend also to the setting of acute MI, a hypothesis which has been tested thus far only for abciximab. Adjunctive abciximab therapy was evaluated in the RAPPORT [59] and CADILLAC [60] trials during primary balloon angioplasty and in the ISAR-2 [61], ADMIRAL [38], CADILLAC [60] and ACE [62] trials during stenting. In general, the magnitude of reduction in 30-day acute ischemic endpoints (death, reinfarction or urgent repeat revascularization) in these trials of acute MI (50–60% relative risk reductions) was similar to that

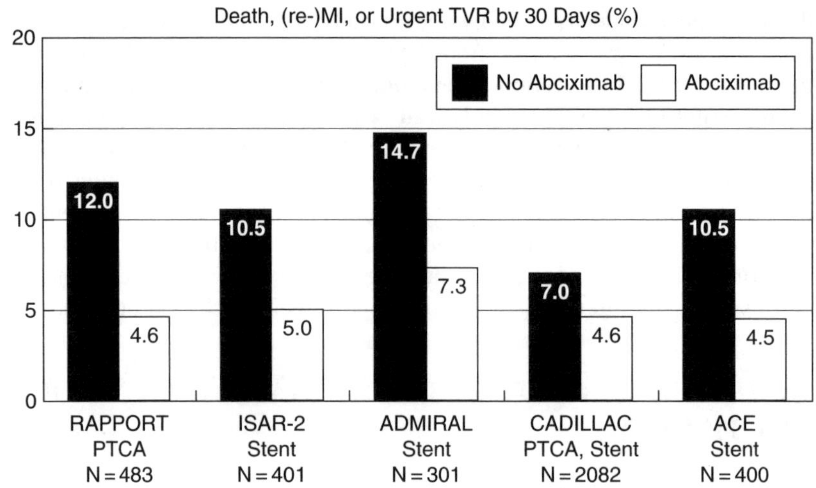

Figure 4.5 Composite 30-day endpoint (death, myocardial infarction, or target vessel revascularization) event rates for the 5 trials of abciximab during primary percutaneous coronary revascularization for acute myocardial infarction. PTCA = balloon angioplasty, TVR = target vessel revascularization

observed in other PCI trials for more elective indications (Figure 4.5). Trends toward reductions in late mortality were also observed. Pooled results of the body of randomized trial data from acute MI studies are concordant with those from other GP IIb/IIIa interventional studies and supports the efficacy of abciximab in reducing acute ischemic events during primary PCI [63].

The clinical benefit of abciximab has been linked in part to observed improvements in infarct-vessel patency [38]. In one trial, complete epicardial vessel patency prior to revascularization performing PCI was present in 16.8% vs 5.4% of patients receiving abciximab and placebo (p-value $= 0.01$), respectively. A significant patency advantage persisted in the abciximab group even immediately after the revascularization procedure. Reductions in reocclusion rates have also been observed [60]. Data regarding the treatment effect of abciximab relative to the timing of administration were supportive of the importance of achieving patency prior to revascularization. Of the 300 patients in the ADMIRAL trial, 78 (26%) were randomized and administered the study drug in the ambulance or emergency department, while the remainder received placebo or abciximab in the intensive care unit or catheterization laboratory. Early administration was associated with an amplification of the treatment effect of abciximab: the 30-day composite endpoint occurred in 21.1% vs 2.5% of patients receiving early assignment to placebo or abciximab, respectively, compared with rates of 12.4% vs 8.3% among those randomized in the intensive care or catheterization units.

Further insights into the mechanisms of benefit of abciximab during PCI for acute MI were derived from a placebo-controlled trial of 200 patients [64]. Measurements of Doppler wire flow velocity and left ventricular function were performed immediately after successful stenting and at 14-day follow-up. Although stent placement was successful with achievement of epicardial vessel patency in nearly all patients, improvements in infarct-vessel peak flow velocity were significantly greater among abciximab-treated patients and correlated with significantly greater improvements in infarct zone wall motion and higher global left ventricular function. These results suggest that abciximab exerts a beneficial effect beyond that in the epicardial artery, and that intense platelet inhibition by GP IIb/IIIa blockade in this setting may improve tissue level microvascular reperfusion and thus enhance myocardial salvage. Similar findings have been observed in studies with eptifibatide during elective stenting [65]. Another study demonstrated that abciximab may reduce platelet–leukocyte interactions and limit microvascular inflammation during reperfusion therapy [66].

GP IIB/IIIA INHIBITORS AS AN ADJUNCT TO FIBRINOLYTIC THERAPY

Preclinical studies demonstrated that GP IIb/IIIa antagonists accelerate reperfusion and potently inhibit reocclusion and cyclic flow variations in animal models of coronary thrombolysis. Phase II clinical trials tested various doses of abciximab, eptifibatide or lamifiban administered either in a delayed fashion or concurrently with full-dose fibrinolytic therapy in patients with acute MI [67–70]. Consistent trends towards improved early [68] or late [67] angiographic infarct vessel patency were observed with administration of GP IIb/IIIa antagonists with fibrinolytic agents. Moreover, combination therapy was associated with improvements in the speed and stability of reperfusion as assessed by continuous electrocardiographic monitoring [68, 69]. Bleeding complications, however, tended to be increased by combination therapy in these studies, in particular with SK [69].

Subsequent trials focused on the hypothesis that by inhibiting platelet activation induced by exogenous plasminogen activators and directly disaggregating the platelet thrombus, adjunctive use of GP IIb/IIIa antagonists may allow administration of *reduced* doses of fibrinolytic agents during acute MI. It was hoped that such an approach might accelerate and enhance early patency, improve tissue level microvascular reperfusion, prevent reocclusion, and diminish bleeding complications. Angiographic trials evaluated various dose combinations of fibrinolytic agents, GP IIb/IIIa inhibitors and heparin (or enoxaparin) among patients with acute MI. Within the limits of relatively small sample sizes and multiple dosing groups, these trials in general suggested improvements in early epicardial vessel patency with a half-dose fibrinolytic agent plus a full-dose GP IIb/IIIa antagonist compared with standard full-dose fibrinolytic monotherapy [56, 57, 71]. Improvements in complete coronary patency rates at 60 min ranged from 10 to 20 absolute percentage points. Additionally, the proportion of patients with resolution of electrocardiographic ST-segment elevations was greater with combination therapy, suggesting enhanced microvascular tissue level reperfusion beyond epicardial vessel recanalization [72]. The combination of abciximab and reduced-dose SK was associated with increased bleeding (mirroring the experience in earlier trials) [57].

Combination therapy has thus far been evaluated in only one large-scale mortality trial, GUSTO V, in which over 16,000 patients were randomized to receive either abciximab plus half-dose reteplase or conventional full-dose reteplase [73]. Combination therapy was associated with only a non-significant reduction in mortality at 30 days, from 5.9% to 5.6% (p-value = 0.45), and mortality rates were identical (8.4%) in the two treatment arms by 1 year [74]. There was evidence of more complete and stable reperfusion among patients treated with abciximab plus half-dose reteplase, however, with significant reductions in rates of reinfarction (3.5% vs 2.3%, p-value <0.0001), recurrent ischemia (12.8% vs 11.3%, p-value = 0.004), or urgent PCI within the first 6 h (8.6% vs 5.6%, p-value <0.0001). Nevertheless, although intracranial hemorrhage rates were the same in the two treatment groups (0.6%), combination therapy was associated with a doubling in rates of non-intracranial bleeding complications. Support for these findings was derived from the subsequent ASSENT-3 trial, in which half-dose tenecteplase plus abciximab was compared with tenecteplase monotherapy [75]. Mortality was not improved with combination therapy, although the beneficial effect of abciximab on reinfarction and urgent PCI coupled with the adverse effects on bleeding complications were similar to those observed in GUSTO V. Given the marginal clinical benefits and increased hemorrhagic risk associated with combination fibrinolytic and GP IIb/IIIa inhibitor therapy, particularly in elderly patients, this strategy has never been adopted into practice as a means of pharmacologic reperfusion for acute MI.

'Facilitated PCI' is an approach to merging the best aspects of pharmacologic and mechanical approaches to myocardial reperfusion, whereby fibrinolytic or antithrombotic agents are administered immediately upon a patient's presentation with acute infarction to 'bridge the gap' until primary PCI can be carried out [76]. The goal of this strategy is to achieve at least some degree of coronary recanalization and microvascular reperfusion, and thus limit myocardial necrosis, during the time delay required to bring patients to the catheterization laboratory and perform definitive revascularization. One randomized trial has compared two different pharmacologic approaches to facilitated PCI – abciximab or the combination of abciximab plus half-dose reteplase [77]. As expected, patients who had received combination therapy had higher rates of coronary patency than those treated with abciximab alone (40% vs 18%, respectively), but this advantage did not translate into improved clinical outcome after PCI. Myocardial infarct size was no different between the two groups, and ischemic complications (death, reinfarction or stroke) and bleeding rates trended in favor of abciximab monotherapy. A central limitation of this study is that it did not test the concept of facilitated PCI *per se*, as there was no control group of patients who underwent PCI without pharmacologic pretreatment. Such trials are currently underway.

4.6 SAFETY OF GP IIB/IIIA INHIBITORS

BLEEDING

The major potential safety issue with this as well as other classes of agents directed against platelet function or coagulation is that of bleeding. The findings of the first trial of this class of therapy, EPIC, highlighted the potential for hemorrhagic risk with these agents. Most bleeding with GP IIb/IIIa antagonists in this and subsequent trials was at sites of vascular access, although spontaneous gastro-intestinal and genito-urinary bleeding also occurred; long-term sequelae were infrequent. Importantly, pooled analysis of the trials indicate that rates of intracranial hemorrhage do *not* appear to be increased [78]. The improvement in the safety profile of these agents subsequent to the EPIC experience shows that modification of conjunctive anticoagulant therapy with heparin by weight adjustment and dose reduction is a key intervention in abrogating excess bleeding risk. Early removal of vascular sheaths and meticulous care of the access site are also likely important means of avoiding hemorrhage. Bleeding may nevertheless be a concern in certain groups of patients, such as those who receive GP IIb/IIIa blockade as an unplanned or 'bailout' intervention in the setting of full-dose heparinization or those undergoing 'rescue' angioplasty for failed reperfusion after full-dose thrombolysis. Partial reversal of heparinization with protamine in the former situation and very careful heparin dose-reduction and ACT monitoring in the latter will likely improve the balance between risk and benefit in these patients.

For patients who develop refractory or life-threatening bleeding, the antiplatelet effect of abciximab may be reversed by discontinuation of drug infusion and by platelet transfusion after the ~10–30 min required for clearance of circulating drug. After introduction of new platelets into the circulation, abciximab redistributes from old to new platelets, reducing the mean level of receptor blockade. In experimental studies, transfusion of the equivalent of 10 U of platelets in primates treated with abciximab led to prompt reduction in mean receptor blockade from 80–90% to less than 70%, near normalization of bleeding times, and partial (~30%) recovery of platelet aggregation [79]. Platelet transfusions should rarely be necessary with the rapidly reversible agents eptifibatide and tirofiban, but theoretically would not be effective during the ~2 h required for elimination of high concentrations of these agents from the circulating plasma phase.

EMERGENCY CORONARY BYPASS SURGERY

There has been concern about the risk of excessive peri-operative bleeding if patients require urgent coronary artery bypass surgery for failed angioplasty after administration of a GP IIb/IIIa inhibitor. The rapidly reversible agents eptifibatide and tirofiban should present little in the way of peri-operative bleeding risk in this regard; platelet aggregation and bleeding times return to normal following discontinuation of both of these agents within a few hours, the time period required for coronary artery bypass to be performed. Despite its more prolonged duration of action, however, antecedent treatment with abciximab should not be considered a contraindication to necessary emergency surgical revascularization. In a detailed study of surgical outcomes among 85 patients requiring urgent coronary surgery in the EPILOG and EPISTENT trials, abciximab therapy was not associated with a major increase in peri-operative blood loss [80]. Platelet transfusions were administered more frequently (in part prophylactically) to patients who had received abciximab, but the need for other blood products was the same in the abciximab and placebo groups. Although surgical re-exploration for bleeding tended to be more frequent in patients who had received abciximab, surgical cross clamp, cardiopulmonary bypass and closure times were not prolonged and the utilization of optimal mammary artery conduits was not impaired. Moreover, ischemic events tended to be less frequent in abciximab-treated patients. Thus, hemorrhagic risk may be modestly increased by abciximab in the event of urgent coronary bypass surgery, but is unlikely to be associated with excess mortality or important morbidity. Conventional procedures for intra-operative ACT-guided heparin dosing and selective application of platelet transfusions appear appropriate for the management of these patients.

THROMBOCYTOPENIA

Thrombocytopenia occurs infrequently following GP IIb/IIIa inhibition, but may be precipitous and profound (platelet count $<20{,}000/\text{mm}^3$); the excess risk of profound thrombocytopenia associated with abciximab (0.4–1.1%) appears to be higher than with eptifibatide (0–0.2%) or tirofiban (0.1–0.3%). Thrombocytopenia in this setting is not a benign event. In a pooled analysis of 7290 patients in the EPIC, EPILOG and EPISTENT trials, 178 (2.4%) developed thrombocytopenia, with an independent association observed with abciximab therapy (odds ratio 1.75) [81]. Even with the analysis confined to the 126 patients without antecedent coronary bypass surgery, those with thrombocytopenia had significantly higher rates of major and minor hemorrhage (33% versus 9%, *p*-value <0.001), red cell transfusions (21% versus 5%, *p*-value <0.001) and 30-day mortality (4.8% versus 0.6%, *p*-value <0.001) than did patients without thrombocytopenia. Perhaps somewhat surprisingly, however, bleeding complications and mortality were *less* frequent if thrombocytopenia occurred in patients who had been randomized to abciximab than if thrombocytopenia was in the context of placebo administration.

The mechanism of thrombocytopenia associated with GP IIb/IIIa inhibitors is unknown. Thrombocytopenia occurring after administration of a GP IIb/IIIa agent can usually be differentiated from that due to the heparin-induced thrombocytopenia syndrome by the early and precipitous onset, generally within 1 to 24 h after administration of the GP IIb/IIIa inhibitor [82], as well as by the absence of thrombotic complications. There is little evidence of ongoing platelet clearance following discontinuation of the GP IIb/IIIa antagonist, and most patients experience an increase in platelet count of about 20–30,000/mm^3 per day (the rate of bone marrow production). Unlike heparin-induced thrombocytopenia, platelet transfusions are a safe and protective therapy for profound thrombocytopenia with or without serious bleeding induced by GP IIb/IIIa inhibitors. Platelet counts should be measured within the first 2–4 h after administering these agents and followed for the duration of therapy.

READMINISTRATION

Approximately 5–6% of patients will develop a human anti-chimeric antibody (HACA) response to abciximab; no antibody response has been observed with eptifibatide, tirofiban or lamifiban. A prospective registry found no instances of hypersensitivity or anaphylactic reactions following abciximab readministration in 500 patients, and efficacy of the agent in reducing ischemic complications appeared to be similar with readministration as with first-time use [83]. The rates of profound thrombocytopenia (platelet count $<20{,}000/\text{mm}^3$) following readministration was somewhat higher, however, than expected with first-time administration. Moreover, in contrast to the typically rapid resolution of thrombocytopenia seen with first-time administration, a protracted time course of thrombocytopenia for up to one week was observed in these patients following readministration. The presence or absence of a positive HACA titer did not appear to be predictive of a lack of clinical effectiveness, development of thrombocytopenia or other sequelae in patients undergoing readministration.

4.7 SUMMARY

Platelet GP IIb/IIIa receptor blockade represents a significant advance in the practice of interventional cardiology and the management of acute coronary syndromes. These agents potently inhibit arterial thrombus formation and reduce ischemic complications in these settings. The benefit of this therapy is of greatest magnitude among patients who are ultimately revascularized. Ongoing studies are assessing the incremental benefit of these agents among patients treated with new antagonists of platelet activation pathways or inhibitors of thrombin and other components of the coagulation cascade.

REFERENCES

[1] Falk, E., (1991) Coronary thrombosis: pathogenesis and clinical manifestations. *Am J Cardiol*, 68:28B–35B.

[2] Friedman, M.F., Van der Bovenkamp, E., (1996) The pathogenesis of a coronary thrombus. *Am J Pathol*, 48:19–44.

[3] Lewis, H.D.J., Davis, J.W., Archibald, D.G., *et al.*, (1983) Protective effects of aspirin against acute myocardial infarction and death in men with unstable angina: results of the Veterans Administration Cooperative Study. *N Eng J Med*, 309:396–403.

[4] Cairns, J.A., Gent, M., Singer, J., *et al.*, (1985) Aspirin, sulfinpyrazone, or both in unstable angina. *N Eng J Med*, 313:1369–75.

[5] Theroux, P., Ouimet, H., McCans, J., *et al.*, (1988) Aspirin, heparin, or both to treat acute unstable angina. *N Eng J Med*, 319:1105–11.

[6] RISC Group, (1990) Risk of myocardial infarction and death during treatment with low dose aspirin and intravenous heparin in men with unstable coronary artery disease. *Lancet* 336:827–30.

[7] Schwartz, L., Bourassa, M.G., Lesperance, J., Aldridge, H.E., Kazim, F., Salvatori, V.A., Henderson, M., Bonan, R., David, P.R. (1988) Aspirin and dipyridamole in the prevention of restenosis after percutaneous transluminal coronary angioplasty. *N Eng J Med*, 318:1714–19.

[8] Antiplatelet Trialists' Collaboration, (1994) Collaborative overview of randomised trials of antiplatelet therapy — I: Prevention of death, myocardial infarction, and stroke by prolonged antiplatelet therapy in various categories of patients. *Br Med J*, 308:81–106.

[9] Coller, B.S., (1990) Platelets and thrombolytic therapy. *N Eng J Med*, 322(1):33–42.

[10] Coller, B.S., (1995) Blockade of platelet GPIIb/IIIa receptors as an antithrombotic strategy. *Circulation*, 92:2373–80.

[11] Tcheng, J.E., Ellis, S.G., George, B.S., *et al.*, (1994) Pharmacodynamics of chimeric glycoprotein IIb/IIIa integrin antiplatelet antibody Fab 7E3 in high-risk coronary angioplasty. *Circulation*, 90:1757–64.

[12] Kleiman, N.S., Raizner, A.E., Jordan, R., *et al.*, (1995) Differential inhibition of platelet aggregation induced by adenosine diphosphate or a thrombin receptor-activating peptide in patients treated with bolus chimeric 7E3 Fab: implications for inhibition of the internal pool of GPIIb/IIIa receptors. *J Am Coll Cardiol*, 26:1665–71.

[13] Mascelli, M.A., Worley, S., Veriabo, N.J., *et al.*, (1997) Rapid assessment of platelet function with a modified whole-blood aggregometer in percutaneous transluminal coronary angioplasty patients receiving anti-GP IIb/IIIa therapy. *Circulation*, 96:3860–6.

[14] Mascelli, M.A., Lance, E.T., Damaraju, L., *et al.*, (1998) Pharmacodynamic profile of short-term abciximab treatment demonstrates prolonged platelet inhibition with gradual recovery from GP IIb/IIIa receptor blockade. *Circulation*, 97:1680–8.

[15] Harrington, R.A., Kleiman, N.S., Kottke-Marchant, K., *et al.*, (1995) Immediate and reversible platelet inhibition after intravenous administration of a peptide glycoprotein IIb/IIIa inhibitor during percutaneous coronary intervention. *Am J Cardiol*, 76:1222–7.

[16] Kereiakes, D.J., Kleiman, N.S., Ambrose, J., *et al.*, (1996) Randomized, double-blind, placebo-controlled dose-ranging study of tirofiban (MK-383) platelet IIb/IIIa blockade in high risk patients undergoing coronary angioplasty. *J Am Coll Cardiol*, 27:536–42.

[17] Abdelmeguid, A.E., Topol, E.J., Whitlow, P.L., *et al.*, (1996) Significance of mild transient release of creatine kinase — MB fraction after percutaneous coronary intervention. *Circulation*, 94:1528–36.

[18] Harrington, R.A., Lincoff, A.M., Califf, R.M., *et al.*, (1995) Characteristics and consequences of myocardial infarction after percutaneous coronary intervention: insights from the coronary angioplasty versus excisional atherectomy trial (CAVEAT). *J Am Coll Cardiol*, 25: 1693–9.

[19] Kong, T.Q., Davidson, C.J., Meyers, S.N., *et al.*, (1997) Prognostic implication of creatine kinase elevation following elective coronary artery interventions. *JAMA*, 277:461–6.

[20] Tardiff, B.E., Califf, R.M., Tcheng, J.E., *et al.*, (1996) Post-intervention cardiac enzyme elevations: prognostic significance in IMPACT II (abstr). *J Am Coll Cardiol*, 27:83A.

[21] Topol, E.J., Ferguson, J.J., Weisman, H.F., *et al.*, (1997) Long-term protection from myocardial ischemic events in a randomized trial of brief integrin 3 blockade with percutaneous coronary intervention. *JAMA*, 278:479–84.

[22] Phillips, D.R., Teng, W., Arfstent, A., *et al.*, (1997) Effect of Ca^{2+} on GP IIb-IIIa interactions with Integrilin. Enhanced GP IIb-IIIa binding and inhibition of platelet aggregation by reductions in the concentration of ionized calcium in plasma anticoagulated with citrate. *Circulation*, 96:1488–94.

[23] Tcheng, J.E., Talley, J.D., O'Shea, J.C., *et al.*, (2001) Clinical pharmacology of higher-dose eptifibatide in percutaneous coronary intervention: results of the PRIDE study. *Am J Cardiol*, 88:1097–102.

[24] Simon, D.I., Liu, C.B., Ganz, P., *et al.*, (2001) A comparative study of light transmission aggregometry and automated bedside platelet function assays in patients undergoing percutaneous coronary intervention and receiving abciximab, eptifibatide, and tirofiban. *Catheter Cardiovasc Interv*, 52:425–32.

[25] Kereiakes, D.J., Broderick, T.M., Roth, E.M., *et al.*, (1999) Time course, magnitude, and consistency of platelet inhibition by abciximab, tirofiban, and eptifibatide in patients with unstable angina pectoris undergoing percutaneous coronary intervention. *Am J Cardiol*, 84:391–5.

[26] Valgimigli, M., Percoco, G., Barbieri, D., *et al.*, (2004) The additive value of tirofiban administered with the high-dose bolus in the prevention of ischemic complications during high-risk coronary angioplasty. *J Am Coll Cardiol*, 44(1):14–19.

[27] EPIC investigators, (1994) Use of a monoclonal antibody directed against the platelet glycoprotein IIb/IIIa receptor in high-risk coronary angioplasty. *N Eng J Med*, 330:956–61.

[28] Aguirre, F.V., Topol, E.J., Ferguson, J.J., *et al.*, (1995) Bleeding complications with the chimeric antibody to platelet glycoprotein IIb/IIIa integrin in patients undergoing percutaneous coronary intervention. *Circulation*, 91:2882–90.

[29] Lincoff, A.M., Tcheng, J.E., Califf, R.M., *et al.*, (1997) Standard versus low dose weight-adjusted heparin in patients treated with the platelet glycoprotein IIb/IIIa receptor antibody fragment abciximab (c7E3 Fab) during percutaneous coronary revascularization. *Am J Cardiol*, 79:286–91.

[30] EPILOG investigators, (1997) Platelet glycoprotein IIb/IIIa blockade with abciximab with low-dose heparin during percutaneous coronary revascularization. *N Eng J Med*, 336:1689–96.

[31] EPISTENT investigators, (1998) Randomised placebo-controlled and balloon-angioplasty-controlled trial to assess safety of coronary stenting with use of platelet glycoprotein IIb/IIIa blockade. *Lancet*, 352:87–92.

[32] IMPACT II investigators, (1997) Randomized placebo-controlled trial of effect of eptifibatide on complications of percutaneous coronary intervention: IMPACT II. *Lancet*, 349:1422–8.

[33] ESPRIT investigators, (2000) Novel dosing regimen of eptifibatide in planned coronary stent implantation (ESPRIT): a randomised, placebo-controlled trial. *Lancet*, 356:2037–44.

[34] RESTORE investigators, (1997) Effects of platelet glycoprotein IIb/IIIa blockade with tirofiban on adverse cardiac events in patients with unstable angina or acute myocardial infarction undergoing coronary angioplasty. *Circulation*, 96:1445–53.

[35] Topol, E.J., Moliterno, D.J., Herrmann, H.C., *et al.*, (2001) Comparison of two platelet glycoprotein IIb/IIIa inhibitors, tirofiban and abciximab, for the prevention of ischemic events with percutaneous coronary revascularization. *N Eng J Med*, 344:1888–94.

[36] ERASER investigators, (1999) Acute platelet inhibition with abciixmab does not reduce in-stent restenosis (ERASER Study). *Circulation*, 100:799–806.

[37] Lincoff, A.M., Califf, R.M., Moliterno, D.J., *et al.*, (1999) Complementary clinical benefits of coronary-artery stenting and blockade of platelet glycoprotein IIb/IIIa receptors. *N Eng J Med*, 341:319–27.

[38] Montalescot, G., Barragan, P., Wittenberg, O., *et al.*, (2001) Platelet glycoprotein IIb/IIIa inhibition with coronary stenting for acute myocardial infarction. *N Eng J Med*, 344:1895–903.

[39] Mehilli, J., Kastrati, A., Schuhlen, H., *et al.*, (2004) Randomized Clinical Trial of Abciximab in Diabetic Patients Undergoing Elective Percutaneous Coronary Interventions After Treatment With a High Loading Dose of Clopidogrel. *Circulation*, 110(24):3627–35.

[40] Chen, W., Kaul, U., Leung, S., *et al.*, (2005) A randomized, double-blind, placebo-controlled trial of abciximab for prevention of in-stent restenosis in diabetic patients after coronary stenting: results of the ASIAD (Abciximab in Stenting Inhibits restenosis Among Diabetics) trial. *J Invasive Cardiol*, 17(10):534–8.

[41] Chaves, A.J., Sousa, A.G., Mattos, L.A., *et al.*, (2004) Volumetric analysis of in-stent intimal hyperplasia in diabetic patients treated with or without abciximab. *Circulation*, 109(7): 861–6.

[42] Anderson, K.M., Califf, R.M., Stone, G.W., *et al.*, (2001) Long-term mortality benefit with abciximab in patients undergoing percutaneous coronary intervention. *J Am Coll Cardiol*, 37(8):2059–65.

[43] O'Shea, J.C., Buller, C.E., Cantor, W.J., *et al.*, (2002) Long-term efficacy of platelet glycoprotein IIb/IIIa integrin blockade with eptifibatide in coronary stent intervention. *JAMA*, 287:618–21.

[44] Kastrati, A., Mehilli, J., Schulhlen, H., *et al.*, (2004) A clinical trial of abciximab in elective percutaneous coronary intervention after pretreatment with clopidogrel. *N Eng J Med*, 350:232–8.

[45] Lincoff, A.M., Bittl, J.A., Harrington, R.A., *et al.*, (2003) Bivalirudin and provisional glycoprotein IIb/IIIa blockade compared with heparin and planned glycoprotein IIb/IIIa blockade during percutaneous coronary intervention. The REPLACE-2 trial. *JAMA*, 289: 853–63.

[46] Lincoff, A.M., Kleiman, N.S., Kereiakes, D.J., *et al.*, (2004) Long-term efficacy of bivalirudin and provisional glycoprotein IIb/IIIa blockade vs heparin and planned glycoprotein IIb/IIIa blockade during percutaneous coronary revascularization. REPLACE-2 randomized trial. *JAMA*, 292:696–703.

[47] Lincoff, A.M., Califf, R.M., Anderson, K.M., *et al.*, (1997) Evidence for prevention of death and myocardial infarction with platelet membrane glycoprotein IIb/IIIa receptor blockade by c7E3 Fab (abciximab) among patients with unstable angina undergoing percutaneous coronary revascularization. *J Am Coll Cardiol*, 30:149–56.

[48] PURSUIT trial investigators, (1998) Inhibition of platelet glycoprotein IIb/IIIa with eptifibatide in patients with acute coronary syndromes. *N Eng J Med*, 339:436–43.

[49] PRISM study investigators, (1998) A comparison of aspirin plus tirofiban with aspirin plus heparin for unstable angina. *N Eng J Med*, 338:1498–505.

[50] PRISM PLUS study investigators, (1998) Inhibition of the platelet glycoprotein IIb/IIIa receptor with tirofiban in unstable angina and non-Q-wave myocardial infarction. *N Eng J Med*, 338:1488–97.

[51] PARAGON investigators, (1998) International, randomized, controlled trial of lamifiban (a platelet glycoprotein IIb/IIIa inhibitor, heparin, or both in unstable angina). *Circulation*, 97:2386–95.

[52] GUSTO IV-ACS investigators, (2001) Effect of glycoprotein IIb/IIIa receptor blocker abciximab on outcome in patients with acute coronary syndromes without early coronary revascularisation: the GUSTO IV-ACS randomised trial. *Lancet*, 357:1915–24.

[53] PARAGON-B investigators, (2002) Randomized, placebo-controlled trial of titrated intravenous lamifiban for acute coronary syndromes. *Circulation*, 105:316–21.

[54] Roffi, M., Chew, D.P., Mukherjee, D., *et al.*, (2002) Platelet glycoprotein IIb/IIIa inhibition in acute coronary syndromes. Gradient of benefit related to the revascularization strategy. *Eur Heart J*, 23(18):1441–8.

[55] van den Merkhof, L.F., Zijlstra, F., Olsson, H., *et al.*, (1999) Abciximab in the treatment of acute myocardial infarction eligible for primary percutaneous transliminal coronary angioplasty. *J Am Coll Cardiol*, 33(6):1528–32.

[56] SPEED trial investigators, (2000) Randomized trial of abciximab with and without low-dose reteplase for acute myocardial infarction. *Circulation*, 101:2788–94.

[57] Antman, E., Guigliano, R., Gibson, C., *et al.*, Abciximab facilitates the rate and extent of thrombolysis results of the thrombolysis in myocaridal infarction (TIMI) 14 trial. *Circulation*, 99:2720–32.

[58] Cutlip, D.E., Cove, C.J., Irons, D., *et al.*, (2001) Emergency room administration of eptifibatide before primary angioplasty for ST elevation acute myocardial infarction and its effect on baseline coronary flow and procedure outcomes. *Am J Cardiol*, 88:62–4.

[59] Brener, S.J., Barr, L.A., Burchenal, J.E.B, *et al.*, (1998) A randomized, placebo-controlled trial of platelet glycoprotein IIb/IIIa blockade with primary angioplasty for acute myocardial infarction. *Circulation*, 98:734–41.

[60] Stone, G.W., Grines, C.L., Cox, D.A., *et al.*, (2002) Comparison of angioplasty with stenting, with or without abciximab, in acute myocardial infarction. *N Eng J Med*, 346(13):957–66.

[61] Neumann, F., Kastrati, A., Schmitt, C., *et al.*, (2000) Effect of glycoprotein IIb/IIIa receptor blockade with abciximab on clinical and angiographic restenosis rate after the placement of coronary stents following acute myocardial infarction. *J Am Coll Cardiol*, 35(4):915–21.

[62] Antoniucci, D., Rodriguez, A., Hempel, A., *et al.*, (2003) A randomized trial comparing primary infarct artery stenting with or without abciximab in acute myocardial infarction. *J Am Coll Cardiol*, 42(11):1879–85.

[63] Kandzari, D.E., Hasselblad, V., Tcheng, J.E., *et al.*, (2004) Improved clinical outcomes with abciximab therapy in acute myocardial infarction: a systematic overview of randomized clinical trials. *Am Heart J*, 147(3):457–62.

[64] Neumann, F.J., Blasini, R., Schmitt, C., *et al.*, (1999) Effect of glycoprotein IIb/IIIa receptor blockade on recovery of coronary flow and left ventricular function after the placement of coronary artery stents in acute myocardial infarction. *Circulation*, 98:2695–701.

[65] Gibson, C.M., Cohen, D.J., Cohen, E.A., *et al.*, (2001) Effect of eptifibatide on coronary flow reserve following coronary stent implantation (an ESPRIT substudy). Enhanced Suppression of the Platelet IIb/IIIa Receptor with Integrilin Therapy. *Am J Cardiol*, 87(11): 1293–5.

[66] Neumann, F.J., Zohlnhofer, D., Fakhoury, L., *et al.*, (1999) Effect of glycoprotein IIb/IIIa receptor blockade on platelet-leukocyte interaction and surface expression of the leukocyte integrin Mac-1 in acute myocardial infarction. *J Am Coll Cardiol*, 34:1420–6.

[67] Kleiman, N.S., Ohman, E.M., Kereiakes, D.J., *et al.*, (1991) Profound platelet inactivation with 7E3 shortly after thrombolytic therapy for acute myocardial infarction: preliminary results of the TAMI 8 trial (abstr). *Circulation*, 84(4):II–522.

[68] Ohman, E.M., Kleiman, N.S., Gacioch, G., *et al.*, (1997) Combined acclerated tissue-plasminogen activator and platelet glycoprotein IIb/IIIa integrin receptor blockade with integrilin in acute myocardial infarction. Results of a randomized, placebo-contolled, dose-ranging trial. *Circulation*, 95:846–54.

[69] PARADIGM investigators, (1998) Combining thrombolysis with the platelet glycoprotein IIb/IIIa inhibitor lamifiban: Results of the platelet aggregation receptor antagonist dose investigation and reperfusion gain in myocardial infarction (PARADIGM) trial. *J Am Coll Cardiol*, 32: 2003–10.

[70] Ronner, E., Kesteren, H.A., Zijnen, P., *et al.*, (2000) Safety and efficacy of eptifibatide versus placebo in patients receiving thrombolytic therapy with streptokinase for acute myocardial infarction. A phase II dose escalation, randomized, double-blind study. *Eur Heart J*, 21:1530–6.

[71] Brener, S.J., Zeymer, W., Adgey, A.A.J., *et al.*, (2002) Eptifibatide and low-dose tissue plasminogen activator in acute myocardial infarction. The Integrilin and Low-Dose Thrombolysis in Acute Myocardial Infarction (INTRO AMI) trial. *J Am Coll Cardiol*, 39:377–86.

[72] de Lemos, J.A., Antman, E.M., Gibson, C.M., *et al.*, (2000) Abciximab improves both epicardial flow and myocardial reperfusion in ST-elevation myocardial infarction: observations from the TIMI 14 trial. *Circulation*, 101:239–43.

[73] The GUSTO V investigators, (2001) Reperfusion therapy for acute myocardial infarction with fibrinolytic therapy or combination reduced fibrinolytic therapy and platelet glycoprotein IIb/IIIa inhibition: the GUSTO V randomised trial. *Lancet*, 357:1905–14.

[74] Lincoff, A.M., Califf, R.M., Van de Werf, F., *et al.*, (2002) Mortality at 1 year with combination platelet glycoprotein IIb/IIIa inhibition and reduced-dose fibrinolytic therapy vs conventional fibrinolytic therapy for acute myocardial infarction. GUSTO V randomized trial. *JAMA*, 288:2130–5.

[75] ASSENT-3 (Assessment of Safety and Efficacy of a New Thrombolytic Regimen) investigators, (2001) Efficacy and safety of tenecteplase in combination with enoxaparin, abciximab, or unfractionated heparin: the ASSENT-3 randomised trial in acute myocardial infarction. *Lancet*, 358:605–13.

[76] Herrmann, H.C., Moliterno, D.J., Ohman, E.M., *et al.*, (2000) Facilitation of early percutaneous coronary intervention after reteplase with or without abciximab in acute myocardial infarction. Results from the SPEED (GUSTO-4 Pilot) trial. *J Am Coll Cardiol*, 36:1489–96.

[77] Kastrati, A., Mehilli, J., Schlotterbeck, K., Dotzer, F., Dirschinger, J., Schmitt, C., Nekolla, S.G., Seyfarth, M., Martinoff, S., Markwardt, C., Clermont, G., Gerbig, H.W., Leiss, J., Schwaiger, M., Schomig, A. (2004) Early administration of reteplase plus abciximab versus abciximab alone in patients with acute myocardial infarction referred for percutaneous coronary intervention: a randomized trial. *JAMA*, 291:947–54.

[78] Akkerhuis, K.M., Deckers, J.W., Lincoff, A.M., *et al.*, (2001) Risk of stroke associated with abciximab among patients undergoing percutaneous coronary intervention. *JAMA*, 286:78–82.

[79] Wagner, C.L., Cunningham, M.R., Wyand, M.S., *et al.*, (1995) Reversal of the antiplatelet effects of chimeric 7E3 Fab treatment by platelet transfusion in cynomolgous monkeys (abstr). *Thromb Haemost*, 73:1313.

[80] Lincoff, A.M., LeNarz, R.A., Despotis, G.J., *et al.*, (2000) Abciximab and bleeding complications during coronary surgery: results from the EPILOG and EPISTENT trials. *Ann Thorac Surg*, 70:516–26.

[81] Kereiakes, D.J., Berkowitz, S.D., Lincoff, A.M., *et al.*, (2000) Clinical correlates and course of thrombocytopenia during percutaneous coronary intervention in the era of abciximab glycoprotein IIb/IIIa blockade. *Am Heart J*, 140:74–80.

[82] Berkowitz, S.D., Harrington, R.A., Rund, M.M., *et al.*, (1997) Acute profound thrombocytopenia after c7E3 Fab (abciximab) therapy. *Circulation*, 95:809–13.

[83] Tcheng, J.E., Kereiakes, D.J., Lincoff, A.M., *et al.*, (2001) Abciximab readministration. Results of the ReoPro Readministration Registry. *Circulation*, 104:870–5.

5 Unfractionated Heparin

5.1 INTRODUCTION

The generation of thrombin at the site of local vascular injury is a pivotal step in the development of intravascular thrombus, a process that is integral to the pathogenesis of UA and NSTEMI (known collectively as the ACS), STEMI and VTE. The wide range of thrombin's activities including the conversion of fibrinogen to fibrin, upregulation of coagulation factors, promotion of platelet aggregation and promotion of smooth muscle cell proliferation contribute to the development and maintenance of a thrombogenic milieu. Although an endogenous inhibitor of thrombin's pro-coagulant activity, antithrombin (AT), exists, its activity is overwhelmed in the pathologic setting.

Unfractionated heparin (UH), an indirect antithrombin, remains the most widely employed antithrombin therapy today (Table 5.1). The utility of UH has been demonstrated in patients across the spectrum of CV disease ranging from a primary role in decreasing ischemic events in ACS, as an adjunct to fibrinolysis in STEMI, and in the acute management of VTE, to name a few examples. Although UH has demonstrated its value, the associated risk of hemorrhagic complications, the interpatient variability in anticoagulant response and HIT, the 'Achilles' heel' of UH therapy, have prompted the search for effective alternative agents such as LMWH and DTI. This chapter will serve to discuss the pharmacology of the UH as well as to review the evidence supporting its use in acute ischemic syndromes and in VTE.

Table 5.1 Clinical indications for UH use

Cardiovascular indications
Early treatment of ACS
Early treatment of acute MI
PCI
Cardiopulmonary bypass
Vascular surgery
Venous thrombembolic indications
Acute treatment of DVT
Acute treatment of PE
Prevention of VTE

Management Strategies in Antithrombotic Therapy Arman T. Askari, Adrian W. Messerli and A. Michael Lincoff

5.2 PHARMACOLOGY

MECHANISM OF ACTION

UH is a heterogeneous mixture of sulfated mucopolysaccharides possessing molecular weights ranging from 3000 to 30,000 with a mean of 15,000 (Figure 5.1) [1]. UH exerts its anticoagulant effects through several mechanisms including interactions with AT, interactions with heparin cofactor II (HCII) and interactions directly with factor Xa (clinically not important) with the latter two contributing to the anticoagulant effects only at supratherapeutic concentrations [2, 3]. Binding with AT occurs through a unique pentasaccharide sequence present in approximately one-third of UH fragments. The interaction of UH with AT inactivates a number of coagulation enzymes including thrombin (factor IIa), as well as factor IXa, Xa, XIa and XIIa. Thrombin and factor Xa are most responsive to inactivation, with the UH-AT complex accelerating their inactivation approximately 1000-fold [4]. Inhibition of factor Xa can occur through interaction with pentasaccharide-containing UH fragments of any length bound to AT; however, inhibition of thrombin requires that UH fragments at least 18 saccharide residues long (including the pentasaccharide component) and AT bind to it forming a tertiary complex. Because almost all fragments of UH are at least 18 saccharide residues in length, UH exerts equivalent inhibition of both factor Xa (thrombin generation) and thrombin (thrombin activity).

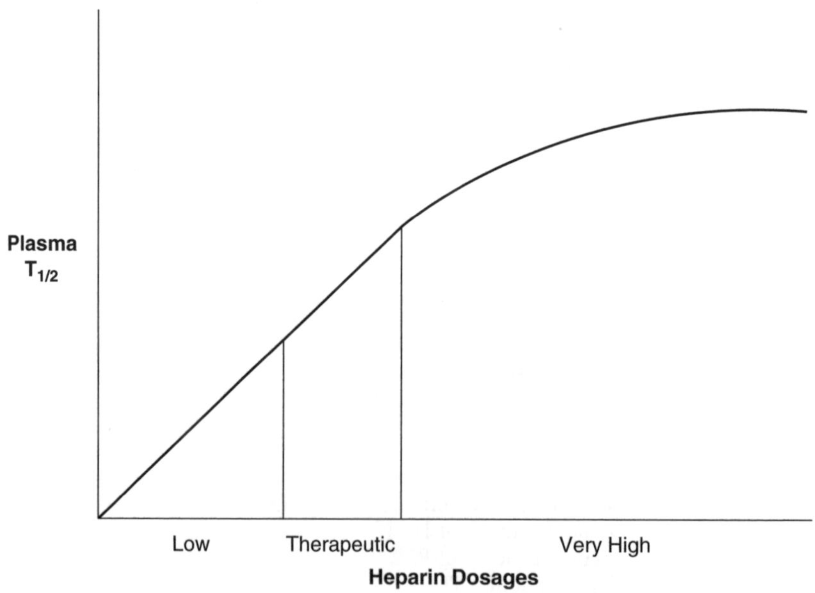

Figure 5.1 Demonstration of the clearance of UH from plasma. At Low doses of UH, clearance is primarily via saturable mechanisms. Therapeutic doses of heparin are cleared by a combination of the rapid, saturable mechanism and the slower, nonsaturable dose-independent mechanism of renal clearance. Very high doses of heparin are cleared predominantly through the slower nonsaturable mechanism of clearance

The interaction of heparin with HCII provides an AT-independent mechanism of thrombin inactivation [2]. This pathway requires UH at least 24 saccharide units in length but does not require the 'unique' pentasaccharide sequence. This pathway is thought to be operative at higher concentrations of UH than the AT-mediated pathway as well as in cases of AT deficiency.

Although still incompletely understood, the antithrombotic actions of UH may, in part, be related to the stimulation of tissue factor pathway inhibitor (TFPI) release from endothelial cells [5]. One of the many antithrombotic effects of TFPI involves binding with and inactivating factor Xa. This TFPI–factor Xa complex subsequently functions to regulate the extrinsic coagulation pathway by inactivating factor VIIa [6]. Although theoretically important, this may actually be a double-edged sword, as the degree of TFPI release induced by UH may, in part, explain the transient prothrombotic state related to thrombin generation and the clinical events that occur during treatment with UH and following its abrupt cessation [7–9]. As will be discussed in subsequent chapters, this is one limitation not as operative with alternative anticoagulants, such as LMWH and DTI, that make them attractive alternatives to UH within the spectrum of thromboembolic diseases.

PHARMACOKINETICS AND PHARMACODYNAMICS

UH is not absorbed through the gastrointestinal mucosa and, therefore, must be given parenterally either by continuous intravenous (IV) infusion or by subcutaneous (SC) injection. Therapeutic levels of anticoagulation can be achieved with either route, but if immediate anticoagulation is necessary IV administration is preferred as the onset of action of SC UH generally occurs within 20–60 min. In addition, the dose of UH should be increased approximately 10% when given subcutaneously to account for the lower bioavailability than with IV delivery [10]. Although therapeutic levels of anticoagulation can be achieved with high-dose SC injections divided twice daily [11], the higher incidence of subtherapeutic anticoagulation compared with IV infusion and the resultant recurrent thrombotic events [10] have reserved this route primarily for administration of prophylactic doses of UH. However, patients can be adequately anticoagulated with UH given via the SC route should the need arise [12, 13].

Once within the bloodstream, UH binds to plasma proteins such as vitronectin and fibrinogen, to proteins secreted by platelets such as platelet factor 4 and to proteins secreted by endothelial cells such as vWf [14]. This avid non-specific protein binding of UH is felt to contribute to its poor bioavailability and variable anticoagulation [15]. In addition, the binding to platelet proteins also contributes to the immunogenicity of UH and to activation of platelets which may result in increased risk of the development of HIT and thrombosis. Coupled with its short half-life, this also translates into the need for IV administration as well as frequent monitoring and dose adjustments with UH.

UH is cleared through the combination of a rapid saturable and a slower non-saturable mechanism (Figure 5.1) [16–18]. The saturable, dose-dependent, phase of UH clearance results from interactions with the reticulo-endothelial system during which it is depolymerized [18]. The non-saturable phase of UH clearance is primarily through renal excretion. At therapeutic doses, UH is predominantly cleared via the rapid saturable mechanism, which accounts for the non-linear response and the apparent prolonged biological half-life to increasing doses of UH. The half-life of the anticoagulant activity in humans is approximately 1, 1.5 and 2. h at doses of 100, 200 and 400 U/kg, respectively. The half-life of UH may be shortened in patients with pulmonary embolism and prolonged in patients with hepatic cirrhosis or end-stage renal disease [19].

HEPARIN MONITORING

Because of UH's often unpredictable pharmacokinetics and its narrow therapeutic range, therapy with this agent requires laboratory monitoring for proper dosing [20]. The methods used to monitor the level of anticoagulation achieved by the administration of UH depend on the clinical situation and the dosing utilized. The activated partial thromboplastin time (aPTT) is used to monitor the level of anticoagulation when usual therapeutic doses are used while the activated clotting time (ACT) is used to monitor higher levels of anticoagulation such as that seen with cardiopulmonary bypass or PCI [21–24]. Historically, given that an aPTT between 1.5 and 2.5 times control values was associated with improved outcomes, this range of anticoagulation has been deemed 'therapeutic' [21]. However, the currently available laboratory techniques for monitoring UH anticoagulation are not only numerous, but also heterogeneous [25], resulting in variability in monitoring UH anticoagulation.

This variability in UH monitoring results from differences between thromboplastin reagents and coagulation instruments [26–30]. At therapeutic heparin levels measured by anti-factor Xa activity, various thromboplastin reagents produce aPTT ratios that range from 1.6 to more than 6 times control values [25, 28]. Thus, it is understandable that a standard recommendation of achieving an aPTT 1.5 to 2.5 times control may result in grossly under or overestimating the level of anticoagulation achieved with UH and in untoward clinical outcomes. As a means of minimizing this risk, it is recommended that each institution standardize their aPTT assay by correlating it with therapeutic anti-factor Xa levels.

Despite its limitations, the aPTT remains the most common method used to monitor the anticoagulant response to heparin. The aPTT should be assessed 6 h after an IV bolus of UH and the subsequent dosing adjusted accordingly. To facilitate timely therapeutic levels several dosing nomograms have been developed such as that demonstrated in Table 5.2 [31] and Table 5.3 [32]. The failure to achieve therapeutic levels of anticoagulation may be associated with recurrent clinical events and with increased morbidity and mortality [10, 11]. It is prudent to remember that none of these nomograms pertain to all aPTT reagents and the 'therapeutic' range should be adapted to the particular agent used.

Table 5.2 A weight-based dosing nomogram for thrombotic disorders. Adapted from Raschke *et al.* [31]

aPTT	UH dose
Initial dose	80 U/kg bolus, then 18 U/kg per h
<35 s	80 U/kg bolus, then increase by 4 U/kg per h
35–45 s	40 U/kg bolus, then increase by 2 U/kg per h
46–70 s	Therapeutic range*
71–90 s	Decrease infusion by 2 U/kg per h
>90 s	Hold infusion × 1 h, then decrease infusion by 3 U/kg per h

* The therapeutic range should be assessed at every institution by correlation with anti-factor Xa levels between 0.3 and 0.7 U/mL

Table 5.3 A weight-based UH dosing nomogram for ACS. Adapted from Becker *et al.* [32]

aPTT (seconds)	bolus	Infusion adjustment (U/kg per h)
<35	70 U/kg additional	+3
35–49	35 U/kg additional	+2
50–70	Therapeutic range*	0
71–90	0	−2
>100	Hold infusion for 30 min	−3

Initial dose: 60 U/kg bolus and 12 U/kg per h infusion

* The therapeutic range should be assessed at every institution by correlation with anti-factor Xa levels between 0.3 and 0.7 U/mL

5.3 CLINICAL USES OF UH

That thrombin generation plays a pivotal role in the genesis of pathologic thrombosis across the spectrum of cardiovascular disease ranging from the acute coronary syndromes to venous thromboembolic disease has facilitated the expansion of the field of available antithrombotic agents. The emergence of several agents including LMWH and DTI have been born out of a need to address the limitations of UH. Despite its shortcomings, UH has weathered this onslaught of attempts to replace it as the most widely utilized antithrombotic agent.

UH IN IHD

UH is used for the management of several cardiovascular diseases, either alone or, more commonly, in conjunction with antiplatelet agents (e.g. aspirin, clopidogrel and GP IIb/IIIa inhibitors), fibrinolytic agents or both. Although large, randomized, controlled trials assessing the efficacy of UH are scant, a substantial body of literature, primarily observational, has accrued. The role of UH in PCI, in medical therapy for ACS/NSTEMI, and within the realm of STEMI is, primarily, to decrease recurrent ischemic events by decreasing thrombus formation. Despite its ability to decrease recurrent events, UH has not been shown to substantially impact mortality.

UH DURING PCI

Classically associated with two major limitations, abrupt vessel closure and restenosis, routine PCI has experienced markedly improved outcomes through the routine use of adjunct pharmacotherapies such as antithrombin and antiplatelet agents and through advances in technology including intracoronary stents [33–35]. UH is the most frequently used thrombin inhibitor during PCI, although other AT-dependent agents (e.g. LMWH) [36] and AT-independent agents (e.g. hirudin, bivalirudin and argatroban) [37] have also been studied and are commonly employed in clinical practice. Intravenous UH is used during PCI to prevent arterial thrombus formation at the site of vessel wall injury as well as on the equipment used for coronary interventions [38]. The efficacy of UH in patients with ACS presenting for PCI has also been demonstrated as sole therapy [39] or in combination with antiplatelet agents [40–42].

HEPARIN MONITORING AND DOSING DURING PCI

In order to balance the risk of hemorrhage with the benefits imparted by antithrombin therapy, an understanding of procedural monitoring of the level of anticoagulation achieved is essential. The aPTT can provide a somewhat accurate measure of anticoagulation intensity in the clinical setting; however, aPTTs are not useful for this purpose during PCI given the significantly larger doses of UH required to prevent thrombus formation in this setting [43–45]. The bedside test readily available for this purpose is the ACT [45]. Irrespective of the device used for procedural monitoring, Hemo Tec® or Hemochron®, the level of anticoagulation achieved as assessed by the ACT has been correlated with peri-procedural events; inversely with ischemic and directly with hemorrhagic complications [44, 46, 47]. Although the target ACT is usually 250 to 350 sec, one study suggested that the optimal ACT during heparin monotherapy may be in the range of 350 to 375 sec while the ACT with the lowest incidence of bleeding complications was in the range of 325 to 350 sec [48].

Dosing of UH during PCI depends on several factors including the use of stents, the use of adjunctive anti-platelet agents (i.e. GP IIb/IIIa inhibitors) and the clinical scenario (elective PCI versus PCI in patients with ACS). With the availability of intracoronary stents, recent studies have suggested that lower doses of UH may be safe and effective [49]. In a series of 1375 consecutive patients undergoing elective PCI, low-dose bolus UH (5000) was associated with early sheath removal and infrequent ischemic complications within 48 h [49]. Although this regimen may decrease the risk of hemorrhagic complications, the routine use of ACTs to guide therapy remains clinically prudent.

It has been suggested that the use of weight-adjusted UH would offer benefits above those experienced with fixed dosing. However, the benefit of weight-adjusted dosing seems to be primarily related to earlier sheath removal with similar clinical outcomes when used alone [50]. On the other hand, the concomitant use of UH with GP IIb/IIIa inhibitors dictates the use of lower, weight-adjusted dosing. In these cases, similar clinical outcomes can be achieved with fewer bleeding complications with ACTs in the range of >200 sec whether stents are used or not. In a trial of 2064 patients, all of whom received stents, randomly assigned to eptifibatide or placebo prior to PCI the lowest risk of bleeding was seen in patients with an ACT <244 sec with comparable clinical outcomes compared to those with higher ACTs [51]. In addition, low-dose heparin (70 U of heparin per kilogram to a maximum of 7000 U), with additional boluses to maintain an ACT at approximately 200 sec, reduced the incidence of hemorrhagic complications without increasing coronary events in a study of patients primarily undergoing balloon angioplasty [52].

In summary, the following empiric recommendations can be made with respect to anticoagulation during PCI. UH should be administered with either weight-adjusted (70–100 IU/kg) or gender-adjusted (7000 U for women and 8000 U for men) bolus doses to achieve an ACT of 250–350 sec. Weight-adjusted heparin can be used to avoid excessive levels of anticoagulation. When a GP IIb/IIIa inhibitor is used, the heparin bolus should be reduced to 50 to 70 U/kg. In such patients, an ACT of 200 to 250 sec appears to be safe and effective.

DURATION OF UH IN PCI

Whereas prolonged UH for up to 24 h following PCI was previously routine [53], data has emerged that deems this approach unnecessary and associated with increased morbidity (in particular, bleeding) [54]. Since the use of stenting has increased to over 85% of PCIs and since studies have shown a low (0.6%) incidence of post-procedure events with dual antiplatelet therapy, there appears to be little indication for post-procedure heparin in such patients [55].

UH IN THE MANAGEMENT OF ACS/NSTEMI

Intracoronary thrombus remains central to the pathogenesis of the ACS. Although a large-scale, randomized, controlled trial assessing the efficacy of UH in ACS is lacking, several smaller studies have demonstrated the utility of UH in the management of these patients (Table 5.4). When used as the sole antithrombotic agent in ACS, UH has been associated with decreased recurrent angina or recurrent MI [56–59]. In addition, studies have suggested that combining UH and aspirin in ACS results in further benefit and, importantly, serves to reduce the rebound ischemia that occurs following cessation of UH therapy. Expanding upon the role of a multi-pronged approach to the management of ACS, addition of the GP IIb/IIIa inhibitors has been shown to further improve outcomes (Chapter 4).

UH ALONE OR IN COMBINATION WITH ASPIRIN FOR ACS

Several studies have compared UH, aspirin and UH plus aspirin (Table 5.4). Early trials that compared UH to aspirin in patients with ACS revealed mixed results. Whereas one trial demonstrated a significantly decreased rate of MI with UH titrated to aPTT 1.5–2 times control (0.8%) or aspirin 325 mg twice daily (3.3%) compared with placebo (11.9%) [57], another study found that UH (5000 U IV every 6 h for 5 days) was no more effective than aspirin (75 mg/day) [58]. The discrepant results reflect the different modes of UH administration and suggest that intermittent bolus therapy is obsolete. Additional studies comparing UH to aspirin further indicated that UH significantly reduced the rates of MI compared with varying doses of aspirin [60, 61].

Bearing the pathophysiology of ACS in mind, it would seem reasonable to hypothesize that combining UH with aspirin would result in even further benefit compared to either medication alone. However, this has not been definitively established. Two early trials did not show a difference in outcomes between UH plus aspirin compared with aspirin alone [57, 62]. However, neither trial was capable of detecting small differences. On the other hand, a small trial comparing aspirin (162.5 mg/day) to UH (titrated to aPTT 2× control) plus aspirin followed by aspirin plus warfarin provided support for combination therapy [63]. Adding further support, a meta-analysis suggested that the addition of UH to aspirin in patients with ACS decreases the risk of death or MI by 33% over treatment with aspirin alone [64]. The discrepant findings can, in part, be explained by an observation made prior to the use of widespread revascularization for the management of ACS: that an improvement in event rates has been seen during UH administration with a 'catch-up' in event rates following discontinuation of UH.

Further support for the use of UH in ACS can be gleaned from trials of LMWH in this setting. Whereas little incremental benefit of LMWH over UH has been demonstrated in this scenario, compared with placebo, LMWH provide a significant improvement in outcomes. Thus it can be inferred that UH must provide some benefit in this setting [65].

Table 5.4 Trials of UH for the management of ACS

Trial	Type	*N*	Treatment	UH dose	Goal aPTT	ASA dose	Endpoint	Comment
Telford *et al.* [56]	RDBPCT	214	UH Atenolol Placebo UH + atenolol	5000 U every 6 h		NA	Transmural MI	During the trial period, transmural MI developed in 17%, 13%, 2%, and 4% of patients in the placebo, atenolol, heparin, and heparin plus atenolol groups, respectively (p–value = 0.024)
Theroux *et al.* [57]	RDBPCT	479	Placebo UH ASA UH + ASA	1000 U/h Continuous IV infusion × 6 days	1.5–2 × normal	325 mg bid	RA/MI/D	The incidence of MI at a mean follow-up of 6±3 days was significantly reduced in heparin-treated patients (0.8% vs 3.3% with aspirin). The study was not powered to assess the effect of heparin vs aspirin on mortality. Aspirin blunted rebound of UA symptoms after discontinuation of heparin therapy
RISC [58]	RDBPCT	796	Placebo UH ASA UH + ASA	5000 U every 6 h × 5 days	Not stated	75 mg daily	D/MI	Aspirin reduced the event rate in non-Q-wave MI and UA, independently of ECG abnormalities or concurrent drug therapy. Heparin had no significant influence on event rate, although the group treated with aspirin and heparin had the lowest number of events during the initial 5 days
Neri Serneri *et al.* [59]	RDBT	97	UH – intermittent bolus UH – continuous IV ASA + alteplase	6000 U every 6 h 5000 U bolus f/b 1000 U/h IV				On the first days of treatment heparin infusion significantly decreased the frequency of angina (by 84–94%), episodes of silent ischemia (by 71–77%), and the overall duration of ischemia (by 81–86%). Heparin bolus and aspirin were not effective. Alteplase caused small (non-significant) reductions on the first day only

Cohen *et al.* [134]	Pilot trial	93	ASA f/b warfarin UH f/b warfarin ASA + UH f/b warfarin	Titrated to aPTT × 3–4 days	2 × normal	325 mg daily 80 mg daily	D/MI	
Theroux *et al.* [60]	RDBT	484	ASA UH	5000 U bolus then titrated to aPTT	1.5–2.5 × normal	325 mg bid	D/MI	UH was associated with significantly fewer MI than aspirin (0.8% vs 3.7%, respectively)
Cohen *et al.* [63]	PRT	214	ASA ASA + UH f/b ASA + warfarin	Titrated to aPTT × 3–4 days	2 × normal	162.5 mg daily	RA/MI/D	In nonprior aspirin users, combination antithrombotic therapy with aspirin plus anticoagulation significantly reduces recurrent ischemic events in the early phase of UA
Holdright *et al.* [62]	PRT	285	ASA ASA + UH	Titrated to aPTT × 2 days	1.5–2 × normal	150 mg daily		This study suggests that combined therapy with heparin and aspirin compared with aspirin alone makes no difference in the development of in-hospital MI or death, nor does it reduce the development of transient myocardial ischemia
Gurfinkel *et al.* [135]	RDBT	219	ASA ASA + UH ASA + LMWH	400 IU/kg IV daily Titrated to aPTT × 5–7 days 214 UIC/kg SC bid	2 × normal	200 mg daily	RA/MI/UR/D and bleeding	Treatment with aspirin plus a high dose of LMWH during the acute phase of UA was significantly better than treatment with aspirin alone or aspirin plus regular heparin
Neri Serneri *et al.* [61]	PRT	108	IV UH SC UH ASA	Titrated to aPTT 5000–7500 q8h	1.5–2 × normal	325 mg daily	Reduced myocardial ischemia	Aspirin did not significantly affect the incidence of myocardial ischemia. On the first 3 days, infused and SC heparin significantly decreased the frequency of angina, episodes of silent ischemia, and the overall duration of ischemia vs run-in day and aspirin (p-value <0.001 for all variables). The favorable effects of heparin therapy remained evident during follow-up

bid = twice daily; D = death; ECG = electrocardiogram; f/b = followed by; IU = international units; NA = not applicable; PRT = prospective randomized trial; q8h = every eight hours; RA = recurrent angina; RDBPCT = randomized double blind placebo controlled trial; RDBT = randomized double blind trial; UR = urgent revascularization

UH AS AN ADJUNCT IN THE MANAGEMENT OF STEMI

Along the continuum of acute ischemic syndromes, acute STEMI primarily results from cessation of coronary blood flow due to occlusive thrombus formation at the site of a ruptured plaque. Clinical trials assessing the effects of pharmacologic and mechanical reperfusion techniques have demonstrated improved outcomes in patients achieving complete and rapid restoration of antegrade coronary perfusion. As a result, the central paradigm in the management of STEMI has become 'time is myocardium.'

Through effective clot dissolution, fibrinolysis exposes fibrin-bound thrombin. In addition, fibrinolytics have been shown to lead to thrombin generation directly [66]. It would seem reasonable to think that the enhanced fibrinolysis seen with the addition of the indirect AT, UH, in preclinical models [67] would parlay into robust clinical benefit. However, data demonstrating the usefulness of UH in this setting remain limited (Table 5.5). Nevertheless, the rationale for administering UH in patients with STEMI includes preventing ventricular thrombus formation, venous thromboembolism, and cerebral thromboembolism in addition to maintaining patency of the infarct-related artery (IRA).

UH WITHOUT FIBRINOLYTICS IN STEMI

Prior to the fibrinolytic era, antithrombin therapy with UH and oral anticoagulation served to limit ischemic complications and prevent peripheral, cerebral or pulmonary embolization. Although this formed the basis for the use of UH in patients not treated with fibrinolytics, the substantiation of the fibrinolytics era with ISIS-2 called into question the benefit of UH therapy, given the significant mortality benefit with aspirin alone and the marginal risk–benefit ratio with UH added to fibrinolytics [68].

Whereas the combination of aspirin and UH resulted in improved outcomes in patients with ACS, the benefit of combining these agents in patients with STEMI has been more difficult to establish. Observational data from clinical trials of fibrinolytics therapy have revealed conflicting results. Both a lack of a survival benefit [68] and improved survival [69] have been suggested. However, the clinical applicability of these data to present-day management of STEMI is ambiguous, given that the vast majority of patients remain eligible for either fibrinolysis or primary PCI.

UH WITH FIBRINOLYTICS IN STEMI

Clinically relevant data assessing the utility of UH added to a regimen of fibrinolytics alone or fibrinolytics and aspirin remain limited. The majority of the benefit of UH therapy in these patients arises from a decreased incidence of ischemic and thrombotic complications rather than from a mortality benefit. In an early trial of UH without aspirin in patients with STEMI 711 patients were randomized to either subcutaneous UH or no UH beginning within 24 h of the onset of symptoms [70]. SK was given to 433 of these patients admitted within 6 h. In the subgroup receiving SK, transient ischemic episodes and mortality were lower with the addition of UH. An additional benefit of UH was the significantly lower prevalence of left ventricular (LV) thrombus in those that received UH. The clinical applicability of these data to contemporary management of STEMI is negligible given the unequivocal benefit of aspirin and fibrinolytic therapy in these patients.

Table 5.5 Trials of UH in STEMI

Trial	*N*	Reperfusion modality	Treatment groups	UH dose	ASA dose	Endpoint	Comment
ISIS [136]	619	Fibrinolytic – SK	SK Y OR N UH Y OR N ASA Y OR N	5000 U bolus then 1000 U/h for 48 h	325 mg qod × 28 days	D/MI	SK: NS increase in MI (3.9% vs 2.9% placebo); NS decrease in mortality (7.5% vs 9.7% in hospital plus 6.1% vs 8.7% after discharge) ASA: fewer MI (3.2% vs 3.9% placebo, NS), deaths (in hospital: 6.1% vs 10.5%, 2*p* less than 0.05, and after discharge: 7.0% vs 6.9%, NS) UH: fewer MI (2.2% vs 4.9% no UH, NS); no difference in D (in hospital: 8.0% vs 8.5%, NS, and after discharge: 7.0% vs 6.9%, NS)
ISIS-2 [68]	17,187	Fibrinolytic – SK	SK Y OR N ASA Y OR N SK + ASA	UH given to 4295 patients randomized to ASA but no SK	160 mg daily	35-day D	Heparin therapy provided no survival benefit at 35 days (10.9% mortality with IV heparin, 11.2% with SC heparin, and 10.1% with no heparin)
SCATI [70]	711	Fibrinolytic – SK in 433 patients	UH Placebo SK + UH SK + placebo	12,500 U SC bid	NA	In-hospital D, RI, MI	UH associated with decreased mortality. No difference in recurrent ischemia or reinfarction. UH was safe
GISSI-2	12,490	Fibrinolytic SK vs Conventional t-PA	SK + UH SK + placebo t-PA + UH t-PA + placebo	12,500 U SC bid until DC starting at 12 h	300–325 mg daily (all patients)	D + severe ventricular damage	No significant difference in primary endpoint between the two fibrinolytics. UH had no effect on the primary endpoint. Slightly higher bleeding rates with SK + UH
ISIS-3 [71]	41,299	Fibrinolytic – SK vs duteplase vs APSAC	SK APSAC Duteplase ½ UH vs placebo	12,500 SC bid starting at 4 h × 7 daysays or until DC	162 mg daily (all patients)	35-day D	No difference in primary endpoint between fibrinolytics. Duteplase associated with less re-MI. SK associated with less ICH. UH added to ASA associated with less D at 7 days. UH associated with higher bleeding

Table 5.5 (*Continued*)

Trial	*N*	Reperfusion modality	Treatment groups	UH dose	ASA dose	Endpoint	Comment
GUSTO-1 [72]	41,021	Fibrinolytic- SK vs accelerated t-PA	SK + SC UH SK + IV UH t-PA + IV UH SK + t-PA + IV UH	SC = 12,500 U bid starting at 4 h IV = 5000 U bolus then titrated to aPTT 60–85 s	160 mg on admission, then 160–325 mg daily (all patients)	30-day D	Mortality: SK + SC UH, 7.2%; SK + IV UH, 7.4%; t-PA + IV UH, 6.3%; SK + t-PA + IV UH, 7.0%. With SK, no difference between SC or IV UH
LATE [69]	5,711	Fibrinolytic – t-PA	t-PA Y or N; ASA; and UH for later recruits	2860 assigned to placebo received off-protocol UH		35-day D	Lower 35-day mortality in patients receiving off-protocol UH
DUCCS-1 [75]	250	Fibrinolytic – APSAC	APSAC + placebo APSAC + UH	15 U/kg per h start at 4 h then titrated to aPTT 50–90 s	325 mg daily (all patients)	D/RI/MI/IRA patency	Addition of UH was not helpful and was possibly harmful. No difference in primary endpoint. Increased bleeding complications with UH
HART [137]	205	Fibrinolytic – Conventional t-PA	t-PA + UH t-PA + ASA	5000 U bolus then 1000 U/h titrated to aPTT 1.5–2 × normal	80 mg daily	IRA patency within 24 h IRA patency at 7 days 'ischemic complications'	Coronary patency rates associated with t-PA are higher with early concomitant systemic heparin treatment than with concomitant low-dose oral aspirin. IRA patency was associated with higher mean aPTT levels [138]
ECSG-6 [77]	652	Fibrinolytic – Conventional t-PA	t-PA + ASA + UH t-PA + ASA + placebo	5000 U bolus then IV infusion titrated to aPTT	250 mg IV or 300 mg PO, then 75–125 mg qod (all patients)	IRA patency at 48–120 h after fibrinolytics	UH associated with improved patency (83% vs 75%). Patency linked to adequacy of anticoagulation

APSAC = anisoylated plasminogen streptokinase activator complex; bid = twice daily; D = death; DC = discharge; qod = every other day; PO = orally; RI = recurrent ischemia

The added benefit of UH to aspirin in patients receiving fibrinolysis was assessed in the GISSI-2 and ISIS-3 [71] trials. Important considerations for UH therapy also addressed by these trials included the timing and route of administration. In GISSI-2, 20,891 patients were randomized to alteplase or SK, with a subrandomization to subcutaneous UH (12,500 U twice daily) initiated 12 h after fibrinolysis and continued for 7 days or to no UH. The ISIS-3 trial randomized 41,299 patients to SK, duteplase or antistreplase, with a subrandomization carried out to subcutaneous UH (12,500 U twice daily) initiated 4 h after fibrinolysis and continued for 7 days or to no UH. In the combined data set of GISSI-2 and ISIS-3 (totaling over 62,000 patients), the 35-day mortality was 10.0% in the patients receiving subcutaneous UH versus 10.2% in the patients not receiving any subcutaneous UH. Similar outcomes were seen in the GUSTO study, where no difference was seen in the 35-day mortality rate in patients receiving SK plus subcutaneous UH (7.2%) or intravenous UH (7.4%) [72]. The outcomes with respect to route of UH administration when combined with alteplase and aspirin in the GUSTO trial could not be assessed since there was not an arm assessing alteplase plus SC or no UH. Thus, the available information suggests that intravenous UH is probably of no benefit in patients receiving SK plus aspirin but may be helpful in patients receiving t-PA.

OPTIMAL UH DOSING IN STEMI

Although IV UH is commonly used after fibrinolytic therapy, few reports have addressed the relationship between the degree of anticoagulation and clinical outcomes. A subanalysis of the GUSTO-I trial analyzed the relationship between the aPTT and both baseline patient characteristics and clinical outcomes [73]. At 12 h, the aPTT associated with the lowest 30-day mortality, stroke and bleeding rates was 50 to 70 sec. Although the relationship between aPTT and clinical outcome was confounded to some degree by the influence of baseline prognostic characteristics, aPTTs higher than 70 sec were found to be associated with higher likelihood of mortality, stroke, bleeding and reinfarction.

EFFECT OF UH ON IRA PATENCY

A number of trials have assessed the role of UH in establishing and maintaining IRA patency.

When combined with non-fibrin-specific fibrinolytic agents, IV UH did not improve IRA patency rates [74, 75]. Whether UH combined with fibrin-specific agents such as alteplase improves IRA patency remains controversial, in part due to dosing regimens. Whereas UH combined with standard alteplase dosing did not improve IRA patency rates [76], UH combined with accelerated alteplase dosing produced an early, albeit non-sustained, benefit [74]. A potential explanation for these discrepant findings can be found in analysis of the ECSG-6 trial which demonstrated a significant improvement in IRA patency with UH combined with alteplase that was linked to the level of anticoagulation achieved assessed by aPTT [77, 78].

Born out of these trials that suggested better IRA patency when intravenous UH is used as an adjunct, the HEAP pilot study explored whether UH alone could induce reperfusion [79]. In this study, 108 patients with a STEMI were given a single IV bolus of 300 U/kg of UH together with aspirin (160 mg chewed) in the emergency room. Early therapy with high dose UH appeared to be both safe and able to achieve IRA patency in a considerable number of patients, especially in those treated early (<2 h). However, these findings were not reproduced in a subsequent large-scale randomized trial [80].

UH IN VENOUS THROMBOEMBOLIC DISEASE

Prophylaxis of VTE

Although mortality from VTE has decreased over the past 10 to 20 years, it remains a major national health problem, being responsible for 150,000 to 200,000 deaths annually. Despite significant advances in prevention and treatment of VTE, PE remains a common preventable cause of hospital deaths. It is, therefore, imperative to stratify patients according to risk categories and to institute appropriate prophylactic measures.

Prophylaxis of VTE is more effective at preventing the associated morbidity and mortality than is treatment of established disease. UH is indicated for prophylaxis of VTE. However, with the demonstration that LMWHs are easier to administer, do not require monitoring, are associated with less bleeding complications, and impart a lower risk for developing HIT, these agents have become the antithrombotic of choice for this indication. Nevertheless, a role for UH remains.

Low-dose subcutaneous UH

Low-dose UH is usually administered at a dose of 5000 U SC two to three times daily. This regimen has been demonstrated to be effective for the prophylaxis of VTE peri-operatively in patients undergoing moderate-risk general surgical and medical patients. A prospective randomized study found that low-dose UH decreased the incidence of venous thrombosis in patients undergoing a moderate-risk surgical procedure from 16% to 4% and, more importantly, the risk of proximal DVT from 2.9% to 1.0% [81]. In a larger study of 4121 patients, low-dose UH decreased the incidence of fatal pulmonary embolism from 0.7 to 0.1% [82]. These data have been confirmed by meta-analyses that have demonstrated a reduction in all DVT, proximal DVT and PE including fatal PE with low-dose UH in the peri-operative setting [83, 84]. Although shown to be effective in patients undergoing elective hip surgery, it is less effective than warfarin, adjusted-dose UH [84] and LMWH [85].

The utility of low-dose UH for prophylaxis of VTE has also been demonstrated across a broad range of medical patients [86]. When administered to patients following MI, heart failure and central nervous system disorders including stroke, and in patients admitted to the medical intensive care unit, low-dose UH was associated with a decrease in VTE events [87].

Benefits of this regimen for the prophylaxis of VTE include safety, low associated cost and the ease of administration. Whereas minor bleeding events such as wound hematomas occur with slightly increased frequency, the incidence of major bleeding has not been seen with this regimen [84]. In addition, this regimen does not require monitoring of the level of anticoagulation.

Adjusted-dose UH

The concept of adjusted-dose UH for VTE prophylaxis entails administering SC doses to maintain the aPTT in the high normal range. Although this has been shown to be efficacious in patients following total hip arthroplasty, the benefit seen was not as great as that achieved with LMWH [88]. Furthermore, this method of VTE prophylaxis has failed to gain favor as a result of its labor-intensive nature and the associated costs.

Treatment of VTE

Anticoagulation remains the principal treatment for DVT and PE. The anticoagulant regimen used to treat these VTE disorders has continued to evolve. Whereas therapy for both entities historically has been with IV UH in an inpatient setting, the development of strategies aimed at reducing costs without sacrificing safety and efficacy has challenged this dogma. However, owing to the potential morbidity and mortality associated with PE, initial treatment is delivered in a closely monitored setting in all but the most stable cases. Integral to the move towards a less intensive approach to both DVT and PE has been the appearance of the LMWH class of anticoagulants (Chapter 6). Nevertheless, an important role for UH in the treatment of these common and potentially devastating disorders remains.

DVT and PE

The goals of treatment for DVT and PE are to stop clot propagation and prevent clot recurrence, recurrent PEs, and a potential complication of recurrent PEs, pulmonary hypertension. Anticoagulant therapy is indicated for patients with proximal DVT since PE will occur within weeks in up to 50% of untreated patients [89, 90]. Anticoagulation is usually achieved with UH or LMWH overlapped with oral warfarin in the early phase of treatment.

The experiences to date have established that the efficacy of UH rests in the ability to achieve therapeutic levels of anticoagulation, defined as an aPTT >1.5 times normal (range 1.5–2 × normal), within the first 24 h of treatment primarily via continuous IV infusion [10, 31, 91–93]. One trial demonstrated a rate of recurrent VTE of approximately 19% in patients achieving a subtherapeutic level of anticoagulation with UH [10]. In addition, an analysis of three consecutive randomized double-blind trials evaluating initial UH for treatment of proximal vein thrombosis revealed a recurrent VTE rate of 23.3% in patients with a subtherapeutic aPTT compared with 4 to 6% in those whose aPTT exceeded the therapeutic threshold within 24 h [92].

Therapeutic anticoagulation has been shown to be achieved earlier and more successfully using protocol-based UH dosing rather than with physician-directed adjustment [31, 94, 95]. In a prospective randomized controlled trial of 115 patients with DVT, PE, UA or acute arterial insufficiency, the time to achieve therapeutic aPTT was significantly reduced with a weight-based nomogram (Table 5.2). Ninety-seven percent of patients receiving the weight-based dosing regimen had therapeutic aPTT levels (>1.5 × control) compared with 77% of those receiving the standard dosing regimen [31]. This translated into a significantly decreased risk of recurrent VTE among the patients with DVT or PE without an increased risk of bleeding.

For patients with submassive DVT or PE, the administration of UH for 5 days appears to be equivalent in efficacy and safety to 10 days of therapy [96]. A randomized double-blind trial of 199 patients with documented acute proximal DVT compared a 5-day course of IV UH, with warfarin begun on the first day with a conventional 10-day course of IV

UH, with warfarin begun on the fifth day. There was no significant difference in the risk of recurrent VTE between the two groups [96]. The adherence to the shorter duration of therapy can facilitate more expeditious anticoagulation and shorten hospitalization times, and cost, without increased adverse event rates.

5.4 CLINICAL CONSIDERATIONS

HEPARIN RESISTANCE

Not uncommonly, a patient may be encountered who requires unusually high doses of UH (i.e. >35,000 U/day) in order to achieve a therapeutic level of anticoagulation [97, 98]. Patients such as this are termed 'heparin resistant,' a situation that is encountered in up to 25% of patients with VTE [96]. The etiology of heparin resistance appears to be multifactorial given its association with AT deficiency [99], increased UH clearance [100], increased UH binding plasma proteins [101–103], elevated fibrinogen levels [104] and increased levels of factor VIII [97]. In addition, drug-induced heparin resistance has been reported with specific medications such as aprotinin [105] and nitroglycerin [106, 107]. However, that nitroglycerin induces heparin resistance has been called into question [108, 109].

Although felt by some to be a relative laboratory phenomenon [97], heparin resistance has been associated with unusually severe thrombotic or recurrent thrombotic events despite adequate anticoagulation and may result in severe untoward outcomes. In these circumstances, AT concentrate has been used safely and effectively to facilitate therapeutic anticoagulation [110–114]. For example, in patients with heparin resistance undergoing cardiopulmonary bypass the use of AT concentrate has facilitated the achievement of predefined therapeutic anticoagulation [111, 113, 114]. In addition, the only randomized trial of AT concentrate in patients undergoing cardiopulmonary bypass suggested that treating patients with heparin resistance with AT concentrate was more effective and faster for obtaining adequate anticoagulation than using additional heparin [112]. AT concentrate at doses effective at achieving AT levels between 75 and 120% of normal should be utilized [110].

OSTEOPOROSIS

Given its established safety and efficacy during prolonged (>1 month) administration, UH has remained the most widely used anticoagulant. However, prolonged therapy with this agent is not without risk of untoward clinical effects. Clinically significant osteoporosis has been demonstrated in pregnant patients requiring therapy with UH. Radiographic evidence of osteopenia has been reported in 17% of women treated with UH throughout pregnancy [115]. In most cases, the osteopenia resolves within 1 year after delivery; this process however, may not be entirely reversible. Spontaneous osteoporotic vertebral fractures occur in 2–3% of pregnant women receiving UH for 1 month or more [116]. Higher doses of UH and a prolonged duration of treatment may predispose these patients to developing osteoporosis. In addition, the risk of osteoporosis appears be present in non-pregnant patients receiving long-term UH [117], although this remains a suboptimally studied population.

UH appears to mediate its effects on bone density directly. Preclinical studies have suggested that UH decreases the rate of bone formation and accelerates the rate of bone resorption primarily in trabecular bone [118]. This appears to be via direct binding of UH to osteoblasts which, in turn, secrete osteoclast activating factors contributing to the 45% decrease in osteoblasts and the 58% increase in osteoclast surface, respectively. The development of osteoporosis in patients requiring prolonged anticoagulation may be associated with significant morbidity and has contributed to the search for alternative anticoagulants for these patients.

HIT

One of the most devastating complications of UH therapy is the development of HIT, which usually occurs within 5–10 days after the initiation of UH therapy [119]. The reported estimates of the frequency of HIT vary widely. Approximately 10–20% of patients receiving UH will experience a fall in platelet count to less than the normal range or a 50% fall in the platelet count within the normal range beginning within the first few days of therapy and resolving with continued heparin therapy [120]. The majority of these cases are accounted for by a benign form of HIT, termed HIT type I.

The incidence of true immune-mediated HIT, HIT type II, has been variable in the literature and occurs with a frequency of 0.3% to 3% in patients exposed to UH for more than 4 days [119]. Given the clinical nature and complex pathophysiology of this syndrome an entire chapter has been devoted to an in-depth discussion of this entity (Chapter 13).

REBOUND ISCHEMIA

As discussed above, UH possesses the ability to inhibit both thrombin generation and thrombin activity via its AT-dependent inhibition of factor Xa and thrombin, respectively. However, UH is able to inhibit only the soluble fractions of these coagulation proteins. UH is unable to inhibit factor Xa bound to the prothrombinase complex, fibrin-bound thrombin or thrombin bound to subendothelial surfaces [121]. UH binds to both fibrin and the heparin binding sites of thrombin simultaneously, and in doing so protects fibrin-bound thrombin from inactivation by the UH/AT complex [122]. Coupled with depletion of AT by UH administration, the protection of thrombin by fibrin binding results in a locally present prothrombotic milieu. This results in a transient hypercoagulable state and may explain the 'rebound' of ischemic event associated with cessation of UH therapy in patients admitted with acute coronary syndromes.

Several studies of antithrombotic therapy with UH for the treatment of acute coronary syndromes have suggested a 'rebound' in ischemic events following the cessation of UH [7, 8, 123–126]. In general, these studies have demonstrated a recurrence in ischemic events during the period ranging from 9.5 h to approximately 24 h following discontinuation of UH. That this phenomenon is related to thrombin and its effects on platelet aggregation is suggested by the demonstration that anti-platelet agents and LMWH can attenuate or abolish these events [7, 127, 128]. Alternative anticoagulants that target both free and fibrin-bound thrombin such as the direct thrombin inhibitors may eliminate this phenomenon from clinical consideration in the future.

REVERSING HEPARIN ANTICOAGULATION

One characteristic that has allowed UH to remain one of the most widely utilized anticoagulant across the spectrum of cardiovascular thromboembolic disease is the ready availability of an 'antidote.' Given that the anticoagulant effect of UH disappears within hours after discontinuation of the drug, mild bleeding due to UH can usually be controlled without administration of an antagonist. However, if life-threatening hemorrhage occurs, the effect of UH can be reversed quickly by intravenous infusion of the sulfate salt of protamine, a mixture of basic polypeptides isolated from salmon sperm. Protamine binds tightly to UH *in vitro* and thereby neutralizes its anticoagulant effect. The typical dose of protamine sulfate is 1 mg/100 U UH.

Although protamine is used routinely to reverse the anticoagulant effect of UH following cardiac surgery and other vascular procedures, as well as in cases of life-threatening hemorrhage, severe untoward reactions to its use have been reported. A potentially fatal antibody-mediated anaphylactic reaction may occur within minutes after protamine administration [129, 130]. This complication occurs in approximately 1% of patients with diabetes mellitus who have received protamine-containing insulin (neutral protein Hagedorn (NPH) insulin or protamine zinc insulin) but is not limited to this group [130, 131]. A less common non-immunologic reaction consisting of pulmonary vasoconstriction, right ventricular dysfunction and systemic hypotension associated with transient neutropenia may also occur after administration of protamine [132, 133]. The risk of these non-immunologic adverse reactions can be minimized by administering protamine slowly (i.e. over 1–3 min).

5.5 CONCLUSIONS

UH remains the most widely utilized antithrombotic therapy for patients with cardiovascular disease. Despite a myriad of apparent limitations of UH, an improved understanding of the pharmacology and intricacies of monitoring the levels of anticoagulation achieved has made UH a relatively permanent part of the armamentarium to battle thrombotic disorders. Facilitating the continuance of UH as a key anticoagulant are its short half-life, the availability of an antidote and its demonstrated utility across the spectrum of thrombotic disorders. Nevertheless, the quest for the ideal antithrombotic agent with a predictable therapeutic response, short half-life and ready reversibility continues. Although promising, the LMWHs and the DTIs possess limitations of their own that have, at least for the immediate future, also contributed to the staying power of UH.

REFERENCES

[1] Hirsh, J., (1991) Heparin. *N Eng J Med*, 324:1565–74.
[2] Tollefsen, D.M., Majerus, D.W., Blank, M.K., (1982) Heparin cofactor II. Purification and properties of a heparin-dependent inhibitor of thrombin in human plasma. *J Biol Chem*, 257(5):2162–9.
[3] Weitz, J.I., *et al.*, (1999) Vasoflux, a new anticoagulant with a novel mechanism of action. *Circulation*, 99(5):682–9.
[4] Lin, P., Sinha, U., Betz, A., (2001) Antithrombin binding of low molecular weight heparins and inhibition of factor Xa. *Biochim Biophys Acta*, 1526(1):105–13.
[5] Bendz, B., Andersen, T.O., Sandset, P.M., (2000) Dose-dependent release of endogenous tissue factor pathway inhibitor by different low molecular weight heparins. *Blood Coagul Fibrinolysis*, 11(4):343–8.
[6] Huang, Z.F., Wun, T.C., Broze, G.J., Jr., (1993) Kinetics of factor Xa inhibition by tissue factor pathway inhibitor. *J Biol Chem*, 268(36):26950–5.

[7] Theroux, P., *et al.*, (1992) Reactivation of unstable angina after the discontinuation of heparin. *N Eng J Med*, 327(3):141–5.
[8] Granger, C.B., *et al.*, (1995) Rebound increase in thrombin generation and activity after cessation of intravenous heparin in patients with acute coronary syndromes. *Circulation*, 91(7): 1929–35.
[9] Becker, R., *et al.*, (1999) Thrombin generation after the abrupt cessation of intravenous unfractionated heparin among patients with acute coronary syndromes. *J Am Coll Cardiol*, 34:1020–7.
[10] Hull, R.D., *et al.*, (1986) Continuous intravenous heparin compared with intermittent subcutaneous heparin in the initial treatment of proximal-vein thrombosis. *N Eng J Med*, 315(18):1109–14.
[11] Turpie, A.G., *et al.*, (1989) Comparison of high-dose with low-dose subcutaneous heparin to prevent left ventricular mural thrombosis in patients with acute transmural anterior myocardial infarction. *N Eng J Med*, 320(6):352–7.
[12] Pini, M., *et al.*, (1990) Subcutaneous vs intravenous heparin in the treatment of deep venous thrombosis—a randomized clinical trial. *Thromb Haemost*, 64(2):222–6.
[13] Doyle, D.J., *et al.*, (1987) Adjusted subcutaneous heparin or continuous intravenous heparin in patients with acute deep vein thrombosis. A randomized trial. *Ann Intern Med*, 107(4): 441–5.
[14] Hirsh, J., Raschke, R., (2004) Heparin and low-molecular-weight heparin: the Seventh ACCP Conference on Antithrombotic and Thrombolytic Therapy. *Chest*, 126(3 Suppl): 188S–203S.
[15] Manson, L., *et al.*, (1997) The variable anticoagulant response to unfractionated heparin in vivo reflects binding to plasma proteins rather than clearance. *J Lab Clin Med*, 130(6):649–55.
[16] Boneu, B., *et al.*, (1987) Evidence for a saturable mechanism of disappearance of standard heparin in rabbits. *Thromb Res*, 46(6):835–44.
[17] Bjornsson, T.D., Wolfram, K.M., Kitchell, B.B., (1982) Heparin kinetics determined by three assay methods. *Clin Pharmacol Ther*, 31(1):104–13.
[18] Boneu, B., Caranobe, C., Sie, P., (1990) Pharmacokinetics of heparin and low molecular weight heparin. *Baillieres Clin Haematol*, 3(3):531–44.
[19] Hirsh, J., *et al.*, (1976) Heparin kinetics in venous thrombosis and pulmonary embolism. *Circulation*, 53(4):691–5.
[20] Kher, A., *et al.*, (1997) Laboratory assessment of antithrombotic therapy: what tests and if so why? *Haemostasis*, 27(5):211–18.
[21] Basu, D., *et al.*, (1972) A prospective study of the value of monitoring heparin treatment with the activated partial thromboplastin time. *N Eng J Med*, 287(7):324–7.
[22] Rath, B., Bennett, D.H., (1990) Monitoring the effect of heparin by measurement of activated clotting time during and after percutaneous transluminal coronary angioplasty. *Br Heart J*, 63:18.
[23] Varah, N., Smith, J., Baugh, R.F., (1990) Heparin monitoring in the coronary care unit after percutaneous transluminal coronary angioplasty. *Heart Lung*, 19:265.
[24] Nath, F.C., *et al.*, (1993) Heparin monitoring during coronary intervention: activated clotting time versus activated partial thromboplastin time. *Can J Cardiol*, 9(9):797–801.
[25] Kitchen, S., Preston, F.E., (1996) The therapeutic range for heparin therapy: relationship between six activated partial thromboplastin time reagents and two heparin assays. *Thromb Haemost*, 75(5):734–9.
[26] Bjornsson, T.D., Nash, P.V., (1986) Variability in heparin sensitivity of APTT reagents. *Am J Clin Pathol*, 86(2):199–204.
[27] Toulon, P., *et al.*, (1998) Monitoring heparin therapy using activated partial thromboplastin time—results of a multicenter trial establishing the therapeutic range for SILIMAT, a reagent with high sensitivity to heparin. *Thromb Haemost*, 80(1):104–8.
[28] Rosborough, T.K., (1998) Comparing different lots of activated partial thromboplastin time reagent: analysis of two methods. *Am J Clin Pathol*, 110(2):173–7.
[29] Taylor, C.T., Petros, W.P., Ortel, T.L., (1999) Two instruments to determine activated partial thromboplastin time: implications for heparin monitoring. *Pharmacotherapy*, 19(4): 383–7.

[30] Nelson, D.E., (1999) Current considerations in the use of the APTT in monitoring unfractionated heparin. *Clin Lab Sci*, 12(6):359–64.

[31] Raschke, R.A., *et al.*, (1993) The weight-based heparin dosing nomogram compared with a 'standard care' nomogram. A randomized controlled trial. *Ann Intern Med*, 119(9): 874–81.

[32] Becker, R.C., *et al.*, (1999) A randomized, multicenter trial of weight-adjusted intravenous heparin dose titration and point-of-care coagulation monitoring in hospitalized patients with active thromboembolic disease. Antithrombotic Therapy Consortium Investigators. *Am Heart J*, 137(1):59–71.

[33] George, B.S., *et al.*, (1993) Multicenter investigation of coronary stenting to treat acute or threatened closure after percutaneous transluminal coronary angioplasty: clinical and angiographic outcomes. *J Am Coll Cardiol*, 22(1):135–43.

[34] Fischman, D.L., *et al.*, (1994) A randomized comparison of coronary-stent placement and balloon angioplasty in the treatment of coronary artery disease. Stent Restenosis Study Investigators. *N Eng J Med*, 331(8):496–501.

[35] Serruys, P.W., *et al.*, (1994) A comparison of balloon-expandable-stent implantation with balloon angioplasty in patients with coronary artery disease. Benestent Study Group. *N Eng J Med*, 331(8):489–95.

[36] Ferguson, J.J., *et al.*, (2004) Enoxaparin vs unfractionated heparin in high-risk patients with non-ST-segment elevation acute coronary syndromes managed with an intended early invasive strategy: primary results of the SYNERGY randomized trial. *JAMA*, 292(1): 45–54.

[37] Lincoff, A.M., *et al.*, (2004) Comparison of bivalirudin versus heparin during percutaneous coronary intervention (the Randomized Evaluation of PCI Linking Angiomax to Reduced Clinical Events [REPLACE]-1 trial). *Am J Cardiol*, 93:1092–6.

[38] Grayburn, P.A., *et al.*, (1991) In vivo thrombus formation on a guidewire during intravascular ultrasound imaging: evidence for inadequate heparinization. *Cathet Cardiovasc Diagn*, 23(2):141–3.

[39] Laskey, M.A., *et al.*, (1990) Influence of heparin therapy on percutaneous transluminal coronary angioplasty outcome in patients with coronary arterial thrombus. *Am J Cardiol*, 65(3): 179–82.

[40] The EPIC investigators, (1994) Use of a monoclonal antibody directed against the platelet glycoprotein IIb/IIIa receptor in high-risk coronary angioplasty. The EPIC Investigation. *N Eng J Med*, 330(14):956–61.

[41] Randomised placebo-controlled trial of abciximab before and during coronary intervention in refractory unstable angina: the CAPTURE Study, (1997) *Lancet*, 349(9063):1429–35.

[42] Randomised placebo-controlled trial of effect of eptifibatide on complications of percutaneous coronary intervention: IMPACT-II. Integrilin to Minimise Platelet Aggregation and Coronary Thrombosis-II, (1997) *Lancet*, 349(9063):1422–8.

[43] Dougherty, K.G., *et al.*, (1992) Activated clotting times and activated partial thromboplastin times in patients undergoing coronary angioplasty who receive bolus doses of heparin. *Cathet Cardiovasc Diagn*, 26(4):260–3.

[44] Ferguson, J.J., *et al.*, (1994) Relation between procedural activated coagulation time and outcome after percutaneous transluminal coronary angioplasty. *J Am Coll Cardiol*, 23(5): 1061–5.

[45] Bowers, J., Ferguson, J.J., (1994) The use of activated clotting times to monitor heparin therapy during and after interventional procedures. *Clin Cardiol*, 17(7):357–61.

[46] Narins, C.R., *et al.*, (1996) Relation between activated clotting time during angioplasty and abrupt closure. *Circulation*, 93:667–671.

[47] Hillegass, W.B., *et al.*, (2002) Relationship between activated clotting time during percutaneous intervention and subsequent bleeding complications. *Am Heart J*, 144(3):501–7.

[48] Chew, D.P., *et al.*, (2001) Defining the optimal activated clotting time during percutaneous coronary intervention: aggregate results from 6 randomized, controlled trials. *Circulation*, 103(7):961–6.

[49] Koch, K.T., *et al.*, (1997) Safety of low dose heparin in elective coronary angioplasty. *Heart*, 77(6):517–22.

[50] Boccara, A., *et al.*, (1997) A randomized trial of a fixed high dose vs a weight-adjusted low dose of intravenous heparin during coronary angioplasty. *Eur Heart J*, 18(4):631–5.
[51] Tolleson, T.R., *et al.*, (2003) Relationship between heparin anticoagulation and clinical outcomes in coronary stent intervention: observations from the ESPRIT trial. *J Am Coll Cardiol*, 41(3): 386–93.
[52] The EPILOG Investigators, (1997) Platelet glycoprotein IIb/IIIa receptor blockade and low-dose heparin during percutaneous coronary revascularization. *N Eng J Med*, 336(24):1689–96.
[53] Ferguson, J.J., *et al.*, (1995) Results of a national survey on anticoagulation for PTCA. *J Invasive Cardiol*, 7(5):136–41.
[54] Rabah, M., *et al.*, (1999) Heparin after percutaneous intervention (HAPI): a prospective multicenter randomized trial of three heparin regimens after successful coronary intervention. *J Am Coll Cardiol*, 34(2):461–7.
[55] Leon, M.B., *et al.*, (1998) A clinical trial comparing three antithrombotic-drug regimens after coronary-artery stenting. Stent Anticoagulation Restenosis Study Investigators. *N Eng J Med*, 339(23):1665–71.
[56] Telford, A.M., Wilson, C., (1981) Trial of heparin versus atenolol in prevention of myocardial infarction in intermediate coronary syndrome. *Lancet*, 1(8232):1225–8.
[57] Theroux, P., *et al.*, (1988) Aspirin, heparin, or both to treat acute unstable angina. *N Eng J Med*, 319(17):1105–11.
[58] The RISC group, (1990) Risk of myocardial infarction and death during treatment with low dose aspirin and intravenous heparin in men with unstable coronary artery disease. *Lancet*, 336(8719):827–30.
[59] Neri Serneri, G.G., *et al.*, (1990) Effect of heparin, aspirin, or alteplase in reduction of myocardial ischaemia in refractory unstable angina. *Lancet*, 335(8690):615–18.
[60] Theroux, P., *et al.*, (1993) Aspirin versus heparin to prevent myocardial infarction during the acute phase of unstable angina. *Circulation*, 88(5 Pt 1):2045–8.
[61] Neri Serneri, G.G., *et al.*, (1995) Randomised comparison of subcutaneous heparin, intravenous heparin, and aspirin in unstable angina. Studio Epoorine Sottocutanea nell'Angina Instobile (SESAIR) Refrattorie Group. *Lancet*, 345(8959):1201–4.
[62] Holdright, D., *et al.*, (1994) Comparison of the effect of heparin and aspirin versus aspirin alone on transient myocardial ischemia and in-hospital prognosis in patients with unstable angina. *J Am Coll Cardiol*, 24(1):39–45.
[63] Cohen, M., *et al.*, (1994) Combination antithrombotic therapy in unstable rest angina and non-Q-wave infarction in nonprior aspirin users. Primary end points analysis from the ATACS trial. Antithrombotic Therapy in Acute Coronary Syndromes Research Group. *Circulation*, 89(1):81–8.
[64] Oler, A., *et al.*, (1996) Adding heparin to aspirin reduces the incidence of myocardial infarction and death in patients with unstable angina. A meta-analysis. *JAMA*, 276(10):811–15.
[65] Califf, R.M., (2005) Simple principles of clinical trials remain powerful. *JAMA*, 293(4):489–91.
[66] Lee, C.D., Mann, K.G., (1989) Activation/inactivation of human factor V by plasmin. *Blood*, 73(1):185–90.
[67] Cercek, B., *et al.*, (1986) Enhancement of thrombolysis with tissue-type plasminogen activator by pretreatment with heparin. *Circulation*, 74:583–587.
[68] ISIS-2 (Second International Study of Infarct Survival) Collaborative Group, (1988) Randomised trial of intravenous streptokinase, oral aspirin, both, or neither among 17,187 cases of suspected acute myocardial infarction: ISIS-2. *Lancet*, 2(8607):349–60.
[69] Late Assessment of Thrombolytic Efficacy (LATE) study with alteplase 6–24 h after onset of acute myocardial infarction, (1993) *Lancet*, 342(8874):759–66.
[70] The SCATI (Studio sulla Calciparina nell'Angina e nella Trombosi Ventricolare nell'Infarto) Group, (1989) Randomised controlled trial of subcutaneous calcium-heparin in acute myocardial infarction. *Lancet*, 2(8656):182–6.
[71] ISIS-3 (Third International Study of Infarct Survival) Collaborative Group, (1992) ISIS-3: a randomised comparison of streptokinase vs tissue plasminogen activator vs anistreplase and of aspirin plus heparin vs aspirin alone among 41,299 cases of suspected acute myocardial infarction. *Lancet*, 339(8796):753–70.

[72] The GUSTO investigators, (1993) An international randomized trial comparing four thrombolytic strategies for acute myocardial infarction. *N Eng J Med*, 329(10):673–82.

[73] Granger, C.B., *et al.*, (1996) Activated partial thromboplastin time and outcome after thrombolytic therapy for acute myocardial infarction: results from the GUSTO-I trial. *Circulation*, 93(5):870–8.

[74] The GUSTO angiographic investigators, (1993) The effects of tissue plasminogen activator, streptokinase, or both on coronary-artery patency, ventricular function, and survival after acute myocardial infarction. *N Eng J Med*, 329(22):1615–22.

[75] O'Connor, C.M., *et al.*, (1994) A randomized trial of intravenous heparin in conjunction with anistreplase (anisoylated plasminogen streptokinase activator complex) in acute myocardial infarction: The Duke University Clinical Cardiology Study (DUCCS)1. *J Am Coll Cardiol*, 23: 11–18.

[76] Topol, E.J., *et al.*, (1989) A randomized controlled trial of intravenous tissue plasminogen activator and early intravenous heparin in acute myocardial infarction. *Circulation*, 79:281–6.

[77] de Bono, D.P. and on behalf of the European Cooperative Study Group (ECSG-6), (1992) Effect of early intravenous heparin on coronary patency, infarct size, and bleeding complications after alteplase thrombolysis: results of a randomised double blind European Cooperative Study Group (ECSG-6). *Br Heart J*, 67:122–8.

[78] Arnout, J., *et al.*, (1992) Correlation between level of heparinization and patency of the infarct-related coronary artery after treatment of acute myocardial infarction with alteplase (rt-PA). *J Am Coll Cardiol*, 20(3):513–19.

[79] Verheugt, F.W., *et al.*, (1998) High dose bolus heparin as initial therapy before primary angioplasty for acute myocardial infarction: results of the Heparin in Early Patency (HEAP) pilot study. *J Am Coll Cardiol*, 31(2):289–93.

[80] Liem, A., *et al.*, (2000) High dose heparin as pretreatment for primary angioplasty in acute myocardial infarction: the Heparin in Early Patency (HEAP) randomized trial. *J Am Coll Cardiol*, 35(3):600–4.

[81] Gallus, A.S., *et al.*, (1976) Prevention of venous thrombosis with small, subcutaneous doses of heparin. *JAMA*, 235(18):1980–2.

[82] Prevention of fatal postoperative pulmonary embolism by low doses of heparin. An international multicentre trial, (1975) *Lancet*, 2(7924):45–51.

[83] Clagett, G.P., Reisch, J.S., (1988) Prevention of venous thromboembolism in general surgical patients. Results of meta-analysis. *Ann Surg*, 208(2):227–40.

[84] Collins, R., *et al.*, (1988) Reduction in fatal pulmonary embolism and venous thrombosis by perioperative administration of subcutaneous heparin. Overview of results of randomized trials in general, orthopedic, and urologic surgery. *N Eng J Med*, 318(18):1162–73.

[85] Hirsh, J., Levine, M., (1989) Prevention of venous thrombosis in patients undergoing major orthopaedic surgical procedures. *Br J Clin Pract Suppl*, 65:2–8.

[86] Halkin, H., *et al.*, (1982) Reduction of mortality in general medical in-patients by low-dose heparin prophylaxis. *Ann Intern Med*, 96(5):561–5.

[87] Harenberg, J., Roebruck, P., Heene, D.L., (1996) Subcutaneous low-molecular-weight heparin versus standard heparin and the prevention of thromboembolism in medical inpatients. The Heparin Study in Internal Medicine Group. *Haemostasis*, 26(3):127–39.

[88] Leyvraz, P.F., *et al.*, (1991) Prevention of deep vein thrombosis after hip replacement: randomised comparison between unfractionated heparin and low molecular weight heparin. *Br Med J*, 303(6802):543–8.

[89] Alpert, J.S., Dalen, J.E., (1994) Epidemiology and natural history of venous thromboembolism. *Prog Cardiovasc Dis*, 36(6):417–22.

[90] Mannucci, P.M., Poller, L., (2001) Venous thrombosis and anticoagulant therapy. *Br J Haematol*, 114(2):258–70.

[91] Brandjes, D.P., *et al.*, (1992) Acenocoumarol and heparin compared with acenocoumarol alone in the initial treatment of proximal-vein thrombosis. *N Eng J Med*, 327(21):1485–9.

[92] Hull, R.D., *et al.*, (1997) Relation between the time to achieve the lower limit of the APTT therapeutic range and recurrent venous thromboembolism during heparin treatment for deep vein thrombosis. *Arch Intern Med*, 157(22):2562–8.

[93] Hull, R.D., *et al.*, (1997) The importance of initial heparin treatment on long-term clinical outcomes of antithrombotic therapy. The emerging theme of delayed recurrence. *Arch Intern Med*, 157(20):2317–21.

[94] Elliott, C.G., *et al.*, (1994) Physician-guided treatment compared with a heparin protocol for deep vein thrombosis. *Arch Intern Med*, 154(9):999–1004.

[95] Kershaw, B., *et al.*, (1994) Computer-assisted dosing of heparin. Management with a pharmacy-based anticoagulation service. *Arch Intern Med*, 154(9):1005–11.

[96] Hull, R.D., *et al.*, (1990) Heparin for 5 days as compared with 10 days in the initial treatment of proximal venous thrombosis. *N Eng J Med*, 322(18):1260–4.

[97] Levine, M.N., *et al.*, (1994) A randomized trial comparing activated thromboplastin time with heparin assay in patients with acute venous thromboembolism requiring large daily doses of heparin. *Arch Intern Med*, 154(1):49–56.

[98] Anand, S.S., Brimble, S., Ginsberg, J.S., (1997) Management of iliofemoral thrombosis in a pregnant patient with heparin resistance. *Arch Intern Med*, 157(7):815–6.

[99] Olson, J.D., *et al.*, (1998) College of American Pathologists Conference XXXI on laboratory monitoring of anticoagulant therapy: laboratory monitoring of unfractionated heparin therapy. *Arch Pathol Lab Med*, 122(9):782–98.

[100] Whitfield, L.R., Lele, A.S., Levy, G., (1983) Effect of pregnancy on the relationship between concentration and anticoagulant action of heparin. *Clin Pharmacol Ther*, 34(1):23–8.

[101] Preissner, K.T., Muller-Berghaus, G., (1987) Neutralization and binding of heparin by S protein/vitronectin in the inhibition of factor Xa by antithrombin III. Involvement of an inducible heparin-binding domain of S protein/vitronectin. *J Biol Chem*, 262(25):12247–53.

[102] Young, E., *et al.*, (1992) Heparin binding to plasma proteins, an important mechanism for heparin resistance. *Thromb Haemost*, 67(6):639–43.

[103] Cosmi, B., *et al.*, (1997) Effect of nonspecific binding to plasma proteins on the antithrombin activities of unfractionated heparin, low-molecular-weight heparin, and dermatan sulfate. *Circulation*, 95(1):118–24.

[104] Cotton, R.C., Shaikh, M.S., Dent, R.V., (1968) Heparin resistance and plasma fibrinogen in elderly subjects with and without occlusive vascular disease. *J Atheroscler Res*, 8(6):959–66.

[105] Fisher, A.R., *et al.*, (1992) Heparin resistance after aprotinin. *Lancet*, 340(8829): 1230–1.

[106] Habbab, M.A., Haft, J.I., (1987) Heparin resistance induced by intravenous nitroglycerin. A word of caution when both drugs are used concomitantly. *Arch Intern Med*, 147(5):857–60.

[107] Becker, R.C., *et al.*, (1990) Intravenous nitroglycerin-induced heparin resistance: a qualitative antithrombin III abnormality. *Am Heart J*, 119(6):1254–61.

[108] Schoenenberger, R.A., *et al.*, (1992) Absence of nitroglycerin-induced heparin resistance in healthy volunteers. *Eur Heart J*, 13(3):411–14.

[109] Berk, S.I., *et al.*, (1993) Effect of intravenous nitroglycerin on heparin dosage requirements in coronary artery disease. *Am J Cardiol*, 72(5):393–6.

[110] Schwartz, R.S., *et al.*, (1989) Clinical experience with antithrombin III concentrate in treatment of congenital and acquired deficiency of antithrombin. The Antithrombin III Study Group. *Am J Med*, 87(3B):53S–60S.

[111] Kanbak, M., (1999) The treatment of heparin resistance with Antithrombin III in cardiac surgery. *Can J Anaesth*, 46(6):581–5.

[112] Williams, M.R., *et al.*, (2000) A randomized trial of antithrombin concentrate for treatment of heparin resistance. *Ann Thorac Surg*, 70(3):873–7.

[113] Lemmer, J.H., Jr., Despotis, G.J., (2002) Antithrombin III concentrate to treat heparin resistance in patients undergoing cardiac surgery. *J Thorac Cardiovasc Surg*, 123(2):213–17.

[114] Koster, A., *et al.*, (2003) Management of heparin resistance during cardiopulmonary bypass: the effect of five different anticoagulation strategies on hemostatic activation. J *Cardiothorac Vasc Anesth*, 17(2):171–5.

[115] Dahlman, T., Lindvall, N., Hellgren, M., (1990) Osteopenia in pregnancy during long-term heparin treatment: a radiological study post partum. *Br J Obstet Gynaecol*, 97(3):221–8.

[116] Dahlman, T.C., (1993) Osteoporotic fractures and the recurrence of thromboembolism during pregnancy and the puerperium in 184 women undergoing thromboprophylaxis with heparin. *Am J Obstet Gynecol*, 168(4):1265–70.

[117] Ginsberg, J.S., *et al.*, (1990) Heparin effect on bone density. *Thromb Haemost*, 64(2):286–9.

[118] Muir, J.M., *et al.*, (1996) Histomorphometric analysis of the effects of standard heparin on trabecular bone in vivo. *Blood*, 88(4):1314–20.

[119] Warkentin, T.E., (2004) Heparin-induced thrombocytopenia: diagnosis and management. *Circulation*, 110(18):e454–8.

[120] Harenberg, J., Jorg, I., Fenyvesi, T., (2002) Heparin-induced thrombocytopenia: pathophysiology and new treatment options. *Pathophysiol Haemost Thromb*, 32(5–6):289–94.

[121] Weitz, J.I., *et al.*, (1990) Clot-bound thrombin is protected from inhibition by heparin-antithrombin III but is susceptible to inactivation by antithrombin III-independent inhibitors. *J Clin Invest*, 86(2):385–91.

[122] Becker, D.L., *et al.*, (1999) Exosites 1 and 2 are essential for protection of fibrin-bound thrombin from heparin-catalyzed inhibition by antithrombin and heparin cofactor II. *J Biol Chem*, 274(10):6226–33.

[123] Kontny, F., (1997) Reactivation of the coagulation system: rationale for long-term antithrombotic treatment. *Am J Cardiol*, 80(5A):55E–60E.

[124] Hansen, J.B., *et al.*, (2000) Rebound activation of coagulation after treatment with unfractionated heparin and not with low molecular weight heparin is associated with partial depletion of tissue factor pathway inhibitor and antithrombin. *Thromb Res*, 100(5):413–17.

[125] Bahit, M.C., *et al.*, (2001) Reactivation of ischemic events in acute coronary syndromes: results from GUSTO-IIb. Gobal Use of Strategies To Open occluded arteries in acute coronary syndromes. *J Am Coll Cardiol*, 37(4):1001–7.

[126] Bijsterveld, N.R., *et al.*, (2003) Recurrent cardiac ischemic events early after discontinuation of short-term heparin treatment in acute coronary syndromes: results from the Thrombolysis in Myocardial Infarction (TIMI) 11B and Efficacy and Safety of Subcutaneous Enoxaparin in Non-Q-Wave Coronary Events (ESSENCE) studies. *J Am Coll Cardiol*, 42(12): 2083–9.

[127] Lauer, M.A., *et al.*, (2001) Attenuation of rebound ischemia after discontinuation of heparin therapy by glycoprotein IIb/IIIa inhibition with eptifibatide in patients with acute coronary syndromes: observations from the platelet IIb/IIIa in unstable angina: receptor suppression using integrilin therapy (PURSUIT) trial. *Circulation*, 104(23):2772–7.

[128] Antman, E.M., *et al.*, (2002) Enoxaparin is superior to unfractionated heparin for preventing clinical events at 1-year follow-up of TIMI 11B and ESSENCE. *Eur Heart J*, 23(4): 308–14.

[129] Shikuma, L.R., Eyer, S.D., Zaske, D.E., (1988) Protamine sulfate and fatal anaphylactoid shock. *Drug Intell Clin Pharm*, 22(3):211–13.

[130] Weiss, M.E., *et al.*, (1989) Association of protamine IgE and IgG antibodies with life-threatening reactions to intravenous protamine. *N Eng J Med*, 320(14):886–92.

[131] Ellerhorst, J.A., Comstock, J.P., Nell, L.J., (1990) Protamine antibody production in diabetic subjects treated with NPH insulin. *Am J Med* Sci, 299(5):298–301.

[132] Lowenstein, E., *et al.*, (1983) Catastrophic pulmonary vasoconstriction associated with protamine reversal of heparin. *Anesthesiology*, 59(5):470–3.

[133] Lowenstein, E., Zapol, W.M., (1990) Protamine reactions, explosive mediator release, and pulmonary vasoconstriction. *Anesthesiology*, 73(3):373–5.

[134] Cohen, M., *et al.*, (1990) Usefulness of antithrombotic therapy in resting angina pectoris or non-Q-wave myocardial infarction in preventing death and myocardial infarction (a pilot study from the Antithrombotic Therapy in Acute Coronary Syndromes Study Group). *Am J Cardiol*, 66(19):1287–92.

[135] Gurfinkel, E.P., *et al.*, (1995) Low molecular weight heparin versus regular heparin or aspirin in the treatment of unstable angina and silent ischemia. *J Am Coll Cardiol*, 26(2): 313–18.

[136] ISIS (International Studies of Infarct Survival) pilot study group, (1987) Randomized factorial trial of high-dose intravenous streptokinase, of oral aspirin and of intravenous heparin in acute myocardial infarction. *Eur Heart J*, 8(6):634–42.

[137] Hsia, J., *et al.*, (1990) A comparison between heparin and low-dose aspirin as adjunctive therapy with tissue plasminogen activator for acute myocardial infarction. Heparin-Aspirin Reperfusion Trial (HART) Investigators. *N Eng J Med*, 323(21):1433–7.

[138] Hsia, J., *et al.*, (1992) Heparin-induced prolongation of partial thromboplastin time after thrombolysis: relation to coronary artery patency. *J Am Coll Cardiol*, 20:31–5.

6 Low-Molecular-Weight Heparins

6.1 INTRODUCTION

Intravascular thrombus formation remains the bane of cardiovascular disease. With the understanding that thrombin plays a pivotal role in coordinating and regulating hemostasis, numerous investigations across the spectrum of cardiovascular diseases including STEMI, NSTEMI and UA, as well as venous thromboembolic disease, have assessed the efficacy of various antithrombotic regimens. Until recently, UH has been the backbone of these investigations as well as the AT of choice for the management of vascular thrombosis. Despite its role as the prototypical anticoagulant over the past several decades, several limitations of UH have been recognized, prompting the search for alternative compounds.

The LMWHs as a class have emerged as a viable alternative to UH (Table 6.1). The safety and efficacy of LMWH have been demonstrated in a number of trials spanning the spectrum of atherothrombotic cardiovascular diseases [1–9]. This chapter will discuss the pharmacology of the LMWHs as well as review the evidence supporting their use in ACS and in VTE.

6.2 COMPARISONS BETWEEN UH AND LMWH

MECHANISM OF ACTION

UH is a heterogeneous mixture of sulfated mucopolysaccharides possessing molecular weights ranging from 3000 to 30,000 with a mean of 15,000 [10]. LMWHs, in contrast, are produced from UH through controlled enzymatic or chemical depolymerization processes which yield fragments with a mean molecular weight of approximately 5000 (Table 6.1) [11]. Similar to UH, LMWHs exert their anticoagulant effects by binding with AT through a unique pentasaccharide sequence present in approximately one-third of UH fragments and in 15–25% of LMWH fragments. The interaction of UH with AT results accelerates the AT-mediated inactivation of both factor Xa and thrombin (IIa) approximately 1000-fold [12]. Inhibition of factor Xa can occur through interaction with pentasaccharide-containing UH fragments of any length bound to AT; however, inhibition of thrombin requires that UH fragments of at least 18 saccharide residues (including the pentasaccharide component) and AT bind to it forming a tertiary complex. Because almost all fragments of UH are at least 18 saccharide residues in length, UH exerts equivalent inhibition of both factor Xa

Management Strategies in Antithrombotic Therapy Arman T. Askari, Adrian W. Messerli and A. Michael Lincoff

Table 6.1 Selected LMWHs

Generic name	Trade name	Manufacturer	Molecular weight (Da)	Xa:IIa	$t_{1/2}$ (after SC dosing)	FDA approved Indications
Ardeparin	Normiflo	Wyeth-Ayerst	6000	1.9	3–4 h	Yes DVT prophylaxis
Dalteparin	Fragmin Fragmine Fragmin P Forte	Pfizer	6000	2.7	3–5 h	Yes 1) Prophylaxis and treatment of DVT in patients undergoing hip replacement surgery, in patients undergoing abdominal surgery, and in medical patients with acute illness. 2) Prevention of ischemic complications in UA and NSTEMI
Enoxaparin	Lovenox Clexane 40 Clexane Forte Klexane	Aventis Pharmaceuticals	4200	3.8	4.5 h	Yes 1) Prophylaxis and treatment of DVT in patients undergoing hip or knee replacement surgery, in patients undergoing abdominal surgery, and in medical patients with acute illness 2) Inpatient treatment DVT with or without PE, when administered in conjunction with warfarin 3) Outpatient treatment of acute DVT without PE 4) Prophylaxis of ischemic complications of UA and NSTEMI when administered with aspirin
Nadroparin	Fraxiparine	Sanofi	4500	3.6	3–5 h	Not commercially available in US
Tinzaparin	Innohep or Logiparin	Pharmion Corporation	4500	1.9	3–4 h	Yes Treatment of DVT with or without PE (inpatient), when administered in conjunction with warfarin

US = United States

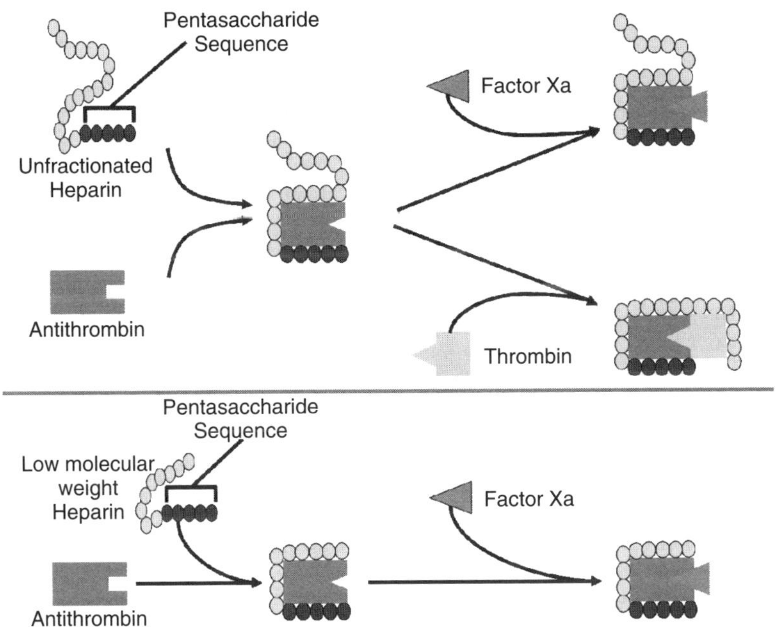

Figure 6.1 Binding of UH with Antithrombin III and Thrombin Requires at least 18 saccharide units including the pentasaccharide essential for Antithrombin III binding. Only a small percentage of LMWH are long enough to bind both antithrombin III and thrombin, accounting for the greater antiXa:antiIIa ratio. A full colour version of this figure can be found in the colour plate section of this book.

(thrombin generation) and thrombin (thrombin activity). However, LMWH exert a predominant inhibitory effect on factor Xa, as fewer than 50% of LMWH chains are 18 saccharide residues in length (Figure 6.1). This accounts for the observed predominant inhibition of thrombin generation (factor Xa activity) and the observed anti-Xa:anti-IIa ratios of between 2:1 and 4:1 with LMWHs [13]. The greater anti-Xa effect over the anti-IIa effect is thought to contribute to the observed benefit of LMWH compared with UH in early trials [5, 6].

One of the many antithrombotic effects of TFPI involves binding with and inactivating factor Xa. This TFPI–factor Xa complex subsequently functions to regulate the extrinsic coagulation pathway by inactivating factor VIIa [14]. Although still incompletely understood, the antithrombotic actions of both UH and LMWH may, in part, be related to their stimulation of TFPI release from endothelial cells [15]. This may explain the persistence of an anti-thrombotic state, at a time when anti-Xa activity is no longer detectable, 12 h after administration of LMWH [16]. On the other hand, the greater degree of TFPI release induced by UH than by LMWH [17] may also explain the transient pro-thrombotic state related to thrombin generation and the clinical events that occur during treatment with UFH and following its abrupt cessation [18–20]. In addition to the differences in the mechanism of action compared with UH, the LMWHs possess several unique features that have resulted in their attractiveness as an alternative, if not preferred, AT agent across the spectrum of atherothrombotic diseases (Table 6.2).

Table 6.2 Comparison of UH and LMWHs

UH	LMWH
Non-specific protein binding [22] Variable anticoagulation Requires monitoring Requires frequent dose adjustment Poor bioavailability (~30%)	**Less non-specific protein binding** [22] Monitoring unnecessary Dose adjustment unnecessary Improved bioavailability (>90%)
Short plasma half-life (~1 h) [11] Requires continuous intravenous infusions	**Long Plasma half-life (~3–6 h)** [21] Allows for subcutaneous administration
Depletes TFPI [17, 141] Decreased attenuation of the tissue factor pathway of coagulation Rebound hypercoagulability	**Less TFPI depletion** [15, 17] Less rebound hypercoagulability
Not effective on clot-bound thrombin or Xa [142] Pro-thrombogenic Rebound thrombosis following cessation	**Effective on clot-bound Xa** [143]
Increased interaction with platelets [144] Neutralization by platelet factor 4 Increased immunogenicity Increased platelet activation Increased risk of bleeding, HIT, thrombosis	**Less platelet activation** [144] Not neutralized by platelet factor 4
No effect on vWF [145] Increased vWF in ACS Increased potential for thrombosis	**Attenuates the increase of vWF in ACS** [145]
Ratio of Xa:IIa specificity [11] 1:1	**Ratio of Xa:IIa specificity** [11] 2–4 : 1

PHARMACOKINETICS AND PHARMACODYNAMICS

Both UH and LMWH require either IV or SC administration, owing to their poor absorption from the gastrointestinal tract. When administered subcutaneously, the antithrombotic effect is evident within 30 min and approaches 100% with LMWH as compared with the more variable and prolonged absorption of UH [21].

Mechanisms exist that may account for the pharmacokinetic differences between UH and LMWH. UH binds to plasma proteins such as vitronectin and fibrinogen, to proteins secreted by platelets such as platelet factor 4 and to proteins secreted by endothelial cells such as von Willebrand factor (vWf) [13]. This avid non-specific protein binding of UH is felt to contribute to its poor bioavailability and variable anticoagulation. In addition, the binding to platelet proteins also contributes to the immunogenicity of UH and to activation of platelets which may result in increased risk of thrombosis and the development of HIT. Coupled with its short half-life, this also translates into the need for IV administration as well as frequent monitoring and dose adjustments with UH. LMWH possess a decreased propensity to bind to plasma proteins and platelets, resulting in improved bioavailability, a more predictable anticoagulant effect and the feasibility of SC administration without the need for frequent monitoring and dose adjustment [22, 23].

UH is mainly cleared by a cellular mechanism while LMWH is essentially cleared by a renal mechanism. Contributing to the prolonged half-life of LMWH is a decreased interaction with macrophages, the cellular constituent of UH clearance. After IV and SC injection, clearance of LMWH is significantly longer than for UH lasting approximately 3–4 h [24]. While the half-life of anti Xa activity persists longer with LMWH than with UH, the half-life of anti-IIa activity is similar for LMWH and UH, reflecting the more rapid clearance of longer heparin chains.

6.3 CLINICAL USES OF LMWH

The central role of thrombin in pathogenesis of thrombotic vascular disease has dictated the search for a potent antithrombotic agent with minimal toxicity and/or bleeding complications. As demonstrated in the preceding sections, the LMWHs as a class possess properties that have contributed to their burgeoning popularity for the management of IHD and VTE. It is important to note, however, that the individual LMWHs vary with respect to their anti-Xa: anti-IIa ratios, molecular weights and half-lives, along with several additional properties that may account for the variable clinical responses and approved indications for each agent (Table 6.1). Nevertheless, a substantial body of literature has accrued within the field of cardiovascular medicine that supports the use of LMWHs.

LMWH IN IHD

Whereas UH has traditionally been the antithrombotic agent of choice for patients undergoing PCI, LMWH is an alternative option particularly well suited for individuals who present with ACS. While efficacious, the limitations of LMWHs in the PCI setting include the difficulty in monitoring the level of anticoagulation, the potential for increased risk of bleeding complications primarily at the arteriotomy site and incomplete reversibility with protamine should bleeding become an issue. However, the favorable characteristics of LMWH compared with UH have prompted several trials of LMWH with or without GP IIb/IIIa inhibitors in patients undergoing elective or urgent PCI.

LMWH during PCI

Several trials of LMWHs have been performed to assess the utility of these agents during PCI (Table 6.3). Whether the LMWH was reviparin [9], enoxaparin [25–28] or dalteparin [29], the feasibility of these agents as a substitute for UH in patients undergoing PCI has been consistently suggested. In addition, no increase in hemorrhagic complications was seen with any of these agents compared with UH.

These small pilot trials and registries assessed the route of LMWH delivery in patients undergoing PCI. The limited experience using IV LMWH in PCI has been associated with elevated anticoagulation levels and the potential for delayed sheath removal. Choussat *et al.* evaluated the safety and efficacy of a low-dose (0.5 mg/kg) IV enoxaparin regimen in 242 consecutive patients undergoing elective PCI [27]. They observed that this dose of enoxaparin was safe and effective, achieving a pre-specified target level of anticoagulation which allowed early sheath removal in the vast majority of patients undergoing PCI. The NICE registries

Table 6.3 Trials of LMWH in patients undergoing PCI

Trial	Study population	LMWH (Dose)	Control	*N*	Primary efficacy endpoint	Timing of outcome	LMWH (%)	Control (%)	Timing of PCI relative to last LMWH dose	Supplemental peri-procedural anticoagulant
Without GP IIb/IIIa inhibitors										
Rabah *et al.* [25]	Elective PCI	Enoxaparin (1 mg/kg IV × 1 dose)	UH	60	TIMI 3 Flow	Post-PCI	97	93	Immediately	None
					Ischemic complications	30 days	0	10		
REDUCE [9]	Elective PCI	Reviparin (7000 U IV bolus + infusion)	UH	612	D/MI/R	30 weeks	33.3	32	Immediately	10,500 U IV over first 24 h then 3500 U SC QD × 28 days
PEPCI [53]	Elective PCI	Enoxaparin (1 mg/kg SC bid)	NA	40	D/MI/UR	30 days	5.4	NA	8–12 h	0.3 mg/kg IV
NICE 1 [26]	Elective or urgent PCI	Enoxaparin (1 mg/kg IV × 1 dose)	NA	828	D/MI/UR	30 days	7.7	NA	Immediately	None
Choussat *et al.* [27]	Elective PCI	Enoxaparin (0.5 mg/kg IV × 1 dose)	NA	242	D/MI/UR	30 days	2.5	NA	Immediately	None
ESSENCE/TIMI-11B [58]	UA/NSTEMI	Enoxaparin (1 mg/kg SC bid ±30 mg IV bolus)	UH	924	D/MI	43 days	3.3	5.9	Physician discretion after 24 h	UH at discretion of investigator
Collet *et al.* [59]	UA/NSTEMI	Enoxaparin (1 mg/kg SC bid)	NA	132	D/MI	30 days	3.0	NA	4-8 h	None
FRISC II [48]	UA/NSTEMI	Dalteparin (120 IU/kg bid)	NA	1222	D/MI	6 months	9.4	NA	≤12 h pre-PCI	NA

With GP IIb/IIIa inhibitors										
SYNERGY [50]	UA/NSTEMI	Enoxaparin (1 mg/kg SC bid)	UH	10,000	D/MI	30 days	14	14.5	6-8 h	0.3 mg/kg IV if >8 h from last SC dose
NICE 4 [30]	Elective or urgent PCI	Enoxaparin (0.75 mg/kg IV × 1 dose) (Abciximab)	NA	818	D/MI/UR	30 days	6.8	NA	Immediately	NA
Kereiakes *et al.* [29]	Elective or urgent PCI	Dalteparin (40 IU/kg IV×1 dose; 60 IU/kg IV×1 dose) (Abciximab)	NA	103	D/MI/UR	IH	11.1	NA	Immediately	NA
							17.1	NA		
CRUISE [28]	Elective or urgent PCI	Enoxaparin (0.75 mg/kg IV×1 dose) (Eptifibatide)	UH	261	D/MI/UR	48 h	8.5	7.6	Immediately	NA
NICE 3 [41]	UA/NSTEMI	Enoxaparin (1 mg/kg SC bid) (Tirofiban, Eptifibatide, or abciximab)	NA	283	D/MI/RI	30 days	11.3	NA	Physician discretion	NA

bid = twice daily; D = death; IH = in hospital; QD = once daily; NA = not assessed; UR = urgent revascularization provided data regarding enoxaparin as a procedural anticoagulant compared with historical controls. NICE-1 assessed the efficacy and safety of IV enoxaparin administered to 828 patients undergoing elective or urgent PCI. Major adverse cardiac events were observed in 7.7% of patients with comparable bleeding complications to historical controls.

The combination of LMWH and GP IIb/IIIa inhibitors during elective or urgent PCI has been evaluated by two registries [26, 30] and, more recently, two trials [28, 29] (Table 6.3). Enoxaparin combined with Integrilin for patients undergoing elective PCI was shown to be feasible and safe [28]. Similarly, the combination of dalteparin and abciximab during PCI also appears promising, not only in elective PCI but also in patients with UA/NSTEMI [29]. These trials suggested a more consistent antithrombotic effect of LMWH during PCI without an increase in hemorrhagic complications. Emerging data also suggests that LMWHs can be utilized as stand-alone therapy or in conjunction with PCI for patients with ACS.

LMWH and the medical management of ACS

Rupture of a vulnerable atherosclerotic plaque followed by local thrombosis resulting in varying levels of occlusion of the culprit artery is the usual inciting event in an ACS. Ultimately, the goals of therapy for an ACS are to prevent progression of intracoronary thrombus, to promote atherosclerotic plaque stabilization and to decrease the risk of subsequent ischemic events. UH combined with aspirin has previously been the backbone of antithrombotic therapies for the management of ACS [31–33]. However, as outlined above, UH possesses several characteristics that have impeded its advancement as the ideal antithrombotic agent.

Born out of the limitations of UH, several studies have assessed the utility of both short-term and long-term administration of LMWH in patients with ACS (Table 6.4). Studies comparing short-term LMWH with placebo have demonstrated the superior efficacy of LMWH in this patient population [7, 34, 35]. On the other hand, administration of LMWH for more than 7 days does not provide any additional benefit compared with placebo [36]. In addition, the efficacy and safety of LMWH alone [5, 6, 37, 38] and when combined with GP IIb/IIIa inhibitors [39–44] compared with UH has been demonstrated.

Trials comparing LMWH with placebo

The FRISC trials

In the FRISC trial, 1506 patients with UA/NSTEMI were randomly assigned SC dalteparin (120 IU/kg twice daily for 6 days then 7500 IU once daily for the next 35–45 days) or placebo injections [35]. The primary endpoint, the rate of death and new MI within 6 days, occurred less frequently in patients who received dalteparin (1.8% vs 4.8%, p-value = 0.001, respectively). This trial demonstrated the benefit of dalteparin for the acute management of patients with UA/NSTEMI. However, long-term efficacy of dalteparin treatment was not demonstrated.

FRISC-II randomized 2267 patients to either dalteparin (120 IU/kg twice daily) or placebo for 3 months following at least 5 days of treatment with open-label dalteparin [7]. Whereas a significant decrease in the primary endpoint, death or MI, was observed with dalteparin compared with placebo at 30 days (3.1% vs 5.9%, p-value = 0.002, respectively), the difference observed at 3 months was no longer significant (6.7% vs 8.0%, p-value = 0.17,

Table 6.4 LMWH without GP IIb/IIIa inhibitors in ACS: UA/NSTEMI

Trial	Duration of therapy	LMWH dose	Control	*N*	Primary endpoint	LMWH (%)	Control (%)	Absolute difference (%) (*p*-value)
Dalteparin								
FRIC [146]	6 days	120 IU/kg SC bid	UH 5000 IU bolus + 1000 IU/h (aPTT 1.5 × control)	1482	D/MI/RA	9.3	7.6	1.7 (NS)
	40 days	7500 IU SC qd	Placebo		D/MI/RA	12.3	12.3	–
FRISC [35]	6 days	120 IU/kg SC bid	Placebo	1506	D/MI	1.8	4.8	−3 (0.001)
	35–45 days	7500 IU SC qd	Placebo		D/MI/UR	18	23.7	−5.7 (0.005)
FRISC II [7]	3 months after ≥5 days open label dalteparin	120 IU/kg SC bid	Placebo	2267	D/MI (3 months)	10.0	11.2	−1.2 (NS)
Nadroparin								
Gurfinkel *et al.* [34]	5–7 days	214 ICU/kg SC bid	ASA	219	D/MI/UI/RA	22	ASA – 59	−37 (0.00001)
			UH (titrated to aPTT)				UH – 63	−41 (0.00001)
FRAXIS [38]	6 days	86 IU/kg SC bid (ST)	UH 5000 IU bolus + 1250 IU/h (ST)	3468	D/MI/RA (14D)	17.8	18.1	−0.3 (NS)
	14 days	86 IU SC bid (LT)	Placebo (LT)			20	18.1	1.9 (NS)
Enoxaparin								
ESSENCE [5]	2–8 days	1 mg/kg SC bid	UH 5000 U bolus plus infusion (aPTT 55–85 s)	3171	D/MI/RA(14D)	16.6	19.8	−3.2 (0.019)
TIMI 11B [6]	Max 8 days	1 mg/kg SC bid	UH 70 U/kg + 15 U/kg per h (aPTT 1.5–2.5 × control)	3910	D/MI/UR (8 days)	12.4	14.5	−2.1 (0.048)
	43 days		Placebo		D/MI/UR (43 days)	17.3	19.7	−2.4 (0.048)

bid = twice daily; D = death; LT = long term; MB = major bleed respectively). Patients in whom the treatment with dalteparin for more than 5 days may be of benefit include those awaiting revascularization. However, prolonged administration for more than 30 days affords no additional improvement in outcomes.

Trials comparing LMWH and UH without glycoprotein IIb/IIIa inhibitors

Three LMWHs have been compared to UH in patients presenting with ACS. These agents, enoxaparin, nadroparin and dalteparin, not only differ with respect to their molecular weights, anti-Xa:anti-IIa ratio and plasma half-lives (Table 6.1), but also differ in efficacy in comparison with UH (Table 6.4). Given the heterogeneity of the LMWHs, the specific trial designs and the patient populations studied, a brief review of the key findings from each trial will be presented.

Nadroparin (FRAXIS)

The FRAXIS trial assessed the benefit of short-term LMWH therapy with nadroparin compared with UH in 3468 patients with UA/NSTEMI and to determine whether a longer, 2-week LMWH regimen would offer additional clinical benefit. [38]. Patients assigned to nadroparin experienced a comparable rate of the primary composite endpoint, cardiac death, MI, refractory angina or recurrence of unstable angina at day 14, compared with UH (17.8% vs 18.1%, p-value = NS, respectively). Once again, prolonged administration of LMWH did not provide any additional benefit.

Dalteparin (FRIC)

The FRIC study compared the efficacy of the LMWH dalteparin with UH in 1482 patients presenting with an ACS [37]. This trial was composed of two phases: (i) an open, acute phase during which patients were assigned twice daily SC injections of dalteparin or a dose-adjusted IV infusion of UH and (ii) a double-blind prolonged treatment phase between days 6 and 45 comparing dalteparin (7500 IU once daily) with placebo. The administration of dalteparin during the acute phase of the study was associated with similar outcomes with respect to the composite endpoint of death, MI, or recurrent angina compared with UH (9.3% vs 7.6%, p-value = 0.33, respectively). Prolonged administration of dalteparin did not confer additional benefit. Equivalence of dalteparin and UH for the treatment of ACS was thus suggested.

Enoxaparin (ESSENCE)

The ESSENCE trial was a randomized, double-blind, placebo-controlled trial that compared enoxaparin 1 mg/kg twice daily given by SC injection for 2–8 days (median 2.6 days) with UH administered as a continuous IV infusion in 3171 patients with UA/NSTEMI [5]. The primary endpoint, the composite of death, MI or recurrent angina at 14 days, was significantly lower in patients randomized to enoxaparin than in those randomized to UH (16.6% vs 19.8%, p-value = 0.019, respectively). This advantage was sustained at 30 days (19.8% vs 23.3%, p-value = 0.016). Although the benefit of enoxaparin afforded to patients with UA/NSTEMI was primarily a result of less recurrent angina, there was a notable reduction in the risk of both death (19.8% RRR) and MI (25.5% RRR) at 30 days. Also seen was a significant reduction in the need for revascularization at 30 days in patients who received enoxaparin (27.0% vs 32.2% with UH; p-value = 0.001). This was the first large trial to demonstrate improved efficacy of a LMWH over UH in reducing the incidence of ischemic events in patients with UA/NSTEMI.

The initial benefit of enoxaparin in ESSENCE was also demonstrated to be sustained over the long term (1 year) [45]. The incidence of the composite triple endpoint was lower among patients receiving enoxaparin as compared with those receiving UH (32.0% vs 35.7%, *p*-value = 0.022), with a trend toward a lower incidence of the secondary composite endpoint of death or MI (11.5% vs 13.5%, *p*-value = 0.082). At one year, the need for diagnostic catheterization and coronary revascularization was lower in the enoxaparin group (55.8% vs 59.4%, *p*-value = 0.036 and 35.9% vs 41.2%, *p*-value = 0.002, respectively). Consistent with a hypothesized benefit of LMWH over UH, less rebound ischemia was also demonstrated in a substudy of this trial [46].

TIMI-11B

In TIMI-11B, 3910 patients with UA/NSTEMI were randomized to IV UH for 3–8 days followed by SC placebo injections or uninterrupted AT therapy with enoxaparin during both the acute phase (initial 30 mg IV bolus followed by SC injections of 1.0 mg/kg every 12 h) and outpatient phase (injections every 12 h of 40 mg for patients weighing <65 kg and 60 mg for those weighing ≥65 kg) [6]. The primary endpoint (death, MI or urgent revascularization) occurred by 8 days in 14.5% of patients in the UH group and 12.4% of patients in the enoxaparin group (OR 0.83; 95% CI 0.69 to 1.00; *p*-value = 0. 048) and by 43 days in 19.7% of the UFH group and 17.3% of the enoxaparin group (OR 0.85; 95% CI 0.72 to 1.00; *p*-value = 0.048). Consistent with the results observed in the ESSENCE trial, enoxaparin was demonstrated to be superior to UH for reducing a composite of death and serious cardiac ischemic events during the acute management of UA/NSTEMI. Also, consistent with the FRIC and FRAXIS trials, prolonged treatment with enoxaparin did not provide additional benefit.

Summary

These four trials comparing the addition of either LMWH or UH to aspirin have revealed that

- dalteparin and nadroparin offer similar efficacy to UH in patients with ACS
- enoxaparin decreases the composite endpoint of death, MI, and recurrent angina by 12 to 25% at varying time points (48 h to 43 days) following presentation of ACS
- LMWH use in this patient population was safe without an increase in major hemorrhagic events
- prolonged treatment with LMWH in this patient population does not provide any additional benefit.

Of interest is the fact that both dalteparin and nadroparin were equivalent to UH in this patient population despite a significant difference in their anti-Xa:anti-IIa ratio, which raises questions about the validity of this ratio contributing to the benefit of LMWH. On the other hand, the two large trials of enoxaparin as stand-alone therapy in patients with ACS, the ESSENCE trial and the TIMI-11B trial, support the hypothesis that differences in LMWH formulations, such as the anti-Xa:anti-IIa ratio, may account for the improved outcomes with LMWH in this population. The discordant findings between trials may be the result of a real difference between LMWH formulations, or they may be the result of the inherent heterogeneity of these trials. The only comparative trial, the EVET trial, suggests that the inherent properties of the individual LMWH contribute to the variable benefit observed with different LMWH formulations in this patient population [47]. This trial compared the efficacy of enoxaparin with that of tinzaparin in the management of 438 patients with UA/NSTEMI. The primary composite endpoint, recurrent angina, myocardial infarction (or reinfarction) or death at day 7, occurred in 12.3% in the enoxaparin group and 21.1% in the tinzaparin group (p-value = 0.015), suggesting greater benefit of enoxaparin as compared with tinzaparin in the treatment of these patients.

While the data in these trials suggest that LMWHs may afford some incremental benefit over that of UH, several limitations preclude the extrapolation of these data to contemporary practice patterns. These were studies primarily of medical management of patients with ACS. Based on recent clinical trials [48, 49], a substantial proportion of these patients would be treated with an early invasive approach. Furthermore, when these patients were taken to the catheterization laboratory, the majority had their AT therapy crossed over to UH, a practice that has recently been shown to result in worse outcomes [50]. In addition, none of these trials assessed the added benefit of LMWH over UH in patients being treated with a GP IIb/IIIa inhibitor or a thienopyridine, two classes of adjunctive antiplatelet medications that confer additional benefit in these patients [51, 52]. Nevertheless, these data paved the way for further analyses of LMWHs in a more contemporary practice pattern across the spectrum of CV disease.

In an attempt to bridge the clinical and interventional worlds, Martin *et al.* designed a trial to establish a dosing regimen for enoxaparin [53]. In this study 55 patients underwent PCI 8–12 h after a 1 mg/kg SC dose of enoxaparin. All patients received a 0.3 mg/kg IV bolus of enoxaparin at the start of the procedure. The observed anti-Xa levels were within the therapeutic range in 98% of patients 2–8 h after the last SC dose, in 96% of patients following the IV bolus and in 91% of patients for a further 2 h. This study provides an outline of enoxaparin dosing for patients transitioning from the clinical to the interventional service as a function of time from the last administered dose.

LMWH with GP IIb/IIIa inhibitors for medical management of ACS

When administered individually in patients with ACS, platelet GP IIb/IIIa inhibitors and LMWH may reduce adverse events. In a small feasibility trial, the coadministration of tirofiban and enoxaparin was generally well tolerated and a trend towards greater inhibition of platelet aggregation was observed with combination therapy [39]. Since this initial trial, several studies have been performed, primarily intended to assess the safety of the LMWH/GPIIb/IIIa combination in patients with ACS (Table 6.5).

The INTERACT trial randomized 746 high-risk ACS to receive open-label enoxaparin (1 mg/kg subcutaneously twice daily) or UH in addition to eptifibatide [42]. Not only was the combination of enoxaparin and eptifibatide associated with fewer major non-coronary artery bypass surgery-related bleeding events (1.8% vs 4.6% with UH, p-value = 0.03), it was also associated with less ischemia as detected by continuous ECG evaluation (12.7% vs 25.9% with UH, p-value <0.0001). In addition, the secondary endpoint of death or MI at 30 days was significantly lower in the enoxaparin group (5% vs 9%, p-value = 0.031).

The principal findings of these trials have suggested that this combination of antithrombotics for the initial management of ACS is safe without a demonstrable increase in

Table 6.5 LMWH with GP IIb/IIIa inhibitors in ACS: UA/NSTEMI

Trial	Duration of therapy	GP IIb/IIIa inhibitor	LMWH dose	Control	*N*	Primary efficacy endpoint	LMWH (%)	Control (%)	Absolute difference (%) (*p*-value)
Enoxaparin									
ACUTE II [40]	24–96 h	Tirofiban	1 mg/kg SC bid	UH (Titrated to aPTT)	525	D/MI/UR (IH)	9.2	9.0	0.2 (NS)
NICE 3 [41]	24–96 h	Tirofiban, Eptifibatide, or Abciximab	1 mg/kg SC bid	Registry data	671	D/MI/UR (30 days)	11.6	NA	NA
A to Z [60]	7 days	Tirofiban	1 mg/kg SC bid	UH 60 U/kg bolus then 12 U/kg per h (Titrated to aPTT)	3987	D/MI/RI	8.4	9.4	−1.0 (NS)
INTERACT [42]	48 h	Eptifibatide	1 mg/kg SC bid	UH 70 U/kg bolus + 15 U/kg per h (aPTT 1.5–2 × control)	746	Ischemia on ECG	14.3	25.4	−11.1 (0.0002)
						D/MI (30 days)	5.0	9.0	4.0 (0.031)
Dalteparin									
GUSTO IV Dalteparin substudy [43]	5–7 days	Abciximab	120 IU SC bid	UH 70 U/kg bolus (max 5000 U) + 10 U/kg per h (max 800 U/h) titrated to a PTT 50–70 s	5112	D/MI (30 days)	9.6	8.5	1.1 (NS)
PARAGON B [44]	3 days	Lamifiban	LMWH	UH (Titrated to aPTT)	5200	D/MI/SRI (30 days)	10.2	12.2	−2.0 (NS)

bid = twice daily; D = death; ECG = electrocardiogram; LT = long term; MB = major bleed; qd = once daily; RA = recurrent angina; SRI = severe refractory ischemia; ST = short term; UI = urgent intervention; UR = urgent revascularization hemorrhagic complications. Although not powered for clinical endpoints, these trials have implied a comparable event rate between combination groups receiving LMWH and the groups receiving UH.

LMWH combined with PCI in ACS

Given the notable improvement in outcomes with an early invasive approach to the management of patients across the spectrum of ACS [48, 49] there is an important need for an antithrombotic regimen that not only functions as a 'stand-alone' regimen but also provides a seamless interface with the cardiac catheterization laboratory.

One of the most significant contributions to improved outcomes for patients with ACS undergoing PCI has been the development of treatment regimens that not only prevent thrombus formation at the site of arterial injury but also on the surface of instruments utilized. Combined with aspirin, heparin, and clopidogrel GP IIb/IIIa inhibitors have contributed to these improved outcomes across the spectrum of patients undergoing PCI or with ACS [51, 54–56] including those with diabetes [57]. The primary limitation of GP IIb/IIIa inhibitors, however, is one of increased bleeding.

The use of LMWH for the medical management of UA/NSTEMI has been associated with favorable outcomes. Recent analyses have also suggested benefits of LMWH in these patients undergoing PCI. A substudy of the ESSENCE and TIMI-11B trials demonstrated that patients randomized to enoxaparin who underwent PCI, experienced a trend towards improved 43-day outcomes [58]. Similarly, in the FRISC-II trial, dalteparin was shown to be safe and effective when administered for 2–7 days before patients were randomized to either invasive or conservative strategies and no longer than 12 h before PCI [48]. In these trials, however, LMWH was discontinued prior to catheterization and UH was utilized as an adjunctive antithrombotic during PCI.

The utility of enoxaparin as a peri-procedural AT was evaluated in 451 consecutive patients with UA/NSTEMI treated for at least 48 h with SC enoxaparin [59]. There were no in-hospital abrupt closures or urgent revascularizations in any of the PCI patients whop underwent coronary angiography followed by immediate PCI within 8 h of LMWH administration. The death/MI rate at 30 days was 6.2% in the whole population and 3.0% in the PCI cohort. No significant differences in bleeding complications were noted. These data suggest that patients treated with a standard dose of enoxaparin for UA/NSTEMI can safely undergo PCI within 8 h of the last SC injection.

Whether combining enoxaparin with a GP IIb/IIIa inhibitor is as safe or as effective as the current standard combination of UH with GP IIb/IIIa inhibitors for the treatment of ACS was assessed in the A to Z trial [60]. This prospective, international, open-label, randomized, non-inferiority trial of 3987 ACS patients receiving tirofiban compared enoxaparin (1 mg/kg twice daily) with weight-adjusted IV UH. Death, recurrent MI or refractory ischemia at 7 days occurred less frequently in patients with enoxaparin (8.4% vs 9.4% with UH, p-value = NS), meeting the pre-specified criterion for non-inferiority. In addition, the combination of enoxaparin and tirofiban did not impart an increased risk of bleeding (3.0% vs 2.2% UH, p-value = 0.13). Although approximately 60% of patients in each group underwent an 'early invasive' management strategy, this trial was not designed to address the key issue of efficacy and safety of enoxaparin for this purpose.

The safety and efficacy of combined enoxaparin and GP IIb/IIIa inhibitors was evaluated in the most relevant manner in the recent SYNERGY trial, the only definitively powered trial in the current era of early invasive management of patients with ACS [50]. This trial enrolled 10,000 high-risk ACS patients and randomized them to receive either enoxaparin (1mg/kg SC twice daily) or UH (60 U/kg bolus then 12 U/kg per hour adjusted to an aPTT of 50 to 70 sec). More than 90% of patients underwent an early invasive strategy (cardiac catheterization at a median of 21 h from randomization). Of these, patients 47% underwent PCI, 19% had coronary bypass surgery and 57% received a GP IIb/IIIa inhibitor. The primary endpoint of death or MI occurred at a similar rate in the two treatment arms (14.5% vs 14.0% in the UH and enoxaparin arms, respectively, p-value = 0.4), although patients tended to do worse when switched from enoxaparin to UH or vice versa. Major bleeding occurred more frequently among patients receiving enoxaparin (7.6% vs 9.1%, respectively, p-value = 0.008). Notably, enoxaparin provided an adequate level of anticoagulation for patients undergoing early PCI, as demonstrated by the similar proportion of patients experiencing untoward events during invasive management.

Thus, enoxaparin may be used either as the sole anticoagulant or in combination with GP IIb/IIIa inhibitors for patients undergoing PCI. Patients can safely undergo PCI while on SC enoxaparin 1 mg/kg twice daily if it is performed within 8 h following the last administered dose. If PCI is undertaken between 8 and 12 h after the last dose, an additional 0.3 mg/kg dose of enoxaparin should be administered. As recently suggested, switching from enoxaparin to UH in these patients should be avoided. Dalteparin may also be utilized in this setting, although the data supporting this remain limited. If used, dalteparin should be administered at a dose of 120 IU/kg subcutaneously twice daily if PCI is performed within 8 h of the last dose. If performed more than 8 h from the last SC dose, PCI should be preceded by an additional 60 IU/kg IV dose.

LMWH as an Adjunct in Patients with STEMI

The mainstay of therapy for STEMI revolves around a rapid and complete reperfusion approach, either pharmacologic or mechanical. While a multi-pronged strategy to stabilizing the thrombotic process impressively reduces mortality rates following STEMI, substantial morbidity and mortality persists.

Only 50–60% of patients receiving fibrinolytic therapy achieve full angiographic reperfusion [61–63]. Recurrent ischemia occurs in approximately 20–30% of patients, reocclusion in approximately 5–15% and reinfarction in approximately 3–5% [64]. Further, it is noted that a considerable proportion of patients who do achieve TIMI 3 flow ('angiographically normal' perfusion) fail to achieve microvascular, or tissue-level, reperfusion, manifested by persistent ST-segment elevation [65].

The safety and efficacy of two LMWHs, dalteparin and enoxaparin, as an adjunct to fibrinolysis in the setting of a STEMI has been evaluated in several trials to date focusing on such endpoints as LV thrombus formation and subsequent thromboembolism [66], infarct-related artery patency [67–71], and clinical outcomes [8, 72, 73]. In general, these trials have demonstrated improved late coronary artery patency and lower rates of late ischemic events with LMWH compared to UH as an adjunct to fibrinolytic therapy (Table 6.6). Two small trials suggested a benefit of the dalteparin with respect to achieving IRA patency when combined with either SK [70] or tPA [71]. In addition to demonstrating the safety of combined LMWH with fibrinolytics, fewer clinical events were also seen.

Three trials have assessed the efficacy of enoxaparin combined with fibrinolysis with respect to IRA patency and have revealed absolute increases in IRA patency between 1%

Table 6.6 LMWH trials in STEMI

LMWH	Dose	Control Arm	*N*	Duration	Fibrinolytic regimen	Primary endpoint	Timing of outcome	LMWH (%)	Control (%)	Absolute difference (%) (*p*-value)
Dalteparin										
FRAMI [66]	150 IU/kg SC	Placebo	517	Hospitalization	SK	Reduction in LV thrombus and arterial TE	9 days	14.2	21.9	−7.7 (0.02)
BIOMACS [70]	100 IU/kg before SK; 120 IU/kg 12 h after SK SC	Placebo	101	24 h	SK	TIMI 3 flow	20–28 h	68	51	17 (0.10)
ASSENT-PLUS [71]	30 IU/kg IV then 120 IU/kg bid	UH	439	4–7 days	t-PA	TIMI 3 flow	4–7 days	69.3	62.5	6.8 (0.163)
Enoxaparin										
ASENOX [72]	40 mg IV then 1 mg/kg SC bid	UH	412	2–3 days	SK	Mortality	30 days	7.1	8.2	−1.1
Baird *et al*. [74]	40 mg IV then 40 mg SC tid	UH	300	4 days	SK, antistreplase, t-PA	Reperfusion D/MI/RH	Not defined 3 months	79.8 26	75.9 36	(3.9) −10 (0.04)
AMI-SK [69]	30 mg IV then 1 mg/kg SC bid	Placebo	496	3–8 days	SK	TIMI 3 flow	5–10 days	70	58	12 (0.01)

HART-II [67]	30 mg IV then 1 mg/kg SC bid	UH	400	≥–3 days	t-PA	IRA patency	90 min	80.1	75.1	5
ENTIRE-TIMI 23 [68]	±30 mg IV then 1 mg/kg SC bid	UH	483	Max 8 days	TNK, 1/2 TNK with abciximab	TIMI 3 flow-angiographic	60 min	51	50	1 (NS)
						Death/MI – clinical	30 days	4.9	11.3	−6.4 (0.01)
ASSENT-3 [8]	30 mg IV then 1 mg/kg SC bid	UH	4075	Max 7 days	TNK	In-hospital D/MI/RI	30 days	11.4	15.4	−4 (<0.001)
ASSENT-3 PLUS [73]	Pre-hospital 30 mg IV then 1 mg/kg SC bid	UH	1639	Max 7 days	TNK	In-hospital D/MI/RI	30 days	14.2	17.4	−3.2
EXTRACT TIMI-25 [147]	Age <75: 30 mg IV then 1 mg/kg SC bid Age ≥75: no IV bolus then 0.75 mg/kg SC bid	UH	20,506	Max 8 days	TNK – 19.3% Alteplase – 54.7% Reteplase – 5.5% SK – 20.3% None – 0.3%	D/MI	30 days	9.9	12.0	−2.1 (<0.001)

bid = twice daily; D = death; RI = recurrent ischemia; TE = thrombo-embolism; tid = three times a day and 12% [67–69]. In each trial, the addition of enoxaparin (30 mg IV bolus followed by 1 mg/kg subcutaneously twice daily) to either tPA [67], SK [69] or tenecteplase (TNK) [68], improved IRA patency without an increase in major bleeding. These trials also suggested that less reocclusion [67], enhanced tissue level reperfusion [69] and combination with a GP IIb/IIIa inhibitor [68] could be achieved with enoxaparin. The addition of enoxaparin to half-dose TNK and abciximab did result, however, in more hemorrhagic complications [68].

Several additional trials have also assessed the clinical efficacy of enoxaparin as an adjunct to fibrinolysis using SK [72], TNK [8, 71], or either SK, antistreplase or tPA [74]. The use of enoxaparin combined with each of these fibrinolytics resulted in an absolute reduction in clinical events ranging between 1.1% and 10%. Encouragingly, no differences in hemorrhagic complications were observed when enoxaparin was combined with standard-dose fibrinolytics.

The ASSENT-3 trial compared the fibrinolytic agent TNK combined with enoxaparin or abciximab, with TNK plus UH in 6095 patients randomized within 6 h of the onset of an acute MI to single-bolus TNK plus SC enoxaparin, TNK plus UH (48-h infusion, aPTT 50–70 sec), or half-dose TNK plus IV UH and IV abciximab [8]. The combined endpoint of 30-day mortality, in-hospital reinfarction or refractory ischemia was significantly lower in the enoxaparin and abciximab groups (11.4% and 11.1%, respectively; p-value = 0.0001) than in the UFH group (15.4%). Although not powered to assess mortality, this traditional endpoint of fibrinolytic trials was not affected by combining TNK with either enoxaparin or abciximab. Despite a slight increase in hemorrhagic complications with enoxaparin, the incidence of intracranial hemorrhage was similar (0.9%) in each group. The results of this trial suggest that the combination of full-dose TNK and up to 7 days of enoxaparin may be the optimal pharmacologic treatment for patients with acute MI of <6 h [8].

Given that 'time is myocardium,' the ASSENT-3 PLUS trial sought to determine the efficacy of prehospital reperfusion with enoxaparin combined with a fibrinolytic. In this study, 1639 patients with STEMI were randomized to treatment with TNK and either enoxaparin (30 mg intravenously followed by 1 mg/kg twice daily for a maximum of 7 days) or UH (weight adjusted). Although treatment with enoxaparin facilitated timely reperfusion (53% within 2 h from symptom onset), only a trend towards reduced ischemic endpoints (30-day mortality or in-hospital reinfarction, or in-hospital refractory ischemia) was seen [73]. However, an increase in intracranial hemorrhage (2.20% vs 0.97% with UH, p-value = 0.047) was seen primarily in patients older than 75, emphasizing the need for further evaluation of enoxaparin in this setting.

A significant number of patients with STEMI, however, present outside the window of opportunity for reperfusion therapy. Therapeutic options remain limited for these patients as there are currently no specific treatment recommendations for this subgroup. The TETAMI randomized trial sought to demonstrate that enoxaparin was superior to UH and that tirofiban was better than placebo in patients with STEMI who did not receive timely reperfusion [75]. A total of 1224 patients with STEMI ineligible for reperfusion were randomized to enoxaparin, enoxaparin plus tirofiban, UH or UH plus tirofiban. The primary efficacy endpoint, the combined incidence of death, reinfarction or recurrent angina at 30 days, occurred in 15.7% of patients who received enoxaparin vs 17.3% for UH (odds ratio 0.89 [95% CI = 0.66 to 1.21]). This study did not show that enoxaparin reduced ischemic complications compared with UFH in non-reperfused STEMI patients, but instead appeared to have a similar safety and efficacy profile.

LMWH IN VENOUS THROMBOEMBOLIC DISEASE

Prophylaxis of VTE

Although mortality from VTE has decreased since the mid-1980s, it remains a major national health problem, being responsible for 150,000 to 200,000 deaths annually [76, 77]. Despite significant advances in prevention and treatment of VTE, PE remains a common preventable cause of hospital deaths. It is, therefore, imperative to stratify patients according to risk categories and to institute appropriate prophylactic measures (Table 6.7).

LMWHs have been shown to be efficacious in the prophylaxis of VTE and a number of these agents are approved for this indication (Table 6.1). The attraction of LMWHs for VTE prophylaxis is that they can be administered once or twice daily at a constant dose without laboratory monitoring. In addition, a substantially lower risk of HIT with LMWH compared with UH has been suggested [78].

LMWHs have been evaluated for prophylaxis of VTE in several, primarily surgical, situations (Table 6.8). LMWHs have been shown to be as or more efficacious than UH for this indication. However, it should be noted that comparison across trials of patients treated with LMWH prophylaxis is difficult, owing to the variability of the dosing schedules used.

General surgery

Randomized trials have found that LMWHs given either once or twice daily are as effective or more effective than UH in preventing thrombosis [3, 79, 80]. In addition, LMWH use has been associated with similar bleeding risks, although in a study of 3809 patients undergoing

Table 6.7 Risk Categories for VTE. Adapted from Gallus *et al.* [148]

Risk category	Risk of VTE (%)		
	Calf vein thrombosis	Proximal vein thrombosis	Fatal pulmonary embolism
High Risk	40–80	10–20	1–5
General surgery in patients >40 years with recent history of DVT or PE			
Extensive pelvic or abdominal surgery for malignant disease			
Major orthopedic surgery on lower limbs			
Moderate Risk[a]	10–40	2–10	0.1–0.7
General surgery in patients >40 years lasting 30 min or more			
Non-major surgery in patients 40–60 years with no additional risk factors			
Immobilization with major medical illness, including stroke, cardiac disease, chronic respiratory disease, bowel disease, and malignancy			
Low Risk	2	0.4	0.002
Minor surgery in patients <40 years with no additional risk factors			

Table 6.8 Advantages of LMWH and studied agents for prevention and treatment of VTE

Indication	Advantages of LMWH	LMWH studied
Prevention		
General Surgery	At least as effective as low-dose UH but can be given once daily and causes fewer hematomas at injection site	Low Risk Dalteparin, Enoxaparin, Tinzaparin, Nadroparin. High Risk Dalteparin, Enoxaparin
Orthopedic Surgery	More effective than low-dose UH; more effective than warfarin in patients undergoing TKR; no monitoring required	Ardreparin, Dalteparin, Enoxaparin, Nadroparin, Tinzaparin.
Acute Spinal Injury	Apparently effective whereas low-dose UH is not, and higher doses of UH cause excessive bleeding	Enoxaparin.
Multiple Trauma	More effective than UH	Enoxaparin.
Medical Conditions	As effective as low-dose UH but can be given once daily	Dalteparin, Enoxaparin.
Treatment		
VTE	At least as safe and effective as UH but can be given SC without the need for monitoring	Dalteparin, Enoxaparin, Nadroparin, Tinzaparin.
UA	At least as effective as UH but can be given SC without monitoring	Dalteparin, Enoxaparin.

TKR = total knee replacement

major abdominal surgery a trend toward fewer major bleeding episodes was noted with LMWH and significantly fewer wound hematomas [3].

Orthopedic surgery

Major orthopedic surgery involving the lower limbs is associated with a substantial risk of VTE. Approximately 40–80% of patients will develop calf vein DVT and up to 5% will experience a fatal PE (Table 6.7). LMWH have been shown to be both efficacious and safe in these patients.

Hip arthroplasty

Trials have compared LMWH to placebo [81], UH [82–85] and warfarin [86] for the prevention of VTE following hip surgery. Compared to placebo, LMWH administered post-operatively was associated with an approximately 50% reduction in the risk of thrombosis without an increase in bleeding [87]. Furthermore, the safety and efficacy of LMWH (enoxaparin) continued for 1 month following hip replacement surgery has also been demonstrated [81]. In this small randomized trial, VTE occurred less frequently in patients given enoxaparin (18% vs 39% with placebo, p-value <0.001). In addition, a different North American randomized trial has confirmed the benefit of post-discharge thromboprophylaxis using dalteparin for a total of 35 days [88]. Combined with data that suggest that the risk of VTE persists for at least 1 month after hip arthroplasty, LMWH for prophylaxis should be given for at least 1 month [89].

LMWHs have also been shown to be equally or more effective than either low-dose SC UH or adjusted-dose UH (started pre-operatively and continued three times daily to maintain aPTT at upper normal range) [82–85]. In addition, a lower rate of hemorrhagic complications was seen with the usc of LMWH.

When compared with warfarin (adjusted dose for International Normalized Ratio (INR) 2.0–3.0), LMWH have been shown to be as effective in preventing VTE following hip surgery, although minor bleeding episodes were more common [86, 90]. Nevertheless, the use of LMWH in this patient population has been cost-effective [91].

Knee arthroplasty

Although the efficacy of LMWH for thromboprophylaxis in patients undergoing knee arthroplasty has been demonstrated, approximately 30% of these patients will experience a VTE [92–94]. Compared with warfarin, LMWH reduces the incidence of VTE, although only at the expense of a trend towards higher bleeding rates and transfusion requirements in this patient population [95–97]. The optimal duration of LMWH following knee arthroplasty remains poorly defined, but it appears that between 7 and 10 days is sufficient [98].

Acute spinal cord injury

A substantial proportion of people with acute spinal cord injury develop venous thrombosis primarily within the first 2 weeks following the injury [99]. Whereas fixed-dose UH has achieved minimal success in this patient population, adjusted-dose UH has been successful, but with an increased rate of hemorrhagic complications [100]. LMWHs have been shown to be both safe and effective in this patient population. Compared with fixed-dose UH, LMWHs have been associated with a decreased rate of VTE [101]. In addition, LMWHs are associated with a similar rate of VTE as fixed-dose UH plus intermittent pneumatic compression in the acute phase [102] and with decrease in the rate of VTE in rehabilitation phase [103] following spinal cord injury.

Multiple trauma

Thromboembolic complications are frequent in patients with multiple trauma [104]. The efficacy of UH for venous thrombosis prophylaxis has not been established. Based on limited prospective data, LMWH appears to be more effective than UH [105] and at least as effective as compression devices [106] for preventing thromboembolic complications in these patients.

Medical conditions

Venous thromboembolism is a common complication of hospitalized patients, imposing a major clinical and economic burden. Three out of four cases of fatal PE occur in non-surgical settings, but thromboprophylaxis is far less common in medical than in surgical patients. This is mainly attributable to the heterogeneity of non-surgical populations and a lack of high-quality evidence to support specific thromboprophylactic measures. According to one study, the presence of acute infectious disease, an age of more than 75 years, cancer and a history of VTE were independent predictors of VTE in this patient population [107]. Enoxaparin (40 mg once daily for 6–14 days), has been shown to reduce the risk of VTE by 63% without increasing adverse events [108]. This benefit extends to a wide range of medical patients [109]. In addition, a recent meta-analysis suggested LMWH to be as effective as UH in medical patients, with a decrease in risk of bleeding complications [110].

Treatment of VTE

Given the advantageous pharmacologic profile of LMWH, once or twice daily dosing without the need for monitoring, the attraction for using these agents for the treatment of VTE is quite apparent. Numerous trials have demonstrated the safety and efficacy of LMWH for the treatment of VTE. Based on these safety and efficacy trials, four LMWH preparations have received FDA approval for this indication (Table 6.1). LMWH may facilitate outpatient therapy for patients with uncomplicated DVT [111, 112]. LMWHs have also demonstrated utility for use as long-term therapy in elderly patients [113], in patients with cancer [114] and in patients with recurrent VTE despite therapy with warfarin [115, 116].

DVT

The goals of treatment for DVT are to stop clot propagation and prevent clot recurrence, PE and a potential complication of recurrent PEs, pulmonary hypertension. An increased likelihood of facilitating thrombus regression and preventing recurrent thromboembolism in patients with documented DVT has been shown with the LMWH reviparin compared with IV UH [117].

With a high degree of consistency, several LMWH preparations have shown efficacy for the initial treatment of DVT [1, 2, 118, 119]. These trials, comparing LMWH with UH for the treatment of DVT, have demonstrated similar efficacy for LMWH and UH with comparable rates of hemorrhagic complications. In addition, a recent meta-analysis suggested that LMWHs are associated with an improvement in mortality [120].

These agents appear to be cost-effective when utilized as initial therapy for DVT, and become cost-saving when even a minority of patients are treated in the outpatient setting [121]. The ease of administration of LMWH make the outpatient management of patients with uncomplicated DVT feasible and effective as an initial therapy until warfarin is at a therapeutic level [111, 112]. This approach results in an improved quality of life and greater patient satisfaction, and may also result in a substantial cost savings to the healthcare system [121, 122].

The potential for long-term therapy for the treatment of DVT with LMWH also appears to be efficacious and safe. Whereas therapy with warfarin has traditionally been used, the need for monitoring and dose adjustments as well as treatment failures with warfarin, have made LMWHs an attractive alternative. One study demonstrated that long-term LMWH is highly effective and safe when used as long-term therapy for secondary prevention in selected prothrombotic disorders in a series of patients with conditions associated with prior warfarin failure or potential to warfarin therapy (antiphospholipid syndrome) [115]. The utility of LMWH was also demonstrated in patients with cancer as a long-term therapeutic as well as for the treatment of cancer patients who have failed warfarin therapy [114, 116].

The feasibility and safety of LMWH for long-term treatment of DVT has also been seen in elderly patients [113]. Thus, LMWHs offer a viable alternative with potential cost-savings to traditional management of DVT.

Pulmonary embolism

Anticoagulation is the principal treatment for PE. Owing to the potential morbidity and mortality associated with PE, initial treatment is delivered in a closely monitored setting. However, the outpatient treatment of select patients with PE is made feasible with LMWH [123]. Until further data support this initial study, the outpatient treatment of PE can not be advocated.

LMWHs have recently been shown to be as effective as UH for the initial treatment of PE [124–126]. One study randomly assigned 1021 patients with symptomatic DVT, PE or both to treatment with fixed dose, twice daily, SC reviparin, or adjusted-dose IV UH [124]. Pulmonary embolism was present in approximately one-third of patients, and all patients started therapy with an oral coumarin derivative on the first hospital day. No significant differences in recurrent thromboembolic events, major bleeding or mortality were found between the two treatment groups. Two additional studies demonstrated that the LMWH tinzaparin was equivalent to UH in patients with symptomatic [125] and submassive PE [126]. Although one meta-analysis suggested a mortality benefit with LMWH compared to UH in patients with a PE [127], the superiority of LMWH has not been demonstrated in prospective randomized trials.

CLINICAL CONSIDERATIONS

LMWH in patients with chronic kidney disease

While patients with mild to moderate CKD have been treated with LMWH without a significant increase in adverse events, specifically bleeding, their use in patients with severe CKD (creatinine clearance <30 ml/min) and in those on hemodialysis has been associated with increased untoward events. LMWHs administered at fixed-weight doses and without monitoring show unpredictable anticoagulant effects in patients with severe CKD, leading to serious and even fatal adverse incidents [128]. If used in patients with severe CKD, the dose of enoxaparin should be decreased from the standard (1 mg/kg twice daily) to 64% of the standard dose [129, 130].

LMWH in pregnancy

Thromboembolic disease is a rare, but important, complication of pregnancy, which remains a leading non-obstetric cause of maternal death. Until now, UH has been regarded as the drug of choice for the prevention and treatment of VTE during pregnancy. However, because of its significant side effects (osteoporosis and HIT), the inconvenient mode of administration and need for monitoring, UH is now being replaced by LMWH. The efficacy and safety of LMWH in pregnant women has been demonstrated in several trials to date [131–133]. However, consideration should be given to the dosing of LMWHs in pregnant patients owing to their altered pharmacokinetics in this patient population [133, 134].

Despite the demonstration of the safety of LMWHs in pregnant patients, a specific subpopulation of these patients, those with mechanical heart valves, warrants further study before LMWHs are generally accepted. The evidence in the literature regarding the long-term use of LMWH as the only anticoagulant after mechanical heart valve replacement is limited [135]. In addition, treatment 'failures' have been reported [136]. Until further studies are performed assessing the safety of LMWH in this patient population, their use as a sole anticoagulant cannot be recommended.

Is there an antidote for LMWH?

As discussed above, LMWHs possess several characteristics that make them an attractive alternative to the traditional antithrombotics. However, they also possess an 'Achilles heel,' the lack of an antidote. Whereas protamine sulfate can neutralize the activity of UH, it incompletely neutralizes the effects of LMWH [137–139]. Despite the ability of protamine to block LMWH-induced bleeding in animals [140], limited data in humans exists.

6.4 CONCLUSIONS

The LMWHs have been a welcome addition to our antithrombotic armamentarium. Their ease of administration and predictable anticoagulant effect have catapulted them to the forefront of treatment across the spectrum of thrombotic cardiovascular diseases. These agents have proven to be superior to UH for the management of venous thromboembolic disease. In addition, they appear to be useful alternatives to UH in the management of arterial thrombosis across the spectrum of CV disease. However, limitations of these agents, such as their inability to inhibit clot-bound thrombin and their incomplete reversibility, resulting in an excess of bleeding events in arterial thrombotic diseases, preclude their title as the 'ideal' antithrombotic agent. Nevertheless, the LMWHs maintain a strong position as the antithrombotic agent of choice in certain clinical conditions.

REFERENCES

[1] Hull, R.D., *et al.*, (1992) Subcutaneous low-molecular-weight heparin compared with continuous intravenous heparin in the treatment of proximal-vein thrombosis. *N Eng J Med*, 326(15):975–82.

[2] Prandoni, P., *et al.*, (1992) Comparison of subcutaneous low-molecular-weight heparin with intravenous standard heparin in proximal deep-vein thrombosis. *Lancet*, 339(8791):441–5.

[3] Kakkar, V.V., *et al.*, (1993) Low molecular weight versus standard heparin for prevention of venous thromboembolism after major abdominal surgery. The Thromboprophylaxis Collaborative Group. *Lancet*, 341(8840):259–65.

[4] Kay, R., *et al.*, (1995) Low-molecular-weight heparin for the treatment of acute ischemic stroke. *N Eng J Med*, 333(24):1588–93.

[5] Cohen, M., *et al.*, (1997) A comparison of low-molecular-weight heparin with unfractionated heparin for unstable coronary artery disease. Efficacy and Safety of Subcutaneous Enoxaparin in Non-Q-Wave Coronary Events Study Group. *N Eng J Med*, 337(7):447–52.

[6] Antman, E.M., *et al.*, (1999) Enoxaparin prevents death and cardiac ischemic events in unstable angina/non-Q-wave myocardial infarction. Results of the thrombolysis in myocardial infarction (TIMI) 11B trial. *Circulation*, 100(15):1593–601.

[7] The FRISC II investigators, (1999) Long-term low-molecular-mass heparin in unstable coronary-artery disease: FRISC II prospective randomised multicentre study. FRagmin and Fast Revascularisation during InStability in Coronary artery disease. *Lancet*, 354(9180):701–7.
[8] Efficacy and safety of tenecteplase in combination with enoxaparin, abciximab, or unfractionated heparin: the ASSENT-3 randomised trial in acute myocardial infarction (2001) *Lancet*, 358(9282):605–13.
[9] Karsch, K.R., *et al.*, (1996) Low molecular weight heparin (reviparin) in percutaneous transluminal coronary angioplasty. Results of a randomized, double-blind, unfractionated heparin and placebo-controlled, multicenter trial (REDUCE trial). Reduction of Restenosis After PTCA, Early Administration of Reviparin in a Double-Blind Unfractionated Heparin and Placebo-Controlled Evaluation. *J Am Coll Cardiol*, 28(6):1437–43.
[10] Hirsh, J., (1991) Heparin. *N Eng J Med*, 324:1565–74.
[11] Weitz, J.I., (1997) Low-molecular-weight heparins. *N Eng J Med*, 337:688–98.
[12] Lin, P., Sinha, U., Betz, A., (2001) Antithrombin binding of low molecular weight heparins and inhibition of factor Xa. *Biochim Biophys Acta*, 1526(1):105–13.
[13] Hirsh, J., *et al.*, (1998) Heparin and low-molecular-weight heparin: mechanisms of action, pharmacokinetics, dosing considerations, monitoring, efficacy, and safety. *Chest*, 114 (5 Suppl):489S–510S.
[14] Huang, Z.F., Wun, T.C., Broze, G.J., Jr., (1993) Kinetics of factor Xa inhibition by tissue factor pathway inhibitor. *J Biol Chem*, 268(36):26950–5.
[15] Bendz, B., Andersen, T.O., Sandset, P.M., (2000) Dose-dependent release of endogenous tissue factor pathway inhibitor by different low molecular weight heparins. *Blood Coagul Fibrinolysis*, 11(4):343–8.
[16] Alban, S., Gastpar, R., (2001) Plasma levels of total and free tissue factor pathway inhibitor (TFPI) as individual pharmacological parameters of various heparins. *Thromb Haemost*, 85(5):824–9.
[17] Li, Y., *et al.*, (2002) Comparative effects of unfractionated heparin and low molecular weight heparin on vascular endothelial cell tissue factor pathway inhibitor release: a model for assessing intrinsic thromboresistance. *J Thromb Thrombolysis*, 14(2):123–9.
[18] Theroux, P., *et al.*, (1992) Reactivation of unstable angina after the discontinuation of heparin. *N Eng J Med*, 327:141–5.
[19] Granger, C.B., *et al.*, (1995) Rebound increase in thrombin generation and activity after cessation of intravenous heparin in patients with acute coronary syndromes. *Circulation*, 91:1929–1935.
[20] Becker, R.C., *et al.*, (1999) Thrombin generation after the abrupt cessation of intravenous unfractionated heparin among patients with acute coronary syndromes: potential mechanisms for heightened prothrombotic potential. *J Am Coll Cardiol*, 34(4):1020–7.
[21] Bara, L., *et al.*, (1985) Comparative pharmacokinetics of a low molecular weight heparin (PK 10 169) and unfractionated heparin after intravenous and subcutaneous administration. *Thromb Res*, 39(5):631–6.
[22] Young, E., *et al.*, (1994) Ex-vivo and in-vitro evidence that low molecular weight heparins exhibit less binding to plasma proteins than unfractionated heparin. *Thromb Haemost*, 71(3):300–4.
[23] Cosmi, B., *et al.*, (1997) Effect of nonspecific binding to plasma proteins on the antithrombin activities of unfractionated heparin, low-molecular-weight heparin, and dermatan sulfate. *Circulation*, 95(1):118–24.
[24] Bara, L., Samama, M., (1988) Pharmacokinetics of low molecular weight heparins. *Acta Chir Scand Suppl*, 543:65–72.
[25] Rabah, M.M., *et al.*, (1999) Usefulness of intravenous enoxaparin for percutaneous coronary intervention in stable angina pectoris. *Am J Cardiol*, 84(12):1391–5.
[26] Kereiakes, D.J., *et al.*, (2001) Enoxaparin and abciximab adjunctive pharmacotherapy during percutaneous coronary intervention. *J Invasive Cardiol*, 13(4):272–8.
[27] Choussat, R., *et al.*, (2002) A unique, low dose of intravenous enoxaparin in elective percutaneous coronary intervention. *J Am Coll Cardiol*, 40(11):1943–50.
[28] Bhatt, D.L., *et al.*, (2003) Safety of concomitant therapy with eptifibatide and enoxaparin in patients undergoing percutaneous coronary intervention: results of the Coronary Revascularization Using Integrilin and Single bolus Enoxaparin Study. *J Am Coll Cardiol*, 41(1):20–5.

[29] Kereiakes, D.J., *et al.*, (2001) Dalteparin in combination with abciximab during percutaneous coronary intervention. *Am Heart J*, 141(3):348–52.

[30] Young, J.J., Kereiakes, D.J., Grines, C.L., (2000) Low-molecular-weight heparin therapy in percutaneous coronary intervention: the NICE 1 and NICE 4 trials. National Investigators Collaborating on Enoxaparin Investigators. *J Invasive Cardiol*, 12 Suppl E:E14–18; discussion E25–8.

[31] Theroux, P., *et al.*, (1988) Aspirin, heparin, or both to treat acute unstable angina. *N Eng J Med*, 319(17):1105–11.

[32] Theroux, P., *et al.*, (1993) Aspirin versus heparin to prevent myocardial infarction during the acute phase of unstable angina. *Circulation*, 88(5 Pt 1):2045–8.

[33] Cohen, M., *et al.*, (1994) Combination antithrombotic therapy in unstable rest angina and non-Q-wave infarction in nonprior aspirin users. Primary end points analysis from the ATACS trial. Antithrombotic Therapy in Acute Coronary Syndromes Research Group. *Circulation*, 89(1):81–8.

[34] Gurfinkel, E.P., *et al.*, (1995) Low molecular weight heparin versus regular heparin or aspirin in the treatment of unstable angina and silent ischemia. *J Am Coll Cardiol*, 26(2):313–18.

[35] The FRISC study group, (1996) Low-molecular-weight heparin during instability in coronary artery disease, Fragmin during Instability in Coronary Artery Disease (FRISC) study group. *Lancet*, 347(9001):561–8.

[36] Eikelboom, J.W., *et al.*, (2000) Unfractionated heparin and low-molecular-weight heparin in acute coronary syndrome without ST elevation: a meta-analysis. *Lancet*, 355(9219): 1936–42.

[37] Klein, W., *et al.*, (1997) Comparison of low-molecular-weight heparin with unfractionated heparin acutely and with placebo for 6 weeks in the management of unstable coronary artery disease. Fragmin in unstable coronary artery disease study (FRIC). *Circulation*, 96(1):61–8.

[38] Comparison of two treatment durations (6 days and 14 days) of a low molecular weight heparin with a 6-day treatment of unfractionated heparin in the initial management of unstable angina or non-Q wave myocardial infarction: FRAX.I.S. (FRAxiparine in Ischaemic Syndrome), (1999) *Eur, Heart J*, 20(21):1553–62.

[39] Cohen, M., *et al.*, (1999) Combination therapy with tirofiban and enoxaparin in acute coronary syndromes. *Int J Cardiol*, 71(3):273–81.

[40] Cohen, M., *et al.*, (2002) Randomized double-blind safety study of enoxaparin versus unfractionated heparin in patients with non-ST-segment elevation acute coronary syndromes treated with tirofiban and aspirin: the ACUTE II study. The Antithrombotic Combination Using Tirofiban and Enoxaparin. *Am Heart J*, 144(3):470–7.

[41] Ferguson, J.J., *et al.*, (2003) Combining enoxaparin and glycoprotein IIb/IIIa antagonists for the treatment of acute coronary syndromes: final results of the National Investigators Collaborating on Enoxaparin-3 (NICE-3) study. *Am Heart J*, 146(4):628–34.

[42] Goodman, S.G., *et al.*, (2003) Randomized evaluation of the safety and efficacy of enoxaparin versus unfractionated heparin in high-risk patients with non-ST-segment elevation acute coronary syndromes receiving the glycoprotein IIb/IIIa inhibitor eptifibatide. *Circulation*, 107(2):238–44.

[43] James, S., *et al.*, (2002) Safety and efficacy of abciximab combined with dalteparin in treatment of acute coronary syndromes. *Eur Heart J*, 23(19):1538–45.

[44] Mukherjee, D., *et al.*, (2002) Promise of combined low-molecular-weight heparin and platelet glycoprotein IIb/IIIa inhibition: results from Platelet IIb/IIIa Antagonist for the Reduction of Acute coronary syndrome events in a Global Organization Network B (PARAGON B). *Am Heart J*, 144(6):995–1002.

[45] Goodman, S.G., *et al.*, (2000) Randomized trial of low molecular weight heparin (enoxaparin) versus unfractionated heparin for unstable coronary artery disease: one-year results of the ESSENCE Study. Efficacy and Safety of Subcutaneous Enoxaparin in Non-Q-Wave Coronary Events. *J Am Coll Cardiol*, 36(3):693–8.

[46] Goodman, S.G., *et al.*, (2000) Low molecular weight heparin decreases rebound ischemia in unstable angina or non-Q-wave myocardial infarction: the Canadian ESSENCE ST segment monitoring substudy. *J Am Coll Cardiol*, 36(5):1507–13.

[47] Michalis, L.K., *et al.*, (2003) Enoxaparin versus tinzaparin in non-ST-segment elevation acute coronary syndromes: the EVET trial. *Am Heart J*, 146(2):304–10.

[48] The FRISC II investigators. (1999) Invasive compared with non-invasive treatment in unstable coronary-artery disease: FRISC II prospective randomised multicentre study. FRagmin and Fast Revascularisation during InStability in Coronary artery disease. *Lancet*, 354(9180):708–15.

[49] Cannon, C.P., *et al.*, (2001) Comparison of early invasive and conservative strategies in patients with unstable coronary syndromes treated with the glycoprotein IIb/IIIa inhibitor tirofiban. *N Eng J Med*, 344(25):1879–87.

[50] Ferguson, J.J., Califf, R.M., Antman, E.M., Cohen, M., Grines, C.L., Goodman, S., Kereiakes, D.J., Langer, A., Mahaffey, K.W., Nessel, C.C., Armstrong, P.W., Avezum, A., Aylward, P., Becker, R.C., Biasucci, L., Borzak, S., Col, J., Frey, M.J., Fry, E., Gulba, D.C., Guneri, S., Gurfinkel, E., Harrington, R., Hochman, J.S., Kleiman, N.S., Leon, M.B., Lopezsendor, J.L., Pepine, C.J., Ruzyllo, W., Steinhubl, S.R., Teirstein, P.S., Toro-Figueroa, L., White, H., (2004) Enoxaparin vs unfractionated heparin in high-risk patients with non-ST-segment elevation acute coronary syndromes managed with an intended early invasive strategy: primary results of the SYNERGY randamized trial. *JAMA*, 292:45–54.

[51] The PURSUIT Trial Investigators, (1998) Inhibition of platelet glycoprotein IIb/IIIa with eptifibatide in patients with acute coronary syndromes. Platelet Glycoprotein IIb/IIIa in Unstable Angina: Receptor Suppression Using Integrilin Therapy. *N Eng J Med*, 339(7):436–43.

[52] Yusuf, S., *et al.*, (2001) Effects of clopidogrel in addition to aspirin in patients with acute coronary syndromes without ST-segment elevation. *N Eng J Med*, 345(7):494–502.

[53] Martin, J.L., *et al.*, (2004) Reliable anticoagulation with enoxaparin in patients undergoing percutaneous coronary intervention: The pharmacokinetics of enoxaparin in PCI (PEPCI) study. *Catheter Cardiovasc Interv*, 61(2):163–70.

[54] The RESTORE investigators, (1997) Effects of platelet glycoprotein IIb/IIIa blockade with tirofiban on adverse cardiac events in patients with unstable angina or acute myocardial infarction undergoing coronary angioplasty. Randomized Efficacy Study of Tirofiban for Outcomes and REstenosis. *Circulation*, 96(5):1445–53.

[55] The PRISM study investigators. (1998) A comparison of aspirin plus tirofiban with aspirin plus heparin for unstable angina. Platelet Receptor Inhibition in Ischemic Syndrome Management (PRISM). *N Eng J Med*, 338(21):1498–505.

[56] The PRISM-PLUS study investigators, (1998) Inhibition of the platelet glycoprotein IIb/IIIa receptor with tirofiban in unstable angina and non-Q-wave myocardial infarction. Platelet Receptor Inhibition in Ischemic Syndrome Management in Patients Limited by Unstable Signs and Symptoms (PRISM-PLUS). *N Eng J Med*, 338(21):1488–97.

[57] Roffi, M., *et al.*, (2001) Platelet glycoprotein IIb/IIIa inhibitors reduce mortality in diabetic patients with non-ST-segment-elevation acute coronary syndromes. *Circulation*, 104(23): 2767–71.

[58] Fox, K.A., *et al.*, (2002) Comparison of enoxaparin versus unfractionated heparin in patients with unstable angina pectoris/non-ST-segment elevation acute myocardial infarction having subsequent percutaneous coronary intervention. *Am J Cardiol*, 90(5):477–82.

[59] Collet, J.P., *et al.*, (2001) Percutaneous coronary intervention after subcutaneous enoxaparin pretreatment in patients with unstable angina pectoris. *Circulation*, 103(5):658–63.

[60] Blazing, M.A., *et al.*, (2004) Safety and efficacy of enoxaparin vs unfractionated heparin in patients with non-ST-segment elevation acute coronary syndromes who receive tirofiban and aspirin: a randomized controlled trial. *JAMA*, 292(1):55–64.

[61] The GUSTO investigators, (1993) An international randomized trial comparing four thrombolytic strategies for acute myocardial infarction. *N Eng J Med*, 329(10):673–82.

[62] The GUSTO III investigators, (1997) A comparison of reteplase with alteplase for acute myocardial infarction. The Global Use of Strategies to Open Occluded Coronary Arteries. *N Eng J Med*, 337(16):1118–23.

[63] The ASSENT-2 investigators, (1999) Single-bolus tenecteplase compared with front loaded alteplase in acute myocardial infarction: the ASSENT-2 double-blind randomised trial. Assessment of the Safety and Efficacy of a New Thrombolytic. *Lancet*, 354(9180):716–22.

[64] Hudson, M.P., *et al.*, (2001) Early reinfarction after fibrinolysis: experience from the global utilization of streptokinase and tissue plasminogen activator (alteplase) for occluded coronary arteries (GUSTO I) and global use of strategies to open occluded coronary arteries (GUSTO III) trials. *Circulation*, 104(11):1229–35.

[65] de Lemos, J.A., *et al.*, (2000) ST-segment resolution and infarct-related artery patency and flow after thrombolytic therapy. Thrombolysis in Myocardial Infarction (TIMI) 14 investigators. *Am J Cardiol*, 85(3):299–304.
[66] Kontny, F., *et al.*, (1997) Randomized trial of low molecular weight heparin (dalteparin) in prevention of left ventricular thrombus formation and arterial embolism after acute anterior myocardial infarction: the Fragmin in Acute Myocardial Infarction (FRAMI) Study. *J Am Coll Cardiol*, 30(4):962–9.
[67] Ross, A.M., *et al.*, (2001) Randomized comparison of enoxaparin, a low-molecular-weight heparin, with unfractionated heparin adjunctive to recombinant tissue plasminogen activator thrombolysis and aspirin: second trial of Heparin and Aspirin Reperfusion Therapy (HART II). *Circulation*, 104(6):648–52.
[68] Antman, E.M., *et al.*, (2002) Enoxaparin as adjunctive antithrombin therapy for ST-elevation myocardial infarction: results of the ENTIRE-Thrombolysis in Myocardial Infarction (TIMI) 23 Trial. *Circulation*, 105(14):1642–9.
[69] Simoons, M., *et al.*, (2002) Improved reperfusion and clinical outcome with enoxaparin as an adjunct to streptokinase thrombolysis in acute myocardial infarction. The AMI-SK study. *Eur Heart J*, 23(16):1282–90.
[70] Frostfeldt, G., *et al.*, (1999) Low molecular weight heparin (dalteparin) as adjuvant treatment of thrombolysis in acute myocardial infarction—a pilot study: biochemical markers in acute coronary syndromes (BIOMACS II). *J Am Coll Cardiol*, 33(3):627–33.
[71] Wallentin, L., *et al.*, (2003) Low molecular weight heparin (dalteparin) compared to unfractionated heparin as an adjunct to rt-PA (alteplase) for improvement of coronary artery patency in acute myocardial infarction-the ASSENT Plus study. *Eur Heart J*, 24(10):897–908.
[72] Tatu-Chitoiu, G., *et al.*, (2003) Efficacy and safety of a new streptokinase regimen with enoxaparin in acute myocardial infarction. *J Thromb Thrombolysis*, 15(3):171–9.
[73] Wallentin, L., *et al.*, (2003) Efficacy and safety of tenecteplase in combination with the low-molecular-weight heparin enoxaparin or unfractionated heparin in the prehospital setting: the Assessment of the Safety and Efficacy of a New Thrombolytic Regimen (ASSENT)-3 PLUS randomized trial in acute myocardial infarction. *Circulation*, 108(2):135–42.
[74] Baird, S.H., *et al.*, (2002) Randomized comparison of enoxaparin with unfractionated heparin following fibrinolytic therapy for acute myocardial infarction. *Eur Heart J*, 23(8): 627–32.
[75] Cohen, M., *et al.*, (2003) The safety and efficacy of subcutaneous enoxaparin versus intravenous unfractionated heparin and tirofiban versus placebo in the treatment of acute ST-segment elevation myocardial infarction patients ineligible for reperfusion (TETAMI): a randomized trial. *J Am Coll Cardiol*, 42(8):1348–56.
[76] Horlander, K.T., Mannino, D.M., Leeper, K.V., (2003) Pulmonary embolism mortality in the United States, 1979–1998: an analysis using multiple-cause mortality data. *Arch Intern Med*, 163(14):1711–17.
[77] Lilienfeld, D.E., (2000) Decreasing mortality from pulmonary embolism in the United States, 1979–1996. *Int J Epidemiol*, 29(3):465–9.
[78] Warkentin, T.E., *et al.*, (1995) Heparin-induced thrombocytopenia in patients treated with low-molecular-weight heparin or unfractionated heparin. *N Eng J Med*, 332(20):1330–5.
[79] Liezorovicz, A., *et al.*, (1991) Prevention of perioperative deep vein thrombosis in general surgery: a multicentre double blind study comparing two doses of Logiparin and standard heparin. H.B.P.M. Research Group. *Br J Surg*, 78(4):412–16.
[80] Nurmohamed, M.T., *et al.*, (1992) Low-molecular-weight heparin versus standard heparin in general and orthopaedic surgery: a meta-analysis. *Lancet*, 340(8812):152–6.
[81] Bergqvist, D., *et al.*, (1996) Low-molecular-weight heparin (enoxaparin) as prophylaxis against venous thromboembolism after total hip replacement. *N Eng J Med*, 335(10):696–700.
[82] Eriksson, B.I., *et al.*, (1991) Prevention of deep-vein thrombosis and pulmonary embolism after total hip replacement. Comparison of low-molecular-weight heparin and unfractionated heparin. *J Bone Joint Surg Am*, 73(4):484–93.
[83] Levine, M.N., *et al.*, (1991) Prevention of deep vein thrombosis after elective hip surgery. A randomized trial comparing low molecular weight heparin with standard unfractionated heparin. *Ann Intern Med*, 114(7):545–51.

[84] Leyvraz, P.F., *et al.*, (1991) Prevention of deep vein thrombosis after hip replacement: randomised comparison between unfractionated heparin and low molecular weight heparin. *Br Med J*, 303(6802):543–8.
[85] The German Hip Arthroplasty Trial (GHAT) Group, (1992) Prevention of deep vein thrombosis with low molecular-weight heparin in patients undergoing total hip replacement. A randomized trial. *Arch Orthop Trauma Surg*, 111(2):110–20.
[86] Hull, R., *et al.*, (1993) A comparison of subcutaneous low-molecular-weight heparin with warfarin sodium for prophylaxis against deep-vein thrombosis after hip or knee implantation. *N Eng J Med*, 329(19):1370–6.
[87] Torholm, C., *et al.*, (1991) Thromboprophylaxis by low-molecular-weight heparin in elective hip surgery. A placebo controlled study. *J Bone Joint Surg Br*, 73(3):434–8.
[88] Hull, R.D., *et al.*, (2000) Low-molecular-weight heparin prophylaxis using dalteparin extended out-of-hospital vs in-hospital warfarin/out-of-hospital placebo in hip arthroplasty patients: a double-blind, randomized comparison. North American Fragmin Trial Investigators. *Arch Intern Med*, 160(14):2208–15.
[89] Planes, A., *et al.*, (1996) Risk of deep-venous thrombosis after hospital discharge in patients having undergone total hip replacement: double-blind randomised comparison of enoxaparin versus placebo. *Lancet*, 348(9022):224–8.
[90] Colwell, C.W., Jr., *et al.*, (1999) Comparison of enoxaparin and warfarin for the prevention of venous thromboembolic disease after total hip arthroplasty. Evaluation during hospitalization and three months after discharge. *J Bone Joint Surg Am*, 81(7):932–40.
[91] Sarasin, F.P., Bounameaux, H., (2002) Out of hospital antithrombotic prophylaxis after total hip replacement: low-molecular-weight heparin, warfarin, aspirin or nothing? A cost-effectiveness analysis. *Thromb Haemost*, 87(4):586–92.
[92] Leclerc, J.R., *et al.*, (1992) Prevention of deep vein thrombosis after major knee surgery—a randomized, double-blind trial comparing a low molecular weight heparin fragment (enoxaparin) to placebo. *Thromb Haemost*, 67(4):417–23.
[93] Levine, M.N., *et al.*, (1996) Ardeparin (low-molecular-weight heparin) vs graduated compression stockings for the prevention of venous thromboembolism. A randomized trial in patients undergoing knee surgery. *Arch Intern Med*, 156(8):851–6.
[94] Brookenthal, K.R., *et al.*, (2001) A meta-analysis of thromboembolic prophylaxis in total knee arthroplasty. *J Arthroplasty*, 16(3):293–300.
[95] Leclerc, J.R., *et al.*, (1996) Prevention of venous thromboembolism after knee arthroplasty. A randomized, double-blind trial comparing enoxaparin with warfarin. *Ann Intern Med*, 124(7):619–26.
[96] Heit, J.A., *et al.*, (1997) Efficacy and safety of low molecular weight heparin (ardeparin sodium) compared to warfarin for the prevention of venous thromboembolism after total knee replacement surgery: a double-blind, dose-ranging study. Ardeparin Arthroplasty Study Group. *Thromb Haemost*, 77(1):32–8.
[97] Fitzgerald, R.H., Jr., *et al.*, (2001) Prevention of venous thromboembolic disease following primary total knee arthroplasty. A randomized, multicenter, open-label, parallel-group comparison of enoxaparin and warfarin. *J Bone Joint Surg Am*, 83-A(6):900–6.
[98] Heit, J.A., (2001) Low-molecular-weight heparin: the optimal duration of prophylaxis against postoperative venous thromboembolism after total hip or knee replacement. *Thromb Res*, 101(1):V163–73.
[99] Merli, G.J., *et al.*, (1993) Etiology, incidence, and prevention of deep vein thrombosis in acute spinal cord injury. *Arch Phys Med Rehabil*, 74(11):1199–205.
[100] Green, D., (1991) Prevention of thromboembolism after spinal cord injury. *Semin Thromb Hemost*, 17(4):347–50.
[101] Green, D., *et al.*, (1990) Prevention of thromboembolism after spinal cord injury using low-molecular-weight heparin. *Ann Intern Med*, 113(8):571–4.
[102] Spinal cord injury thromboprophylaxis investigators, (2003) Prevention of venous thromboembolism in the acute treatment phase after spinal cord injury: a randomized, multicenter trial comparing low-dose heparin plus intermittent pneumatic compression with enoxaparin. *J Trauma*, 54(6):1116–24; discussion 1125–6.

[103] Spinal cord injury thromboprophylaxis investigators, (2003) Prevention of venous thromboembolism in the rehabilitation phase after spinal cord injury: prophylaxis with low-dose heparin or enoxaparin. *J Trauma*, 54(6):1111–15.

[104] Geerts, W.H., *et al.*, (1994) A prospective study of venous thromboembolism after major trauma. *N Eng J Med*, 331(24):1601–6.

[105] Geerts, W.H., *et al.*, (1996) A comparison of low-dose heparin with low-molecular-weight heparin as prophylaxis against venous thromboembolism after major trauma. *N Eng J Med*, 335(10):701–7.

[106] Ginzburg, E., *et al.*, (2003) Randomized clinical trial of intermittent pneumatic compression and low molecular weight heparin in trauma. *Br J Surg*, 90(11):1338–44.

[107] Alikhan, R., *et al.*, (2004) Risk factors for venous thromboembolism in hospitalized patients with acute medical illness: analysis of the MEDENOX Study. *Arch Intern Med*, 164(9):963–8.

[108] Samama, M.M., *et al.*, (1999) A comparison of enoxaparin with placebo for the prevention of venous thromboembolism in acutely ill medical patients. Prophylaxis in Medical Patients with Enoxaparin Study Group. *N Eng J Med*, 341(11):793–800.

[109] Alikhan, R., *et al.*, (2003) Prevention of venous thromboembolism in medical patients with enoxaparin: a subgroup analysis of the MEDENOX study. *Blood Coagul Fibrinolysis*, 14(4):341–6.

[110] Mismetti, P., *et al.*, (2000) Prevention of venous thromboembolism in internal medicine with unfractionated or low-molecular-weight heparins: a meta-analysis of randomised clinical trials. *Thromb Haemost*, 83(1):14–19.

[111] Levine, M., *et al.*, (1996) A comparison of low-molecular-weight heparin administered primarily at home with unfractionated heparin administered in the hospital for proximal deep-vein thrombosis. *N Eng J Med*, 334(11):677–81.

[112] Koopman, M.M., *et al.*, (1996) Treatment of venous thrombosis with intravenous unfractionated heparin administered in the hospital as compared with subcutaneous low-molecular-weight heparin administered at home. The Tasman Study Group. *N Eng J Med*, 334(11):682–7.

[113] Veiga, F., *et al.*, (2000) Low molecular weight heparin (enoxaparin) versus oral anticoagulant therapy (acenocoumarol) in the long-term treatment of deep venous thrombosis in the elderly: a randomized trial. *Thromb Haemost*, 84(4):559–64.

[114] Lee, A.Y., *et al.*, (2003) Low-molecular-weight heparin versus a coumarin for the prevention of recurrent venous thromboembolism in patients with cancer. *N Eng J Med*, 349(2):146–53.

[115] Bick, R.L., Rice, J., (1999) Long-term outpatient dalteparin (fragmin) therapy for arterial and venous thrombosis: efficacy and safety–a preliminary report. *Clin Appl Thromb Hemost*, 5 Suppl 1:S67–71.

[116] Luk, C., *et al.*, (2001) Extended outpatient therapy with low molecular weight heparin for the treatment of recurrent venous thromboembolism despite warfarin therapy. *Am J Med*, 111(4):270–3.

[117] Breddin, H.K., *et al.*, (2001) Effects of a low-molecular-weight heparin on thrombus regression and recurrent thromboembolism in patients with deep-vein thrombosis. *N Eng J Med*, 344(9):626–31.

[118] Simonneau, G., *et al.*, (1993) Subcutaneous low-molecular-weight heparin compared with continuous intravenous unfractionated heparin in the treatment of proximal deep vein thrombosis. *Arch Intern Med*, 153(13):1541–6.

[119] Lindmarker, P., *et al.*, (1994) Comparison of once-daily subcutaneous Fragmin with continuous intravenous unfractionated heparin in the treatment of deep vein thrombosis. *Thromb Haemost*, 72(2):186–90.

[120] Gould, M.K., *et al.*, (1999) Low-molecular-weight heparins compared with unfractionated heparin for treatment of acute deep venous thrombosis. A meta-analysis of randomized, controlled trials. *Ann Intern Med*, 130(10):800–9.

[121] Gould, M.K., *et al.*, (1999) Low-molecular-weight heparins compared with unfractionated heparin for treatment of acute deep venous thrombosis. A cost-effectiveness analysis. *Ann Intern Med*, 130(10):789–99.

[122] O'Brien, B., *et al.*, (1999) Economic evaluation of outpatient treatment with low-molecular-weight heparin for proximal vein thrombosis. *Arch Intern Med*, 159(19): 2298–304.

[123] Kovacs, M.J., *et al.*, (2000) Outpatient treatment of pulmonary embolism with dalteparin. *Thromb Haemost*, 83(2):209–11.

[124] The Columbus Investigators, (1997) Low-molecular-weight heparin in the treatment of patients with venous thromboembolism. *N Eng J Med*, 337(10):657–62.

[125] Simonneau, G., *et al.*, (1997) A comparison of low-molecular-weight heparin with unfractionated heparin for acute pulmonary embolism. The THESEE Study Group. Tinzaparine ou Heparine Standard: Evaluations dans l'Embolie Pulmonaire. *N Eng J Med*, 337(10):663–9.

[126] Hull, R.D., *et al.*, (2000) Low-molecular-weight heparin vs heparin in the treatment of patients with pulmonary embolism. American-Canadian Thrombosis Study Group. *Arch Intern Med*, 160(2):229–36.

[127] Dolovich, L.R., *et al.*, (2000) A meta-analysis comparing low-molecular-weight heparins with unfractionated heparin in the treatment of venous thromboembolism: examining some unanswered questions regarding location of treatment, product type, and dosing frequency. *Arch Intern Med*, 160(2):181–8.

[128] Farooq, V., *et al.*, (2001) Serious adverse incidents with the usage of low molecular weight heparins in patients with chronic kidney disease. *Am J Kidney Dis*, 43(3):531–7.

[129] Collet, J.P., *et al.*, (2001) Enoxaparin in unstable angina patients with renal failure. *Int J Cardiol*, 80(1):81–2.

[130] Chow, S.L., *et al.*, (2003) Correlation of antifactor Xa concentrations with renal function in patients on enoxaparin. *J Clin Pharmacol*, 43(6):586–90.

[131] Hunt, B.J., *et al.*, (1997) Thromboprophylaxis with low molecular weight heparin (Fragmin) in high risk pregnancies. *Thromb Haemost*, 77(1):39–43.

[132] Pettila, V., *et al.*, (1999) Thromboprophylaxis with low molecular weight heparin (dalteparin) in pregnancy. *Thromb Res*, 96(4):275–82.

[133] Jacobsen, A.F., Qvigstad, E., Sandset, P.M., (2003) Low molecular weight heparin (dalteparin) for the treatment of venous thromboembolism in pregnancy. *Br J Obstet Gynaecol*, 110(2): 139–44.

[134] Casele, H.L., *et al.*, (1999) Changes in the pharmacokinetics of the low-molecular-weight heparin enoxaparin sodium during pregnancy. *Am J Obstet Gynecol*, 181(5 Pt 1):1113–17.

[135] Ginsberg, J.S., *et al.*, (2003) Anticoagulation of pregnant women with mechanical heart valves. *Arch Intern Med*, 163(6):694–8.

[136] Leyh, R.G., *et al.*, (2002) Anticoagulation for prosthetic heart valves during pregnancy: is low-molecular-weight heparin an alternative? *Eur J Cardiothorac Surg*, 21(3):577–9.

[137] Bang, C.J., Berstad, A., Talstad, I., (1991) Incomplete reversal of enoxaparin-induced bleeding by protamine sulfate. *Haemostasis*, 21(3):155–60.

[138] Holst, J., *et al.*, (1994) Protamine neutralization of intravenous and subcutaneous low-molecular-weight heparin (tinzaparin, Logiparin). An experimental investigation in healthy volunteers. *Blood Coagul Fibrinolysis*, 5(5):795–803.

[139] Crowther, M.A., *et al.*, (2002) Mechanisms responsible for the failure of protamine to inactivate low-molecular-weight heparin. *Br J Haematol*, 116(1):178–86.

[140] Van Ryn-McKenna, J., *et al.*, (1990) Neutralization of enoxaparine-induced bleeding by protamine sulfate. *Thromb Haemost*, 63(2):271–4.

[141] Sandset, P.M., Bendz, B., Hansen, J.B., (2000) Physiological function of tissue factor pathway inhibitor and interaction with heparins. *Haemostasis*, 30 Suppl 2:48–56.

[142] Merlini, P.A., *et al.*, (2000) In vivo thrombin generation and activity during and after intravenous infusion of heparin or recombinant hirudin in patients with unstable angina pectoris. *Arterioscler Thromb Vasc Biol*, 20(9):2162–6.

[143] Ernofsson, M., *et al.*, (1998) Low-molecular weight heparin reduces the generation and activity of thrombin in unstable coronary artery disease. *Thromb Haemost*, 79(3): 491–4.

[144] Cella, G., Girolami, A., Sasahara, A.A., (1999) Platelet activation with unfractionated heparin at therapeutic concentrations and comparison with low-molecular-weight heparin and with a direct thrombin inhibitor. *Circulation*, 99(25):3323.

[145] Montalescot, G., *et al.*, (1998) Early increase of von Willebrand factor predicts adverse outcome in unstable coronary artery disease: beneficial effects of enoxaparin. French Investigators of the ESSENCE Trial. *Circulation*, 98(4):294–9.

[146] Klein, W., *et al.*, (1997) Fragmin in unstable angina pectoris or in non-Q-wave acute myocardial infarction (the FRIC Study). *Am J Cardiol*, 80(5A):30E–4E.
[147] Antman, E.M., Morrow, D. A., McCabe, C.H., Murphy, S.A., Ruda, M., Sadowski, Z., Budaj, A., Lopez-Sendon, J.C., Guneri, S., Jiang, F., White, H.D., Fox, K.A., Braunwald, E., (2006) Enoxaparin versus Unfractionated Heparin with Fibrinolysis for ST-Elevation Myocardial Infarction. *N Eng J Med*, 354(14):1477–88.
[148] Gallus, A.S., Salzman, E.W., Hirsch, J., (1994) Prevention of VTE, in *Hemostasis and thrombosis: basic principles and clinical practice* (eds R.W. Colman, J. Hirsch, V.J. Marder), JB Lippincott: Philadelphia, PA. 1331–45.

7 Direct Thrombin Inhibitors

7.1 INTRODUCTION

Thrombin plays a pivotal role in the pathogenesis of arterial and venous thrombosis, serving both as a key enzyme in the soluble coagulation cascade and as a potent activator of platelets, vascular smooth muscle cells and inflammatory leukocytes [1]. Exposure of subendothelial components at sites of vascular injury leads to platelet adhesion and activation, release of tissue factor and initiation of the coagulation cascade, with local conversion of a small quantities of prothrombin to thrombin [2]. This small amount of thrombin then amplifies its own generation by activating platelets and factors V, VIII and XI, leading to formation of the prothrombinase complex on the platelet phospholipid surface and production of a burst of thrombin. Thrombin acts as the terminal enzyme at the convergence of both the classic intrinsic and extrinsic coagulation cascades, converting fibrinogen to fibrin and cross-linking the fibrin mesh through activation of factor XIII. Moreover, thrombin is a key component of the cellular processes of thrombosis, activating platelets through protease-activated receptors (PARs) which mediate shape-change and secretion of thromboxane, serotonin and ADP. Thrombin also activates the cell-surface GP IIb/IIIa integrin receptor, which binds circulating fibrinogen or vWF as the final common pathway of platelet aggregation. Other cellular interactions with thrombin include changes in endothelial vasoreactivity, proliferation of smooth muscle cells, stimulation of cytokine release from inflammatory cells and enhancement of leukocyte and monocyte chemotaxis.

The multifaceted effects of thrombin provide rationale for the central role of thrombin inhibition in effective anticoagulation strategies for vascular diseases. The thrombin molecule has at least three domains that are relevant to the activities of AT agents: the active catalytic site and two exosites at opposite poles of the enzyme. Exosite-1 is the substrate recognition domain, which binds and aligns appropriate peptide bonds to the catalytic regions of the molecule, while exosite-2 is the heparin-binding site.

Heparin, the traditional and most widely used antithrombotic agent, is a mixture of glycosaminoglycan molecules of various polysaccharide chain lengths [3]. Heparin binds to an endogenous anticoagulant known as AT (formerly, antithrombin III), an inhibitor of various serine proteases in the coagulation cascade (Figure 7.1). The interaction between heparin and AT induces a conformation change which increases the activity of AT by several thousand-fold. Subsequently, the heparin–AT complex binds to and inactivates thrombin (as well as other coagulation proteins including factors X, IX and VII). Although heparin is an effective anticoagulant, it has several important limitations (Table 7.1) [4–8]. First, its pharmacokinetics are non-linear, as it binds to a variety of plasma proteins and vascular receptors, which results in unpredictable variability in interpatient and intrapatient dosing. Second, the animal source and manufacturing processes influence the mixture of various

Management Strategies in Antithrombotic Therapy Arman T. Askari, Adrian W. Messerli and A. Michael Lincoff

Table 7.1 Comparison of heparin and DTIs

UH	DTIs
Indirectly (via antithrombin cofactor) inhibits thrombin	Directly inhibits thrombin without cofactor
Reduced potency with AT cofactor deficiency	No dependence upon cofactor
Unable to inhibit thrombin bound to fibrin clot because of steric hindrance	Inhibits thrombin bound to fibrin clot
Unpredictable bioavailability owing to non-specific binding to circulating or vascular proteins	Little or no non-specific binding
Variable potency depending upon distribution of molecular size in natural mixture	Consistent potency
Inhibited by platelet factor 4 and other circulating inhibitors	No circulating inhibitors
Activates platelets	No platelet activation. Inhibits thrombin-mediated pathway of platelet activation
Antibody-mediated HITS	No HIT or cross-reaction with HITS antibodies

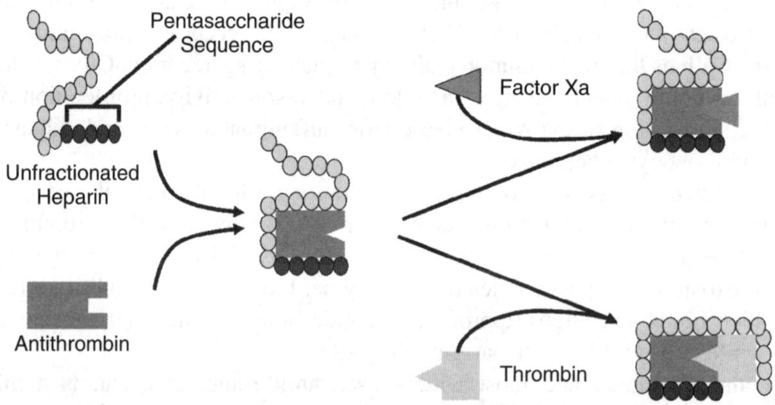

Figure 7.1 Mechanism of action of UH. Interaction of UH with AT is mediated by the pentasaccharide sequence of the drugs. Binding to AT causes a conformational change at its reactive center that accelerates its interaction with factor Xa or thrombin. Adapted from Weitz [53]. A full colour version of this figure can be found in the colour plate section of this book.

size molecules, only one-third of which typically have the unique pentasaccharide sequence necessary for interaction with AT, resulting in variable potency of different preparations. Third, as an indirect thrombin inhibitor, heparin's anticoagulant activity may be impaired in states of AT deficiency [9]. Fourth, heparin is subject to neutralization by various circulating inhibitors, including platelet factor 4 which interferes with the attachment of heparin to AT [10]. Fifth, distinct from its AT effect, heparin also increases the affinity of interaction between thrombin and fibrin by simultaneously binding exosite-2 and fibrin to bridge the two molecules; thrombin thus protected within a fibrin clot cannot be inhibited by the heparin–AT complex owing to the inaccessibility of exosite-2 [4, 11]. This clot-bound thrombin continues to exert a procoagulant and platelet-activating effect. Sixth, heparin itself appears to activate platelets to some extent through a variety of potential mechanisms [8], an effect which has been demonstrated in patients receiving this agent for clinical indications. Seventh, heparin can induce an immunologically mediated HIT in up to 5% of patients, resulting in a paradoxical prothrombotic state [12]. These limitations have prompted investigation of alternative anticoagulants which can more optimally inhibit thrombin's procoagulant effects while simultaneously possessing more favorable pharmacodynamic and pharmacokinetic profiles than heparin.

7.2 OVERVIEW OF DTIs

The DTIs have been developed as an alternative to overcome the limitations of heparin in thrombotic disorders (Table 7.2). Unlike the indirect thrombin inhibitor heparin, DTIs by definition directly bind to and inactivate thrombin [1]. The prototype DTI is hirudin, a molecule derived from the saliva of the medicinal leech (*Hirudo medicinalis*) and the most potent known natural inhibitor of thrombin. Other DTIs under investigation or in clinical use have been synthesized to model the structure or activity of hirudin and have different pharmacokinetic and pharmacodynamic profiles. Bivalent DTIs bind to and block both the active catalytic and the substrate recognition (exosite-1) sites of thrombin, whereas univalent DTIs interact with only the catalytic site (or less commonly with exosite-1) (Figure 7.2).

DTIs have several theoretical advantages over heparin (Table 7.1). Most of these agents do not bind non-specifically to plasma proteins or immobilized receptors, and should thus have more predictable pharmacokinetics and anticoagulant response. There are no known circulating inhibitors of DTIs, nor are they dependent upon the availability or activity of a

Table 7.2 Properties of parenteral DTIs: hirudin, bivalirudin, and argatroban

	Hirudin	Bivalirudin	Argatroban
Type of molecule	65 amino acid polypeptide	20 amino acid peptide	synthetic arginine derivative
Mass (Da)	7000	1980	527
Thrombin binding sites	catalytic, exosite I	catalytic, exosite I	catalytic
Thrombin binding kinetics	irreversible	reversible on proteolytic cleavage	reversible, competitive
Clearance	renal	predominantly endogenous circulating peptidases, minor renal	hepatic
Elimination half-life	60 min	25 min	54 min
Produces antibodies?	yes	no	no

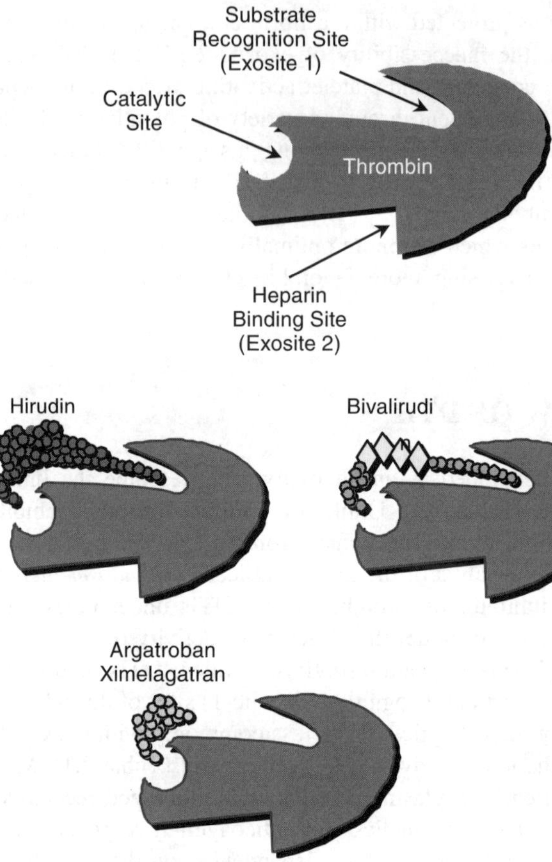

Figure 7.2 Schematic representation of thrombin, showing the different binding patterns of bivalent (hirudin and bivalirudin) and univalent (argatroban and ximelagatran) DTIs. A full colour version of this figure can be found in the colour plate section of this book.

cofactor. They are not subject to the steric hindrance of the heparin–AT complex and are thus able to inactivate clot-bound thrombin. DTIs do not stimulate platelets and, on the contrary, attenuate the potent thrombin-mediated pathway of platelet activation. Finally, they do not cause immune-mediated thrombocytopenia.

In vitro experiments or studies in animal models suggested that DTIs would have superior efficacy compared with heparin in preventing or treating arterial or venous thrombosis in a variety of clinical settings, and preliminary studies in patients seemed similarly promising. The results of large-scale trials during the early 1990s among patients with UA or MI were largely disappointing, however, with DTIs demonstrating only marginal benefit over heparin with regard to protection against ischemic events although with evidence of increased hemorrhagic risk. Clinical use of these agents was thus confined initially to treatment of patients with HIT. More recently, randomized trials have demonstrated the efficacy of at least one of the DTIs as an antithrombotic during percutaneous coronary revascularization, leading to its widespread use as a replacement for heparin and GP IIb/IIIa antagonists in this setting. Ongoing studies are now testing these agents in the contemporary management of acute coronary syndromes, cardiac surgery, atrial fibrillation and venous thromboembolic disorders.

SPECIFIC DTIs

Hirudin is a 65-amino-acid polypeptide (MW 7000 Da) which bivalently binds to thrombin in a 1:1 stoichiometric ratio with very high affinity [1, 13]. This tight binding of hirudin to the thrombin molecule is essentially irreversible. Although hirudin was originally derived from leech saliva, a recombinant form of this agent, *lepirudin*, is now used. Hirudin is cleared or degraded nearly exclusively by the kidneys and has a half-life of approximately 60 min. Systemic clearance can be prolonged for up to several days in states of renal insufficiency. Hirudin is usually administered intravenously, although it has nearly 100% bioavailability after SC injection. Plasma concentrations and aPTTs increase proportionally with intravenous dosing over a range 0.1–0.4 mg/kg. Infusion doses are adjusted to achieve an aPTT ratio of 1.5–2.5 times control; reductions in maintenance dose are required for moderate renal insufficiency, and this agent is contraindicated for patients with creatinine clearance <15 mL/min. Formation of antibodies directed against hirudin have been detected in up to 40% of treated patients, and anaphylactic reactions have been reported. There is some evidence that antihirudin antibodies may prolong its active half-life, leading to drug accumulation. Hirudin is approved for the treatment of HIT.

Bivalirudin (a member of the class of peptides known as hirulogs) is a 20-amino-acid synthetic analog of hirudin (MW 1980 Da), which also bivalently inhibits both the catalytic and substrate recognition sites of thrombin [1, 13, 14). Although the bivalirudin molecule binds with high affinity to thrombin, bivalirudin complexed with thrombin is then cleaved into two fragments by thrombin itself at an arginine–proline bond. These two fragments of bivalirudin only weakly interact with thrombin and lose the ability to block the active site. In contrast to hirudin, then, bivalirudin exhibits reversible pharmacodynamics in its inhibition of thrombin. Plasma levels are linearly related to IV dose, with a half-life of approximately 25 min. As bivalirudin is degraded predominantly by endogenous peptidases in the blood, its clearance is only modestly prolonged by renal insufficiency and dosage adjustments are recommended only for those with moderate to severe renal impairment, although the correlation between the extent of AT activity and ACT values appears weak at high levels of anticoagulation. Antibody or immunologic responses to bivalirudin have not been observed. Bivalirudin is approved for use during percutaneous coronary revascularization.

Argatroban is a synthetic small-molecule derivative of L-arginine. It is a reversible univalent thrombin inhibitor, competitively binding to only the active catalytic site. Unlike hirudin or bivalirudin, approximately half of the intravenous argatroban dose binds to human serum proteins. Argatroban is cleared entirely through hepatic metabolism via pathways that utilize CYP isoenzymes CYP3A4 and CYP3A5 and produce at least four metabolites with varying degrees of anticoagulant activity. Steady-state plasma concentrations are proportional to intravenous dose, and the half-life of argatroban is approximately 54 min. Hepatic impairment is associated with marked reductions in argatroban clearance rates and increases in half-life; renal insufficiency has been shown to have no effect on the pharmacokinetics. ACT and aPTT can be used to measure argatroban's anticoagulant effects, although the strength of correlation between these assays and argatroban concentration is not defined. Argatroban has not been associated with immune-mediated responses in humans. This agent is approved for the treatment of patients with HIT. Other univalent inhibitors of the thrombin active site (*inogatran*) or of exosite-1 (*efegatran*) have been evaluated in early trials but are not under current investigation or available for clinical use [1, 13].

Ximelagatran is the first orally-available direct thrombin inhibitor. It is a pro-drug, which after oral administration is metabolized via esterases to *melagatran*, a competitive univalent inhibitor of the thrombin active enzymatic site [15]. The hepatic P450 enzymes do not participate to an appreciable extent in this pathway of activation, and pharmacokinetics are unaffected by hepatic impairment. Oral bioavailability is approximately 20%. Melagatran is excreted unchanged in the urine with a half-life of 5 h, and clearance is prolonged in patients with renal insufficiency. aPTT can be used to monitor the AT effect of melagatran, although the relationship is non-linear. After oral administration of ximelagatran, aPTT begins to prolong within 20 min, reaches its peak after approximately 2 h, and returns to baseline by 12 h. Ximelagatran has been evaluated in large-scale clinical trials with twice-daily dosing in the settings of venous thromboembolic disease and atrial fibrillation. Despite evidence of clinical efficacy in these investigations and approval by European regulatory agencies in 2003, application for license in the United States was denied by the FDA in 2004 on the basis of the unpredictable occurrence of severe liver injury with ximelagatran therapy. In the pooled trial experience of ~13,000 patients, significant increases in transaminase and bilirubin levels occurred despite routine monitoring in 0.5% of patients (RR = 6.6 compared with warfarin), one-tenth of whom died of causes related to their hepatic failure. Thus, no orally available DIT is currently available in the United States, although other agents are under development.

7.3 CLINICAL USES OF DTIs

DTIs IN ACS

Thrombosis plays a central role in the pathogenesis and complications of ACS – UA and acute MI. Erosion or rupture of the fibrous cap overlying atherosclerotic plaque in the coronary artery leads to exposure of subendothelial components, platelet deposition and activation, local generation of large quantities of thrombin and formation of the platelet-rich fibrin clot. Thrombus formed at the site of plaque rupture may become partially or completely occlusive, leading to downstream myocardial ischemia or infarction. Additionally, embolization of activated platelet–fibrin aggregates impair distal microvascular perfusion through physical obstruction and/or release of platelet vasoconstrictive substances. Antithrombotic agents are the only pharmacologic interventions which have been shown to improve short-term outcome with regard to 'hard' clinical events such as death and myocardial (re-) infarction among patients with ACS.

Acute STEMI

In the majority of patients with acute STEMI, coronary thrombosis will be found to be completely occlusive [16], an observation which led to the paradigm of immediate reperfusion therapy to limit myocardial necrosis, improve ventricular function and reduce subsequent mortality. Adjunctive antiplatelet and AT agents are used to enhance the efficacy of fibrinolytic therapies by accelerating or improving the quality of clot dissolution and by preventing thrombotic reocclusion. Although never subjected to rigorous large-scale randomized trials, heparin is typically administered intravenously for 1–2 days after fibrinolytic therapy with second- and third-generation agents (t-PA, reteplase or TNK) and variably with SK. In animal models of coronary occlusion, administration of hirudin with t-PA was associated with more rapid and complete restoration of coronary blood flow and less cyclical reflow or reocclusion than was heparin [17]. After preliminary clinical studies suggesting the safety of direct thrombin inhibitors with fibrinolysis in this setting, three large-scale randomized trials of hirudin versus heparin were undertaken nearly simultaneously among patients with acute MI: GUSTO-II [18], TIMI 9 [19], and HIT-III trials [20]. These trials were terminated earlier than planned, however, after interim analyses demonstrated higher than expected hemorrhagic rates in the hirudin arms of these studies. Of most concern was the elevated incidence of intracranial bleeding, 1.7–1.8% with hirudin and fibrinolysis in GUSTO-II and TIMI 9, compared with an expected rate of approximately 0.7% from prior large-scale trials of t-PA and SK with heparin. The GUSTO-II and TIMI 9 trials were restarted and successfully completed using substantially lower doses of hirudin (0.6 mg/kg bolus and 0.2 mg/kg per h infusion reduced to 0.1 mg/kg bolus and 0.1 mg/kg per h infusion) [21,22]. GUSTO-IIb enrolled 12,142 patients, of whom 4131 had STEMI (and 8011 had UA or non-Q-wave infarction), while TIMI 9b included 3002 patients, all of whom were treated with fibrinolysis for acute MI (Table 7.3). Although hemorrhagic stroke rates were not elevated by hirudin at the doses used in these trials, significant reductions in ischemic events were not achieved with hirudin compared with heparin. Rates of death or myocardial re-infarction

Table 7.3 Major trials of DTIs in STEMI

		TIMI 9B	GUSTO IIb	HERO-2
Number of patients		3002	4131	17,073
DTI		Hirudin	Hirudin	Bivalirudin
Dose	DTI	0.1 mg/kg bolus 0.1 mg/kg per h×4 days	0.1 mg/kg bolus 0.1 mg/kg per h×3-5 days	0.25 mg/kg bolus 0.5 mg/kg per h×12 h, then 0.25 mg/kg-hr×36 h
	UFH	5000 U bolus 1000 U/h×4 days, aPTT = 55–85 s	5000 U bolus 1000 U/h×3–5 days, aPTT = 60–85 s	5000 U bolus 1000 U/h×48 h, aPTT = 50–75 sec
Fibrinolytic agent		TPA – 64% SK – 36%	TPA – 69% SK – 31%	SK – 100%
Endpoint follow-up		30 days	30 days	96 h
Death (%)	DTI	6.1	5.9	10.8
	UFH	5.0	6.2	10.9
Reinfarction (%)	DTI	4.3	5.0	1.6*
	UFH	5.0	6.0	2.3*
Death or reinfarction (%)	DTI	9.7	9.9	12.6
	UFH	9.3	11.3	13.6
Intracranial hemorrhage (%, in-hospital)	DTI	0.4	0.5	0.6
	UFH	0.7	0.4	0.4
Major bleeding (%, in-hospital)	DTI	3.4	1.1	0.7
	UFH	3.8	1.5	0.5

All p-values = N.S. except *p-value = 0.001

GUSTO = Global Use of Strategies to Open Occluded Coronary Arteries [21]; HERO = Hirulog and Early Reperfusion or Occlusion [23]; TIMI = Thrombolysis and Thrombin Inhibition in Myocardial Infarction [22]

by 30 days among patients with ST elevation in the hirudin vs heparin arms were 9.9% vs 11.3% (p-value = 0.13) in GUSTO-IIb and 9.7% vs 9.5% in TIMI 9B. These disappointing results were amplified by the finding that non-intracranial bleeding events tended to be more frequent with hirudin in these trials, suggesting a narrower than expected therapeutic window with this agent. More recently, the HERO-2 trial demonstrated analogous findings with bivalirudin vs heparin among over 17,000 patients receiving SK for acute MI [23]. Mortality was not improved and bleeding rates were increased among those randomized to bivalirudin, although myocardial re-infarction rates were reduced (2.3% vs 1.6%, p-value = 0.001) in a pattern similar to a trend observed with hirudin in GUSTO-IIb (Table 7.3).

NSTEMI/UA

For patients with acute coronary syndromes without ST segment elevation (UA or 'non-Q-wave' MI), coronary thrombosis is usually not totally occlusive and fibrinolytic therapy has not been shown to provide clinical benefit. In contrast, results of large-scale clinical trials have convincingly demonstrated reductions in ischemic complications rates with antithrombotic therapy with aspirin, thienopyridines, platelet GP IIb/IIIa receptor antagonists, and UH or LMWH. The mechanisms of benefit with these agents in the non-ST-elevation ACS population likely relate to prevention of clot propagation and reduction in distal microvascular embolization.

Phase II studies of hirudin, bivalirudin and argatroban among patients with non-ST-elevation ACS suggested efficacy at least equivalent to that of heparin, with more consistent therapeutic levels of anticoagulation. Only hirudin, however, has thus far been assessed in large-scale pivotal trials, with results that were similar to those in the setting of acute MI (Table 7.4). Among the 8011 patients in the GUSTO-IIb cohort with UA or NSTEMI, rates of death or MI by 30 days were 8.3% vs 9.1% in the hirudin vs heparin arms, respectively (p-value = NS) [21]. Bleeding and transfusion rates were higher with hirudin, and there was a trend toward more frequent intracranial hemorrhages, despite the lack of concomitant fibrinolytic therapy in this group of patients. In the subsequent OASIS-2 trial [24], a higher dose of hirudin (0.4 mg/kg bolus and 0.15 mg/kg per h infusion) was found to have marginal benefit over heparin among 10,141 patients with non-ST-segment ACS: rates of death or MI at 35 days were 6.8% vs 7.7%, respectively (p-value = 0.06). This slight difference in ischemic event rates, however, was again associated with an increased risk of major bleeding complications (1.2% vs 0.7%, p-value = 0.01).

A meta-analysis has been reported of the principal results of 11 trials randomizing in total almost 36,000 patients to DTIs versus heparin for the treatment of ACS [25]. Although the trials used for the analysis included studies of balloon angioplasty during UA (discussed in more detail later), the majority of patients (30,517 of 35,970) had been enrolled in trials of predominantly medical management for acute MI or non-ST-elevation ACS. No differences in mortality or stroke were observed between the treatment regimens, although DTI therapy was associated with an absolute 0.7% reduction (7 events prevented per 1000 patients treated) in the risk of MI which emerged during study drug infusion and was maintained for up to 6 months thereafter. Clinical benefit was seen with bivalent DTIs (hirudin and bivalirudin) but not with univalent inhibitors (argatroban, efegatran, and inogatran). Notably, there was significant heterogeneity in the effect of different DTIs on major bleeding: hirudin was associated with a significant increase in bleeding risk relative

Table 7.4 Major trials of DTIs in non-ST-elevation ACS

		GUSTO IIb	OASIS-2
Number of patients		8011	10,141
DTI		Hirudin	Hirudin
Dose	DTI	0.1 mg/kg bolus 0.1 mg/kg per h × 3–5 days	0.4 mg/kg bolus 0.15 mg/kg per h × 3 days
	UFH	5000 U bolus 1000 U/h × 3–5 days, aPTT = 60–85 s	5000 U bolus 15 U/kg per h × 3 days, aPTT = 60–105 s
Endpoint follow-up		30 days	7 days
Death (%)	DTI	3.7	NR
	UFH	3.9	NR
Reinfarction (%)	DTI	5.6	NR
	UFH	6.4	NR
Death or reinfarction (%)	DTI	8.3	3.6**
	UFH	9.1	4.2**
Intracranial hemorrhage (%, in-hospital)	DTI	0.2*	0
	UFH	0.02*	0
Major bleeding (%, in-hospital)	DTI	1.3*	1.2***
	UFH	0.9*	0.7***

All p-values = NS except *p-value = 0.06, **p-value = 0.066, ***p-value = 0.01
NR = not reported; GUSTO = Global Use of Strategies to Open Occluded Coronary Arteries [21]; OASIS = Organisation to Assess Strategies for Ischemic Syndromes [24]

to heparin (odds ratio 1.28; 95% CI 1.06–1.55), whereas bleeding was significantly reduced with bivalirudin (odds ratio 0.44; 95% CI 0.34–0.56). Intracranial hemorrhage rates were the same with heparin or DTIs, although the three initial studies of 'excessive doses' of hirudin during acute MI (GUSTO-II, TIMI 9, and HIT III – described above) were not included in the analysis.

The findings of this meta-analysis highlighted the impressions derived from the individual trials of DTIs in the setting of ACS, that is of only modest reductions in the risk of MI compared with heparin therapy accompanied by an increase in bleeding complications. As a consequence, DTIs have not been approved or used widely for the management of patients with ACS. Importantly, however, several points limit the broad extrapolation of these results to current clinical practice. First, these trials were carried out in an era of conservative management of ACS, where only a minority of patients underwent early angiography and revascularization; thus, the relative effectiveness of these therapies with aggressive management strategies of coronary revascularization could not be assessed. Second, when percutaneous coronary intervention *was* performed in these trials, it was before the use of coronary stents and small diameter vascular access sheaths. Third, other antithrombotics with proven effectiveness, thienopyridine and GP IIb/IIIa platelet inhibitors, had not yet entered clinical practice at the time of these trials. Fourth, the meta-analysis results were dominated (28,545 of the total 35,970 patients) by the experience with hirudin, an agent which consistently increased bleeding risk. The safety experience with bivalirudin was notably different, motivating continued development of that agent for percutaneous coronary revascularization.

DTIs IN PERCUTANEOUS CORONARY REVASCULARIZATION

Antithrombotic therapy is required during PCI to limit thrombosis at sites of arterial intervention and injury and to prevent the formation of clot around catheters, wires and stents introduced into the vasculature. Although long-term restenosis and revascularization rates have been reduced by advances in equipment design (principally the development of stents), peri-procedural ischemic complications have been favorably impacted only by enhanced antithrombotic therapies. UH had been the standard of adjunctive AT therapy during PCI for that procedure's first 25 years. Since the mid-1990s, significant reductions in peri-procedural complications were achieved with administration of GP IIb/IIIa antagonists [26] and thienopyridine platelet inhibitors [27] in addition to heparin. Improved protection against ischemic complications with the GP IIb/IIIa inhibitors in particular, however, has been associated with increased bleeding risk and substantial cost.

At approximately the same time that early studies were demonstrating the marked efficacy of GP IIb/IIIa blockade with abciximab, two large-scale trials of DTIs as a replacement for heparin during balloon angioplasty garnered substantially less attention in the cardiology community, but nevertheless provided important information regarding the potential benefit of DTI for this indication [28–30]. The primary objective of the first of these, the HELVETICA trial [28], was to determine if hirudin would diminish the risk of restenosis after balloon angioplasty for UA, based upon data in animal models showing reductions in platelet deposition, thrombus formation and subsequent neointimal hyperplasia with this agent following arterial injury. Although HELVETICA failed to demonstrate an effect of hirudin on restenosis, there was evidence of efficacy in reducing acute peri-procedural ischemic complications among the 1141 patients in that study. Death, MI or repeat revascularization occurred within the first 96 h after the angioplasty in 11.0%, 7.9% and 5.6% of patients randomized to heparin, hirudin for 1 day, or hirudin for 4 days, respectively (p-value $= 0.023$) (Figure 7.3). By 7 months, however, the advantage of hirudin over heparin had disappeared, and all ischemic endpoints occurred at similar rates in the three treatment groups. In contrast to trials of hirudin during medical management of ACS, bleeding rates were not increased in HELVETICA, although one patient suffered an intracerebral hemorrhage after 4 days of hirudin therapy.

The second of the early DTI trials in PCI also targeted the acute coronary syndrome population, with 4312 UA patients randomized to receive either bivalirudin or heparin during and for up to 24 h after balloon angioplasty [29, 30]. In this BAT, the risk of death, MI or repeat revascularization in the first 7 days after PCI was significantly reduced from 7.9% to 6.2% in the heparin vs bivalirudin groups, respectively (p-value $= 0.039$), with the benefit of bivalirudin maintained without attenuation over 6 months' follow-up (Figure 7.3). Moreover, treatment with bivalirudin led to a striking reduction in the incidence of clinically significant bleeding, from 9.3% to 3.5% (relative risk reduction 62%, p-value < 0.001). While the finding of a $\sim$20% decrease in ischemic event rates with bivalirudin was overshadowed by the 35–50% reductions seen during the same time period in the PCI trials of abciximab [31], BAT was the first study to suggest that, unlike the experience with GP IIb/IIIa blockade, enhanced antithrombotic efficacy might not invariably be associated with an increased bleeding risk. This favorable safety profile of bivalirudin in contrast to the experience with hirudin was felt to be related to bivalirudin's reversible rather than irreversible thrombin inhibition and its relatively short duration of action [1].

On the basis of the findings in BAT, bivalirudin received regulatory approval as an alternative to heparin during PCI. Broad use of this agent, however, did not occur until a more contemporary trial demonstrated its efficacy relative to heparin with GP IIb/IIIa blockade and in the context of coronary stenting and thienopyridine therapy. Although GP IIb/IIIa inhibitors were clearly effective in suppressing acute ischemic complications of PCI, with a reduction in long-term mortality observed with abciximab as well, use of these agents was not universal during PCI owing to their cost and concerns regarding bleeding. The REPLACE-2 trial therefore compared the 'gold standard' of heparin plus a GP IIb/IIIa inhibitor to treatment with bivalirudin alone, with GP IIb/IIIa blockade administered on a 'provisional' basis only if necessary for a procedural complication [32, 33]. The intent was to determine if GP IIb/IIIa inhibitors could be used selectively rather than routinely by replacing heparin with bivalirudin, thereby reducing medication costs and associated bleeding complications. Reflecting modern clinical practice, stents were used in over 85% of

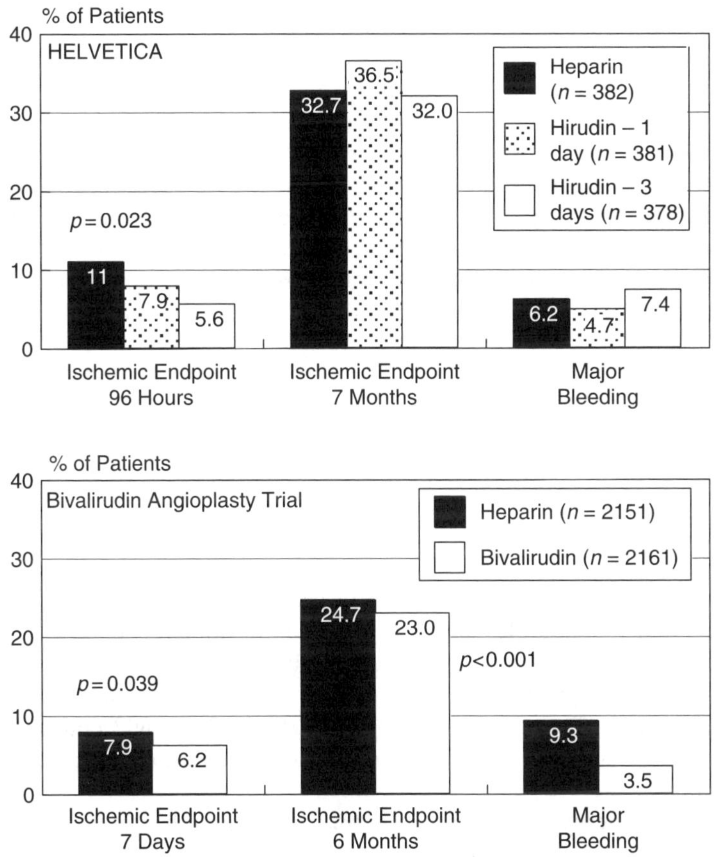

Figure 7.3 Outcomes for ischemic endpoints (composite of death, MI, or repeat revascularization) and major bleeding in early trials of DTIs versus heparin among patients undergoing balloon angioplasty for UA. Top panel – HELVETICA trial of hirudin versus heparin [28]. Bottom panel – Bivalirudin Angioplasty Trial of bivalirudin versus heparin [30]

patients, and virtually all received a thienopyridine platelet inhibitor; provisional GP IIb/IIIa blockade was required in only 7.2% of patients in the bivalirudin arm. Among the more than 6000 patients randomized in that trial, bivalirudin was demonstrated to be non-inferior to the combination of heparin plus GP IIb/IIIa in suppressing acute ischemic complications, with the composite ischemic endpoint of death, MI or urgent repeat revascularization by 30-days occurring in 7.6% and 7.1% of those in the bivalirudin versus heparin plus GP IIb/IIIa arms, respectively (Figure 7.4). Rates of major in-hospital bleeding were significantly reduced with bivalirudin from 4.1% to 2.4% (p-value <0.001), with 60–70% reductions in the risk of vascular access site or retroperitoneal hemorrhages. In a formal economic analysis, bivalirudin therapy was associated with savings in excess of $400 per patient, through a combination of lower drug acquisition costs (provisional GP IIb/IIIa inhibitors were used in only 7.6% of patients in the bivalirudin arm) and reduced expenses associated with bleeding [34]. Other practical advantages of bivalirudin monotherapy related to the logistic convenience of its average 47-min infusion (terminated at the end of the interventional procedure), rather than the 12–18-h infusions of GP IIb/IIIa inhibitors. Over long-term follow-up, the benefit of GP IIb/IIIa blockade with regard to mortality was not lost among patients treated with bivalirudin; mortality rates at 1 year trended to be lower in the bivalirudin arm (1.9% vs 2.5%, hazard ratio 0.78; 95% CI 0.55–1.11; p-value = 0.16), with differences favoring bivalirudin over the combination of heparin plus GP IIb/IIIa blockade particularly marked in high-risk subgroups such as elderly patients, women or those with diabetes mellitus. Subsequent to the publication of the REPLACE-2 findings, bivalirudin is estimated to be used for ~40% of PCI procedures in the United States. Trials are currently underway testing bivalirudin vs heparin-based regimens with or without GP IIb/IIIa blockade in the contemporary management (including an early revascularization strategy) of patients with high-risk acute coronary syndromes, a group that was excluded from enrollment in the REPLACE-2 trial.

DTIs IN HIT

HIT is a potentially life-threatening complication of heparin therapy, resulting from formation of antibodies to the complex of heparin and platelet factor 4 leading to platelet activation, thrombocytopenia, endothelial injury and a marked prothrombotic state [12]. Patients with HIT are at risk for arterial or venous thrombosis and resultant stroke, limb amputation or death. The management of HIT is discussed in detail in Chapter 13. Once HIT becomes manifest, discontinuation of all heparin or LMWH administration is imperative, yet patients require anticoagulation to prevent or treat the thromboembolic complications of HIT and/or their underlying disease processes. Owing to their lack of cross-reactivity with heparin-associated antibodies, DTIs have emerged as essentially the single option for providing anticoagulation in patients with the HIT syndrome. Both hirudin and argatroban are approved for this indication.

Evidence for the efficacy of the lepirudin form of hirudin in this setting was derived from two prospective, historically-controlled studies: the HAT-1 and -2 trials enrolling in total 194 patients [35, 36]. Lepirudin therapy was associated with rapid normalization of platelet counts in ~90% of patients, with all deaths 'judged to be due to the underlying disease rather than to use of lepirudin.' Compared with historical controls, the incidence of the composite endpoint of death, limb amputation or new thromboembolic event was reduced by lepirudin from 52% to 25–32%. Bleeding events also occurred more frequently with

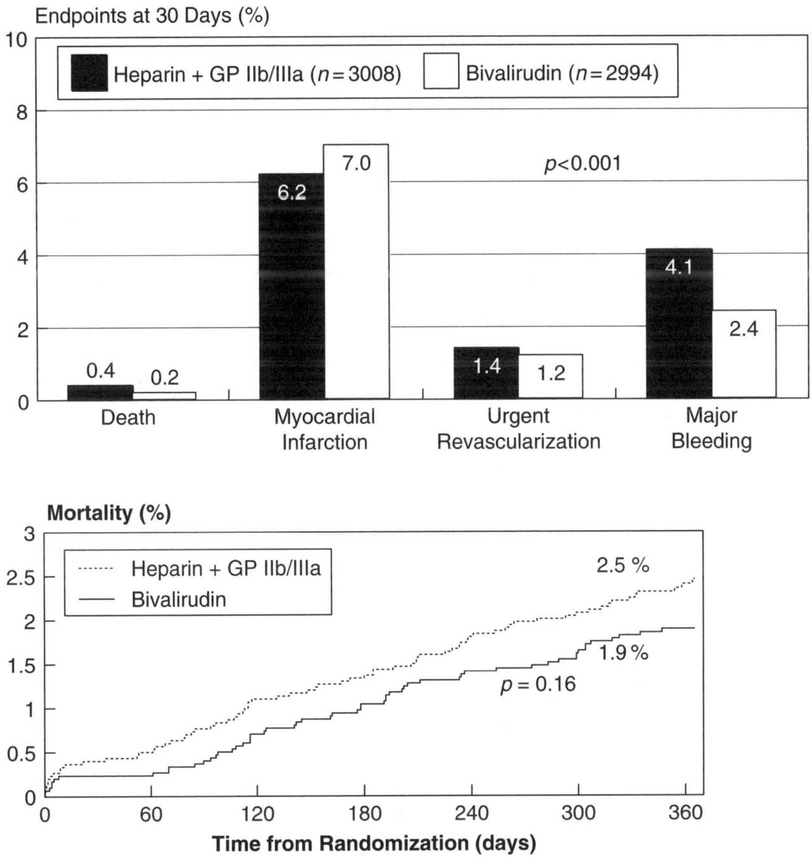

Figure 7.4 Outcomes at 30 days (top panel) and mortality at 1 year (lower panel) in the REPLACE-2 trial comparing heparin with planned glycoprotein GP IIb/IIIa blockade versus bivalirudin and provisional GP IIb/IIIa blockade in patients undergoing elective or urgent percutaneous coronary revascularization [32, 33]

lepirudin therapy than among historical controls (39–45% vs 27%), although transfusion rates were not different.

Similar efficacy in patients with HIT has been observed using argatroban [37]. In a prospective study of 304 patients with HIT or HITTS, platelet counts normalized more quickly in patients receiving argatroban than in historical controls. The composite endpoint was reduced by argatroban as compared with historical controls from 39% to 26% (p-value = 0.014) among the cohort of 160 patients with HIT and from 57% to 44% (p-value = 0.13) among the 144 patients with HITTS. No increase in the risk of bleeding was observed with argatroban. In three other small studies of a total of 91 patients with HIT treated with argatroban during PCI, acute procedural success rates were similar to historical controls *without HIT* (98% vs 94%, respectively), with no differences in major bleeding rates.

The choice between hirudin and argatroban therapy in patients with HIT can be based in part upon the presence of renal (a contraindication to hirudin) or hepatic (a contraindication to argatroban) dysfunction, as well as the extent of institutional experience with either drug. Although bivalirudin has not yet received regulatory approval for the indication of HIT, a prospective multicenter study has been reported of 52 patients with HIT who were treated with bivalirudin during PCI [38]. Procedural success was achieved in 98% of patients, with one major bleeding event after bypass surgery and one death after apparently uncomplicated PCI. Given the lack of contraindications to bivalirudin related to renal or hepatic failure, as well as the widespread experience with this agent during PCI, bivalirudin may emerge as the preferred anticoagulant among patients with HIT.

DTIs IN VENOUS THROMBOEMBOLIC DISORDER

The management of venous thromboembolic disorders, including pulmonary emboli, is discussed in detail in Chapter 12. Parenteral and oral DTIs have been evaluated in this setting, although these agents have yet to become a preferred therapy in clinical practice for this indication.

Hirudin has been shown to be effective for the prevention of venous thromboembolic disorder after total hip replacement in Phase III studies [39–41]. A dose-finding trial established a subcutaneous dose of 15 mg of desirudin twice daily to be effective and safe. Two subsequent phase III trials compared this dose of desirudin to UH (445 patients) or the LMWH enoxaparin (1587 patients). In both trials, desirudin significantly reduced the incidence of venous thromboembolic disorder compared with either UFH 5000 U subcutaneously three times a day (7% vs 23%) or enoxaparin 40 mg subcutaneously once a day (18% vs 26%), while no differences were observed between desirudin and heparin regimens in rates of bleeding complications. In a small dose-finding study of 155 patients with DVT, subcutaneous hirudin appeared to have equivalent efficacy to that of intravenous heparin in preventing DVT progression and new defects on lung ventilation/perfusion scanning [42]. There are no adequate studies of bivalirudin or argatroban for the prevention or treatment of venous thromboembolic disease.

The oral DTI ximelagatran and its active metabolite melagatran have been demonstrated to be effective for both prevention and treatment of VTE. Administration of SC injections of melagatran immediately before surgery followed by oral treatment with ximelagatran has been compared to LMWH for the prevention of VTE following knee or hip surgery. In a large dose-finding study, a dose-related reduction in VTE rates was observed, accompanied by a dose-related increase in bleeding complications [43]. A subsequent phase III trial showed that the melagatran/ximelagatran regimen was superior to enoxaparin for prevention of VTE [20.3% vs 26.7%, respectively, p-value = 0.003), but was associated with significantly more major bleeding events (3.3% vs 1.2%) and transfusions (67% vs 62%) [44]. Ximelagatran has also been compared with warfarin, with either drug started on the morning after total knee replacement. In the first trial of 680 patients, VTE rates were similar in patients randomized to receive ximelagatran 24 mg subcutaneously twice daily vs warfarin (19% vs 26%, respectively, p-value = 0.07), with no difference in bleeding rates [45]. In a subsequent larger study of 2301 patients, a higher dose of ximelagatran (36 mg twice daily) significantly reduced the risk of VTE compared with warfarin (20% vs 28%, respectively, p-value = 0.003), again with no difference in bleeding complications [46].

Two large-scale studies have addressed the potential role for ximelagatran in the secondary prevention and/or treatment of VTE. In the first of these, 1233 patients who had completed a 6-month course of standard anticoagulant therapy for DVT or PE were randomized to receive either ximelagatran 24 mg bid or placebo for the subsequent 18 months [47]. Ximelagatran markedly reduced the incidence of recurrent VTE by 84% (12.6% vs 2.8%, *p*-value <0.001), with no increase in the risk of major or minor bleeding complications. The second trial compared ximelagatran 36 mg bid begun immediately after diagnosis of DVT or PE and for 6 months thereafter to a regimen of enoxaparin for 5–20 days followed by warfarin [48]. No differences between treatment groups were observed in the incidences of recurrent VTE (2.1% vs 2.0%) or bleeding. Thus, although these trials demonstrated the utility of long-term therapy for DVT after the traditional 6-month course of anticoagulation, no advantage of the oral DTI over enoxaparin/warfarin was observed for either efficacy or bleeding risk. Unfortunately, the idiopathic occurrence of severe hepatic injury with ximelagatran has thus far precluded its regulatory approval in the United States, and further examination of the usefulness of chronic oral DTI therapy in this setting must await the availability of other agents.

DTIs AND OTHER POTENTIAL APPLICATIONS

Atrial fibrillation is the strongest risk factor for the development of stroke [49], and the incidence of this common arrhythmia is increasing with an aging population. Although warfarin is effective in reducing the incidence of stroke and thromboembolic complications among patients with atrial fibrillation, compliance with use of this therapy is low due to the difficulties involved in dose titration and coagulation monitoring and the risk of bleeding complications. Ximelagatran has been studied in two pivotal trials among over 7300 patients with non-valvular atrial fibrillation, the SPORTIF-III and -V studies [50, 51]. These two trials had similar designs, comparing ximelagatran 36 mg bid with warfarin targeted to an INR of 2–3. Annual rates of stroke or systemic embolic events were 1.6% vs 2.3% in the ximelagatran vs warfarin arms of SPORTIF-III and 1.6% vs 1.2%, respectively in SPORTIF-V, meeting the specified criteria for non-inferiority. Bleeding rates tended to be slightly lower among patients in the ximelagatran groups, although the difference was not significant in either trial. The risk of bleeding with ximelagatran increased with declining renal function, suggesting that fixed dosing of this renally cleared agent may lead to drug accumulation and adverse effects in patients with diminished creatinine clearance. Thus, apart from the hepatic toxicity of ximelagatran, which has thus far precluded its regulatory approval in the United States, no advantage of this agent over warfarin, aside from the convenience of fixed dosing without monitoring, has been demonstrated in the setting of atrial fibrillation.

Heparin has been used for cardiac surgery since the first operation utilizing cardiopulmonary bypass. Although effective in this setting, limitations include incomplete anticoagulation, heparin resistance, HIT and the need to reverse anticoagulation with protamine, which itself is antigenic. Preliminary investigations have been performed using bivalirudin instead of heparin during cardiac surgery. An important consideration, given that bivalirudin is consumed by thrombin and endogenous peptidases in the blood, is the avoidance of stasis within the cardiopulmonary circuit, cardiac chambers or bypass grafts, which could lead to thrombus formation. The feasibility of using bivalirudin during off-pump coronary artery bypass (OPCAB) surgery was assessed in a single-center randomized pilot trial of

100 patients [52]. Peri-operative blood loss with bivalirudin anticoagulation was similar to that with heparin and protamine (median 793 mL vs 805 mL, respectively), as were rates of blood product transfusions and ischemic events. Follow-up angiography 3 months after surgery provided evidence of improved graft patency with bivalirudin: normal flow was observed in 82% of grafts in bivalirudin-treated patients compared with 67% of grafts in the heparin group (p-value = 0.03). Two multicenter randomized trials of bivalirudin versus heparin during off-pump and on-pump surgery, as well as two uncontrolled registries of bivalirudin in patients with HIT, are currently underway.

7.4 SUMMARY

Mechanistically poised at the juncture between platelet-mediated and soluble coagulation pathways of thrombosis, DTIs are a potent class of agents with several potential advantages over heparin. The most successful clinical application of DTIs to date has been in the field of interventional cardiology, where the reversible inhibitor bivalirudin has been established to provide similar protection against the ischemic complications of PCI as heparin and GP IIb/IIIa blockade, with less bleeding, lower cost and greater ease of use. Bivalirudin may become the antithrombotic regimen of choice for the majority of patients undergoing these procedures. Large-scale investigations are also underway to determine if bivalirudin may improve outcome during the comprehensive management of acute coronary syndromes. The development of orally available DTIs may ultimately prove to enhance the treatment of patients who require chronic anticoagulation for atrial fibrillation, venous thromboembolic disease and other indications.

REFERENCES

[1] Weitz, J.I., Bates, E.R., (2003) Direct thrombin inhibitors in cardiac disease. Cardiovascular Toxicology, 3:13–25.

[2] Mann, K., Butenas, S., Brummel, K., (2003) The dynamics of thrombin formation. *Arterioscler Thromb Vasc Biol*, 23:17–25.

[3] Hirsh, J., Fuster, V., (1994) Guide to anticoagulant therapy. Part 1: Heparin. *Circulation*, 89:1449–68.

[4] Weitz, J.I., Hudoba, M., Massel, D., *et al.*, (1990) Clot-bound thrombin is protected from inhibition by heparin-antithrombin III but is susceptible to inactivation by antithrombin III independent inhibitors. *J Clin Invest*, 86:385–91.

[5] Hirsh, J., (1991) Heparin. *N Eng J Med*, 324:1565–74.

[6] Eitzman, D.T., Chi, L., Saggin, L., *et al.*, (1994) Heparin neutralization by platelet-rich thrombi. Role of platelet factor 4. *Circulation*, 89:1523–29.

[7] Xiao, Z., Theroux, P., (1998) Platelet activation with unfractionated heparin at therapeutic concentrations and comparisons with a low-molecular-weight heparin and with a direct thrombin inhibitor. *Circulation*, 97:251–6.

[8] Sobel, M., Fish, W.R., Toma, N., *etal.*, (2001) Heparin modulates integrin function in human platelets. *J Vasc Surg*, 33:587–94.

[9] Marcianak, E., Gockerman, J.P., (1977) Heparin-induced decrease in circulating antithrombin III. *Lancet*, 2:581–4.

[10] Loscalzo, J., Melnick, B., Handin, R.I., (1985) The interaction of platelet factor four and glycosaminoglycans. *Arch Biochem Biophys*, 240:446–55.

[11] Weitz, J.I., Hudoba, M., (1992) Mechanism by which clot-bound thrombin is protected from inactivation by fluid-phase inhibitors (abstr). *Circulation*, 86:I–413.

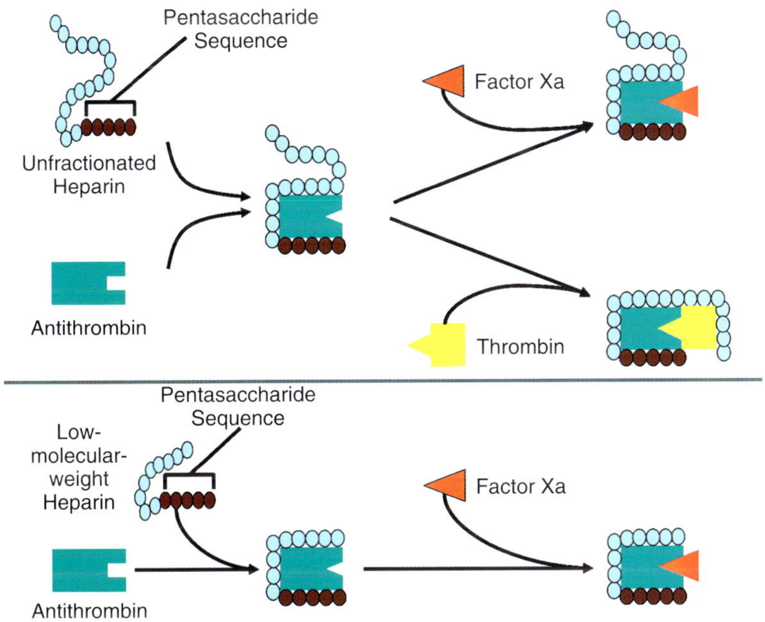

Plates 6.1 & 7.1 Binding of UH with Antithrombin III and Thrombin requires at least 18 saccharide units including the pentasaccharide essential for Antithrombin III binding. Only a small percentage of LMWH are long enough to bind both antithrombin III and thrombin, accounting for the greater antiXa:AntiIIa ratio.

(Top section only) Mechanism of action of UH. Interaction of UH with AT is mediated by the pentasaccharide sequence of the drugs. Binding to AT causes a conformational change at its reactive center that accelerates its interaction with factor Xa or thrombin. Adapted from Weitz JI, N Eng J Med, 1997;337: 688.

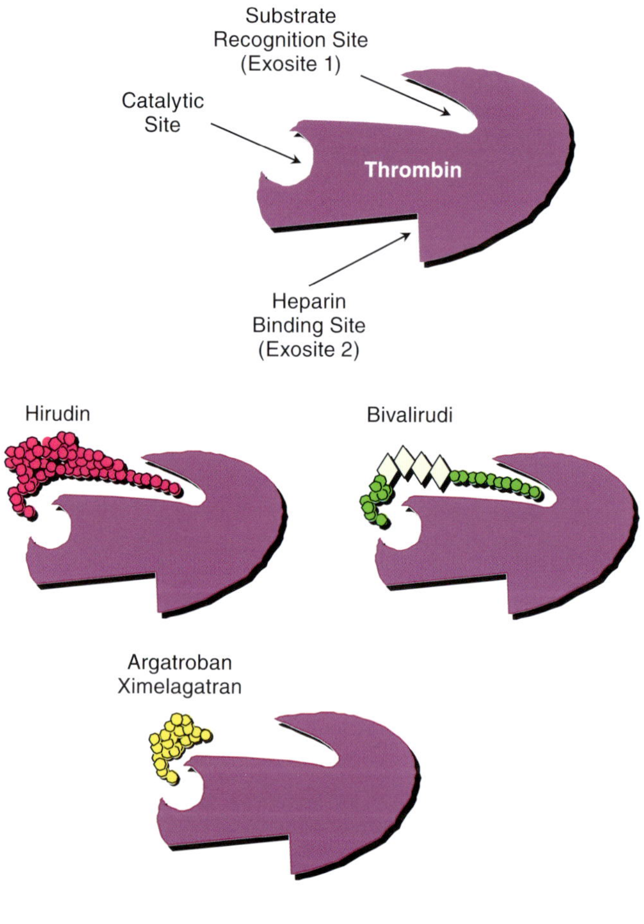

Plate 7.2 Schematic representation of thrombin, showing the different binding patterns of bivalent (hirudin and bivalirudin) and univalent (argatroban and ximelagatran) DTIs.

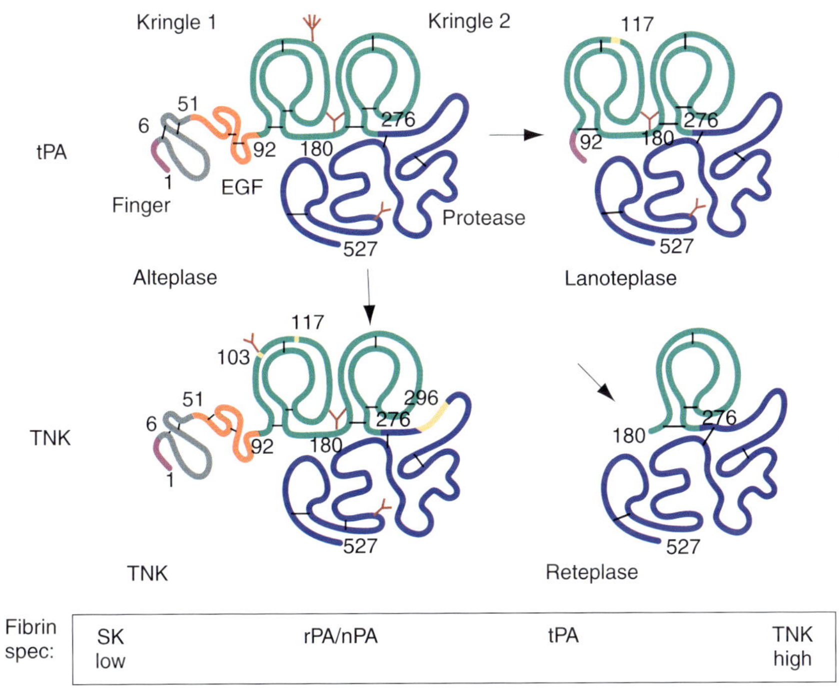

Plate 8.1 Molecular structure of alteplase (tPA), lanoteplase (nPA), reteplase (rPA), and tenecteplase (TNK).

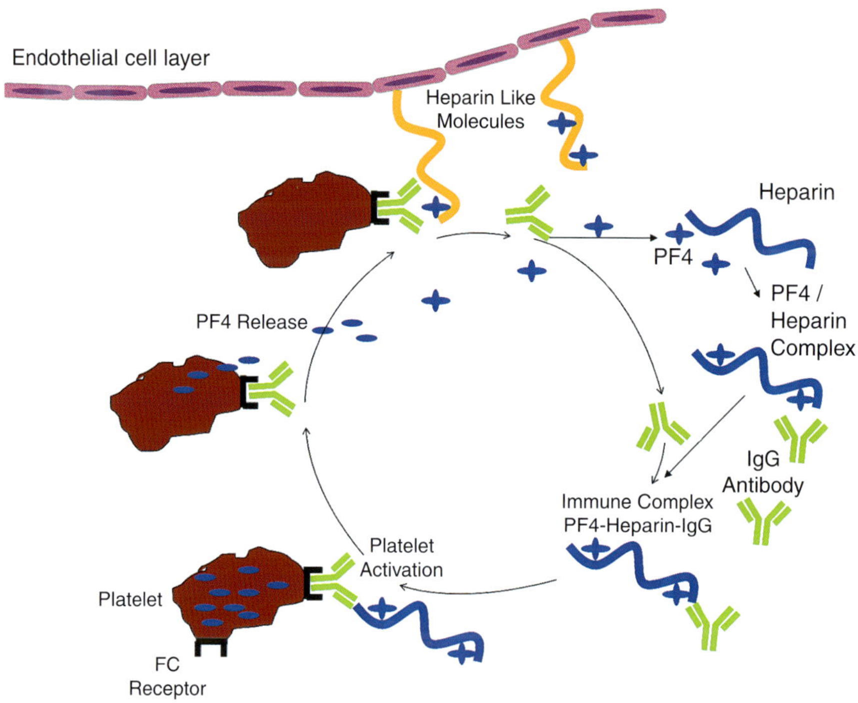

Plate 13.1 Pathogenesis of HIT: Cross-linking of the platelet FcγII receptors by the antibody-heparin/ PF4 complex initiates a cascade of platelet activation, thromboxane biosynthesis, secretion of platelet granular contents including PF4, formation of additional heparin/PF4 complexes, further binding of these complexes by HIT antibody, and ultimately, platelet aggregation.

[12] Warkentin, T.E., Greinacher, A., (2004) Heparin-induced thrombocytopenia: recognition, treatment, and prevention: the Seventh ACCP Conference on Antithrombotic and Thrombolytic Therapy [erratum appears in *Chest*. 2005 Jan; 127(1):416]. *Chest*, 126.

[13] Weitz, J.I., Bates, S.M., (2002) Acute coronary syndromes: a focus on thrombin. *J Invasive Cardiol*, 14:2B–7B.

[14] Maraganore, J.M., Chao, B., Joseph, M.L., *et al.*, (1989) Anticoagulant activity of synthetic hirudin peptides. *J Biol Chem*, 15:8692–8.

[15] Gustafsson, D., Nystrom, J., Carlsson, S., *et al.*, (2001) The direct thrombin inhibitor melagatran and its oral prodrug H 376/95: Intestinal absorption properties,biochemical and pharmacodynamic effects. *Thromb Res*, 101:171–81.

[16] DeWood, M.A., Spores, J., Notske, R., *et al.* (1980) Prevalence of total coronary occlusion during the early hours of transmural myocardial infarction. *N Eng J Med*, 303:897–902.

[17] Kaiser, B., Simon, A., Markwardt, F., (1990) Antithrombin effects of recombinant hirudin in experimental angioplasty and intravascular thrombolysis. *Thromb Haemost*, 63:44–7.

[18] GUSTO IIa Investigators, (1994) Randomized trial of intravenous heparin versus recombinant hirudin for acute coronary syndromes. The Global Use of Strategies To Open occluded coronary arteries (GUSTO) IIa investigators. *Circulation*, 90:1631–7.

[19] Antman, E.M., for the TIMI 9A Investigators, (1994) Hirudin in acute myocardial infarction. Safety report from the thrombolysis and thrombin inhibition in myocardial infarction (TIMI) 9A trial. *Circulation*, 90:1624–30.

[20] Neuhaus, K.L., Essen, R.V., Tebbe, U., *et al.*, (1994) Safety observations from the pilot phase of the randomized r-Hirudin for improvement of thrombolysis (HIT-III) study. A study of the Arbeitsgemeinschaft Leitender Kardiologischer Krankenhausarzte (ALKK). *Circulation*, 90:1638–42.

[21] The GUSTO Investigators, (1996) Global Use of Strategies to Open Occluded Coronary Arteries (GUSTO) IIb Investigators. A comparison of recombinant hirudin with heparin for the treatment of acute coronary syndromes. *N Eng J Med* 335:775–82.

[22] Antman, E.M., for the TIMI 9B Investigators (1996) Hirudin in acute myocardial infarction. Thrombolysis and Thrombin Inhibition in Myocardial Infarction (TIMI) 9B Trial. *Circulation*, 94:911–21.

[23] Hirulog and Early Reperfusion or Occlusion (HERO-2) Trial Investigators, (2001) Thrombin-specific anticoagulation with bivalirudin versus heparin in patients receiving fibrinolytic therapy for acute myocardial infarction: the HERO-2 randomised trial. *Lancet*, 358:1855–63.

[24] Organisation to Assess Strategies for Ischemic Syndromes (OASIS-2) Investigators, (1999) Effects of recombinant hirudin (lepirudin) compared with heparin on death, myocardial infarction, refractory angina, and revascularization procedures in patients with acute myocardial ischaemia without ST elevation: a randomised trial. *Lancet*, 353:429–438.

[25] Direct Thrombin Inhibitors Trialists' Collaborative Group, (2002) Direct thrombin inhibitors in acute coronary syndromes: principal results of a meta-analysis based on individual patients' data. *Lancet*, 359:294–302.

[26] Lincoff, A.M., Califf, R.M., Topol, E.J., (2000) Platelet glycoprotein IIb/IIIa blockade in coronary artery disease. *J Am Coll Cardiol*, 35:1103–15.

[27] Steinhubl, S.R., Berger, P.B., Mann, J.T., *et al.*, (2002) Early and sustained dual oral antiplatelet therapy following percutaneous coronary intervention. A randomized controlled trial. *JAMA*, 288:2411–20.

[28] Serruys, P.W., Herrman, J-P.R, Simon, R., *et al.*, (1995) A comparison of hirudin with heparin in the prevention of restenosis after coronary angioplasty. *N Eng J Med*, 333:757–63.

[29] Bittl, J.A., Chaitman, B.R., Feit, F., *et al.* on behalf of the Bivalirudin Angioplasty Study Investigators, (2001) Bivalirudin versus heparin during coronary angioplasty for unstable or post-infarction angina: final report reanalysis of the Bivalirudin Angioplasty Study. *Am Heart J*, 142:952–9.

[30] Bittl, J.A., Strony, J., Brinker, J.A., *et al.*, (1995) Treatment with bivalirudin (hirulog) as compared with heparin during coronary angioplasty for unstable or postinfarction angina. *N Eng J Med*, 333:764–9.

[31] EPILOG Investigators, (1997) Platelet glycoprotein IIb/IIIa blockade with abciximab with low-dose heparin during percutaneous coronary revascularization. *N Eng J Med*, 336:1689–96.

[32] Lincoff, A.M., Bittl, J.A., Harrington, R.A., *et al.*, (2003) Bivalirudin and provisional glycoprotein IIb/IIIa blockade compared with heparin and planned glycoprotein IIb/IIIa blockade during percutaneous coronary intervention. The REPLACE-2 trial. *JAMA*, 289:853–63.

[33] Lincoff, A.M., Kleiman, N.S., Kereiakes, D.J., *et al.*, (2004) Long-term efficacy of bivalirudin and provisional glycoprotein IIb/IIIa blockade vs heparin and planned glycoprotein IIb/IIIa blockade during percutaneous coronary revascularization. REPLACE-2 randomized trial. *JAMA*, 292:696–703.

[34] Cohen, D.J., Lincoff, A.M., Lavelle, T.A., *et al.*, (2004) Economic evaluation of bivalirudin with provisional glycoprotein IIB/IIIA inhibition versus heparin with routine glycoprotein IIb/IIIa inhibition for percutaneous coronary intervention: Results from the REPLACE-2 trial. *J Am Coll Cardiol*, 44:1792–1800.

[35] Greinacher, A., Volpel, H., Janssens, U., *et al.*, (1999) Recombinant hirudin (lepirudin) provides safe and effective anticoagulation in patients with heparin-induced thrombocytopenia. *Circulation*, 99:73–80.

[36] Greinacher, A., Janssens, U., Berg, G., *et al.*, (1999) Lepirudin (recombinant hirudin) for parenteral anticoagulation in patients with heparin-induced thromobocytopenia. *Circulation*, 100:587–93.

[37] Lewis, B.E., Wallis, D.E., Berkowitz, S.D., *et al.*, (2001) Argatroban anticoagulant therapy in patients with heparin-induced thrombocytopenia. *Circulation*, 103:1838–43.

[38] Mahaffey, K.W., Lewis, B.E., Wildermann, N.M., *et al.*, (2003) The anticoagulant therapy with bivalirudin to assist in the performance of percutaneous coronary intervention in patients with heparin-induced thrombocytopenia (ATBAT) study: main results. *J Invasive Cardiol*, 15:611–16.

[39] Eriksson, B.I., Ekman, S., Kalebo, P., *et al.*, (1996) Prevention of deep-vein thrombosis after total hip replacement: direct thrombin inhibition with recombinant hirudin, CGP 39393 [see comment]. *Lancet*, 347:635–9.

[40] Eriksson, B.I., Wille-Jorgensen, P., Kalebo, P., *et al.*, (1997) A comparison of recombinant hirudin with a low-molecular-weight heparin to prevent thromboembolic complications after total hip replacement [see comment]. *N Eng J Med*, 337:1329–35.

[41] Eriksson, B.I., Ekman, S., Lindbratt, S., *et al.*, (1997) Prevention of thromboembolism with use of recombinant hirudin. Results of a double-blind, multicenter trial comparing the efficacy of desirudin (Revasc) with that of unfractionated heparin in patients having a total hip replacement. *J Bone Joint Surg Am*, 79:326–33.

[42] Heit, J.A., (2003) The potential role of direct thrombin inhibitors in the prevention and treatment of venous thromboembolism. *Chest*, 124:40S–8S.

[43] Eriksson, B.I., Bergqvist, D., Kalebo, P., *et al.*, (2002) Ximelagatran and melagatran compared with dalteparin for prevention of venous thromboembolism after total hip or knee replacement: the METHRO II randomised trial. *Lancet*, 360:1441–7.

[44] Eriksson, B.I., Agnelli, G., Cohen, A.T., *et al.*, (2003) The direct thrombin inhibitor melagatran followed by oral ximelagatran compared with enoxaparin for the prevention of venous thromboembolism after total hip or knee replacement: the EXPRESS study [see comment]. *J Thromb Haemostasis*, 1:2490–6.

[45] Francis, C.W., Davidson, B.L., Berkowitz, S.D., *et al.*, (2002) Ximelagatran versus warfarin for the prevention of venous thromboembolism after total knee arthroplasty. A randomized, double-blind trial [summary for patients in *Ann Intern Med.* 2002 Oct 15; 137(8):I38; PMID: 12379093]. *Ann Int Med*, 137:648–55.

[46] Francis, C.W., Berkowitz, S.D., Comp, P.C., *et al.*, (2003) Comparison of ximelagatran with warfarin for the prevention of venous thromboembolism after total knee replacement [see comment]. *N Eng J Med*, 349:1703–12.

[47] Schulman, S., Wahlander, K., Lundstrom, T., *et al.*, Investigators TI. Secondary prevention of venous thromboembolism with the oral direct thrombin inhibitor ximelagatran [see comment]. *N Eng J Med*, 349:1713–21.

[48] Fiessinger, J.N., Huisman, M.V., Davidson, B.L., *et al.*, (2005) Ximelagatran vs low-molecular-weight heparin and warfarin for the treatment of deep vein thrombosis: a randomized trial [see comment]. *JAMA*, 293:681–9.

[49] Wolf, P.A., Abbott, R.D., Kannel, W.B., (1991) Atrial fibrillation as an independent risk factor for stroke: the Framingham Study. *Stroke*, 22:983–9.

[50] Albers, G.W., SPORTIF Investigators (2004) Stroke prevention in atrial fibrillation: pooled analysis of SPORTIF III and V trials. *Am J Manag Care*, 10.
[51] Sportif Executive Steering Committee for the SPORTIF V Investigators, Albers, G.W., Diener, H.C., *et al.*, (2005) Ximelagatran vs warfarin for stroke prevention in patients with nonvalvular atrial fibrillation: a randomized trial. [see comment]. *JAMA*, 293:690–8.
[52] Merry, A.F., Raudkivi, P.J., Middleton, N.G., *et al.*, (2004) Bivalirudin versus heparin and protamine in off-pump coronary artery bypass surgery. *Ann Thorac Surg*, 77:925–31.
[53] Weitz, J.I., (1997) Low-molecular-weight heparins. *N Eng J Med*, 337:688–98.

8 Fibrinolytic agents

8.1 INTRODUCTION

Although the use of fibrinolytic therapy was first described in 1958 [1], its utility in improving mortality in the setting of an STEMI was not formally suggested until the mid 1980s [2]. Since then a burgeoning body of literature has solidified fibrinolytic therapy as a therapy that revolutionized treatment of these patients. Observations from the initial trials helped define the therapeutic window, limitations and complications of fibrinolysis, as well as the role of adjunctive medications [3–9]. The past decade has focused on methods to further improve the outcomes while minimizing the adverse effects of fibrinolysis. The administration of potent antiplatelet and antithrombin agents with fibrinolytic agents have been assessed in an attempt to break through the 'ceiling' of benefit associated with fibrinolysis [10–23]. The use of fibrinolysis in the setting of STEMI is continuing to evolve with suggestion of improved outcomes when used in a 'facilitated' approach in combination with PCI [24–29]. Although primary PCI has demonstrated superior outcomes compared with fibrinolysis, associated delays in transfer of patients for primary PCI may essentially eliminate its benefits in the United States. Combined with the improved mortality achieved with fibrinolysis, this further supports the role of pharmacologic reperfusion strategies in the current era.

8.2 FIBRINOLYTIC AGENTS FOR STEMI

FIBRINOLYTIC AGENTS

Since the initial benefits of fibrinolytic therapy were demonstrated in the mid-1980s the specific fibrinolytic agents and treatment regimens have continued to evolve. Importantly, fibrinolytic therapy has been shown to restore IRA patency, reduce infarct size, preserve LV function and reduce mortality in patients with STEMI. Furthermore, the current generation of bolus fibrinolytics has been associated with simplified dosing regimens, reduced door-to-needle time, and reduced potential for dosing errors. This has culminated in the lowest mortality rate to date achieved with pharmacologic reperfusion [14, 15]. In addition, irrespective of the fibrinolytic agent used for reperfusion strategies, the efficacy of the fibrinolytic is strongly dependent on the time to therapy and to the degree of both epicardial and tissue-level reperfusion obtained [30–32]. Characteristics of the currently available fibrinolytic agents are listed in Table 8.1.

Management Strategies in Antithrombotic Therapy Arman T. Askari, Adrian W. Messerli and A. Michael Lincoff

Table 8.1 Characteristics of fibrinolytic agents

Agent	Source	Fibrin specificity	Systemic fibrinogen depletion	Antigenic	Effect on plasminogen	Plasma $T_{1/2}$ (min)	Metabolism	Dosing	Heparin Therapy	90-min TIMI 3 flow rates (%)	Cost per dose (US$)
Streptokinase (SK)	Group A streptococci	−	Marked	Yes	Via activator complex	18–23	Hepatic	1.5 million IU IV over 1 h	SC or IV UH	30–35	613
Alteplase (t-PA)	Recombinant, human	++	Mild	No	Direct	4–8	Hepatic	15 mg bolus, then 0.75 mg/kg (max 50 mg) over 30 min, then 0.5 mg/kg (max 35 mg) over 60 min	IV UH	54–60	2974
Reteplase (rPA)	Recombinant, human. Single chain deletion of t-PA	+	Moderate	No	Direct	13–16	Renal	Double bolus (10 U IV over 2 min) 30 min apart	IV UH	∼60	2750
Tenecteplase (TNK)	Recombinant plus point substitutions of t-PA	+++	Minimal	No	Direct	20–24	Hepatic	Single bolus IV For wt <60 kg:30 mg For wt 60–69 kg:35 mg For wt 70–79 kg:40 mg For wt 80–89 kg:45 mg For wt>90 kg:50 mg	IV UH or LMWH	∼60	2833

SK

The ability of SK, an indirect plasminogen activator derived from group A streptococci, to dissolve human thrombus was demonstrated in both preclinical [33] and early clinical studies [2, 34, 35]. Arising out of early clinical studies of SK evolved the time-dependency of reperfusion. For example, one study of intracoronary fibrinolysis with SK demonstrated a consistent decrease in the size of salvaged myocardium with prolonged delays from symptom onset [36]. When looked at from a 'hard-endpoint' (mortality) perspective, the beneficial effects of SK administered to patients with STEMI were enjoyed by those receiving this therapy within 1 h of symptom onset [3], with the benefits extending, albeit in a less robust fashion, to those patients presenting within 6–12 h from symptom onset [37]. What this has been shown to translate into is approximately 30 lives saved per 1000 patients treated within 0–6 h 20 lives saved per 1000 patients treated between 7–12 h from symptom onset [9]. The benefits of a single intravenous infusion of 1.5 million units of SK in prolonging survival of patients with acute myocardial infarction is sustained up to 10 years, with a still-evident trend in favor of the patients admitted earlier [38]. Although SK is not the fibrinolytic agent of choice in the United States, its efficacy in the treatment of STEMI and its extremely low cost have facilitated its persistence worldwide. The early experience with SK (Table 8.2) laid the foundations of the 'reperfusion era' for the management of STEMI.

Alteplase (t-PA)

Tissue plasminogen activator (t-PA), a naturally occurring single-chain serine protease naturally secreted by the vascular endothelium, contains five domains – finger, epidermal growth factor, kringle 1, kringle 2 and serine protease – which are responsible for its pharmacologic properties. In the absence of fibrin, t-PA is a weak plasminogen activator. Fibrin provides a scaffold on which t-PA and plasminogen are held in such a way that the catalytic efficiency for plasminogen activation of t-PA is increased many-fold. Although this fibrin-specificity focuses the delivery of t-PA to sites of active thrombosis, systemic plasminogen activation occurs at clinical doses. Plasma clearance of t-PA is mediated to a varying degree by residues in each of the domains except the serine protease domain, which is responsible for the enzymatic activity of t-PA. Whereas it was originally obtained from the Bowes melanoma cell line, t-PA is now obtained through recombinant DNA techniques.

Given the dramatic reduction in mortality with SK, the focus of treatment strategies for STEMI changed from one of supportive care to one of rapid restoration of antegrade coronary perfusion. Based on a number of angiographic trials comparing IRA patency, which observed superior patency and TIMI grade 3 flow results at both 60 min and 90 min with t-PA compared with SK or antistreplase (APSAC), large-scale randomized trials were performed to determine the relative efficacy of different fibrinolytic agents. However, the earliest fibrinolytic comparison trials failed to show a difference in mortality reduction between SK vs t-PA or SK vs APSAC vs t-PA [5, 7]. It is important to note that these studies used a 3-hour infusion of t-PA together with SC heparin.

The lack of improved outcomes with a more fibrin-specific fibrinolytic agent may have been due, at least in part, to a sub-optimal dosing regimen of t-PA. This was suggested by small angiographic studies, which revealed improved coronary patency rates with an

Table 8.2 Early mortality trials of SK

Trial	N	Age	SK dose	Placebo-blinding	Symptom duration (h)	ECG criteria	ASA given	UH	Follow-up (days)	Major findings
GISSI-1 [3]	11,806	All	1.5 million U over 1 h	No	<12	ST ↑ or ↓	±	±	In-hospital (14–21 days)	↓ mortality with SK
ISAM [128]	1,741	<75 years	1.5 million U over 1 h	Yes	<6	ST ↑	Yes	IV	21	Trend towards ↓ mortality with SK. A similar reduction to that seen in the GISSI-1 trial
ISIS-2 [4]	17,187	All	1.5 million U over 1 h	Yes	<24	None	Randomized	±	35	↓ mortality with SK, ASA; lowest with both
EMERAS [37]	3,568	All	1.5 million U over 1 h	Yes	6–24	None	Yes	±	35	No significant difference in mortality in patients enrolled between 6 and 24 h from symptom onset.

ECG = electrocardiogram; EMERAS = Estudio Multicentrico Estreptoquinasa Republicas de America del Sur; GISSI = Gruppo Italiano per lo Studio della Streptochinasi nell'Infarto Miocardico; ISIS = International Study of Infarct Survival accelerated 90-min regimen of t-PA [39] compared with the traditional 3-hour regimen of t-PA [40], APSAC [41, 42] and SK [43].

Clinical relevance was added to these angiographic data with the GUSTO-I trial [8]. In this trial 41,021 STEMI patients were randomized to SK plus either SC or IV heparin vs accelerated t-PA plus IV heparin. A fourth arm, which randomized patients to a combination of the two fibrinolytic agents plus IV heparin was also included. All patients received aspirin at a dose of 325 mg/day. This trial revealed that the improved IRA perfusion rates translated into a significant improvement in 30-day mortality with the accelerated t-PA regimen compared with SK (6.3% vs 7.3%, respectively, p-value = 0.001). The improvement in mortality was present as early as 24 h after treatment began. In addition, other major complications, such as cardiogenic shock, congestive heart failure and ventricular arrhythmias, were also reduced among patients treated with t-PA. That the benefit of accelerated t-PA was associated with early opening of the IRA was revealed by the relationship between the improved patency at 90 min and the improved survival at both 24 h and at 30 days, further emphasizing the benefits of rapid reperfusion [43, 44].

Although uncommon, the aggressive regimens of fibrinolysis, aspirin and heparin utilized in GUSTO-I were associated with a small, but significant increase in the rate of intracranial hemorrhage. For each of the SK arms, 0.5% of patients suffered an intracranial hemorrhage (ICH) compared with 0.7% of patients treated with accelerated t-PA and 0.9% of patients treated with combination fibrinolytic therapy [8]. However, when comparing the net clinical benefit among the four regimens, accelerated t-PA still provided a clear benefit compared with the other three. The benefit of accelerated t-PA was seen in nearly every subgroup analyzed, including patients with anterior or inferior MI and in young and elderly patients. The absolute benefit was greater in higher-risk patients, for example those with anterior MI.

The search for agents that optimize clinical outcomes while minimizing risk for patients with STEMI has led to the development of the third generation of fibrinolytics using t-PA as the backbone [45] (Figure 8.1). A common feature among these agents is prolonged plasma clearance, allowing them to be administered as a bolus rather than the bolus and double-infusion technique by which accelerated-dose t-PA is administered.

Reteplase (r-PA)

Recombinant plasminogen activator (reteplase, r-PA, Figure 8.1) is a mutant of wild-type t-PA that lacks the kringle 1, finger and epidermal growth factor domains [46]. Because it is produced in *Escherichia coli,* r-PA lacks carbohydrate side chains. These modifications result in preferential activation of fibrin-bound plasminogen, a longer half-life in animals, healthy volunteers and patients, enhanced fibrinolytic potency and lower affinity for endothelial cells [47]. The plasma half-life of reteplase activity is 13–16 min allowing for bolus administration, a property of the third-generation fibrinolytics that has been associated with convenience and with less dosing errors [45].

The clinical efficacy and safety of r-PA was initially compared with SK in the INJECT trial [48]. This European cooperative study compared the efficacy and safety of 10+10 MU of r-PA vs 1.5 MU of SK with concomitant heparin in 6010 patients with an acute MI of less than 12 h duration. Although a non-significant benefit in survival with r-PA was seen at 35 days (9.02% vs. 9.53% with SK), r-PA was deemed at least as effective

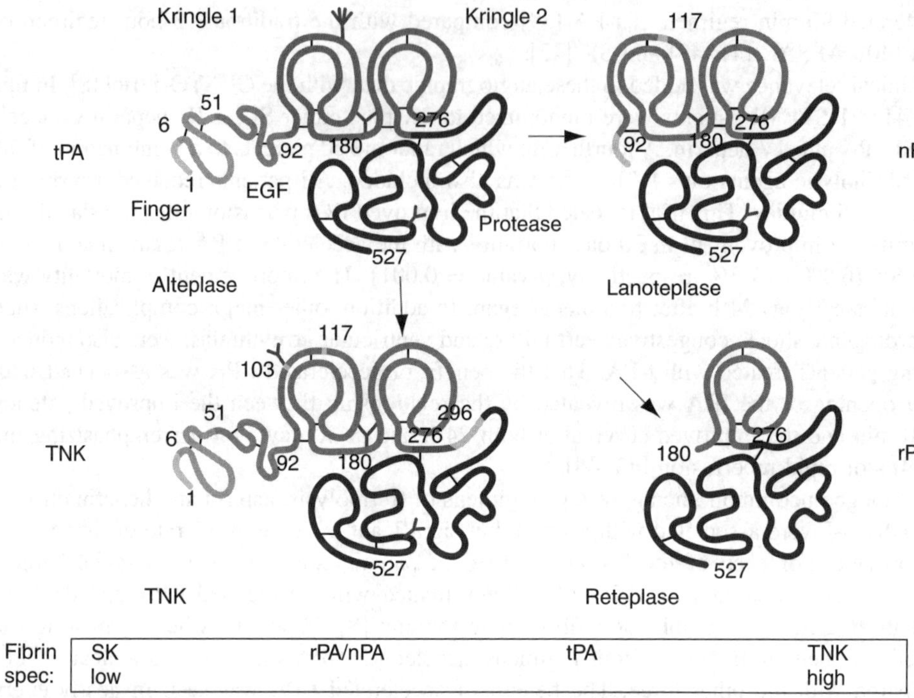

Figure 8.1 Molecular structure of alteplase (tPA), lanoteplase (nPA), reteplase (rPA), and tenecteplase (TNK). A full colour version of this figure can be found in the colour plate section of this book.

as SK by the statistical specifications of the trial. In addition, the incidence of stroke and other bleeding events was similar among the two treatment arms leaving the investigators with the conclusion '...it will be a useful addition to the range of thrombolytic agents available.'

Further enthusiasm for r-PA arose out of angiographic trials that revealed the safety profile and suggested improved patency rates at 60 and 90 min with r-PA compared with the 3-hour regimen [49], and the accelerated regimen of t-PA [50], without an increase risk of bleeding complications. This improvement in patency resulted in improved global and regional left ventricular function and fewer coronary interventions in the RAPID 1 and RAPID 2 trials, respectively.

Born out of the superior angiographic results in pilot studies of acute MI, the GUSTO III trial sought to compare the efficacy and safety of r-PA and t-PA [10]. However, in this trial of 15,059 STEMI patients presenting within 6 h of symptom onset, no significant difference in mortality was seen between the two treatment groups (7.47% reteplase vs 7.24% for alteplase, p-value $= 0.54$). In addition, the incidence of adverse events was near-identical. Despite a lack of superiority of r-PA over t-PA, its favorable safety profile and ease of administration have secured its approval for use in this patient population.

Possible explanations for the dissociation between improved angiographic patency with r-PA and lack of reduction in mortality include: the lower fibrin-specificity translating in a lower rate of TIMI 3 flow at 30 min compared with t-PA [50], higher rates of reocclusion, overestimation of the angiographic advantage in the phase II trials, a higher rate and intensity of platelet activation by r-PA or simply the play of chance. A prospective evaluation of platelet activation and aggregation following revealed that patients treated with r-PA had a significantly higher rate of aggregation in response to various concentrations of ADP, thrombin and collagen than patients treated with t-PA [51]. Furthermore, the r-PA patients also had a significantly higher expression of the GP receptor IIb/IIIa and the platelet–endothelial cell adhesion molecule 1 (PECAM-1). A more recent study in healthy subjects and in patients with coronary artery disease corroborated the superior inhibition of ADP-induced platelet aggregation with t-PA [52]. However, contradictory data are accumulating including a comprehensive evaluation of the effect of r-PA and t-PA on early platelet aggregation, which showed a higher suppression of platelet activation with r-PA than with t-PA. These observations highlight the uncertainty regarding the effect of plasminogen activators on platelet biology and the need for prolonged anti-platelet therapy, particularly 24 h after r-PA in preventing late ischemic events.

Tenecteplase

TNK is a recombinant derivative of t-PA developed by strategic point substitutions resulting in a triple mutant of t-PA with a significantly decreased plasma clearance, increased resistance to PAI-1, and improved fibrin specificity [53]. The lack of susceptibility to inactivation by PAI-1 is an important attribute, because it combats the increased levels of PAI-1 secreted by platelets activated by fibrinolytic agents. The favorable characteristics of TNK compared with t-PA in various experimental thrombosis models helped facilitate the clinical development of TNK [54].

Following the demonstration of the safety and the effective dose range for TNK [55] the efficacy of TNK was compared directly with accelerated t-PA in the angiographic TIMI 10B trial [56]. Eight hundred eighty-six patients with acute STEMI were randomly allocated to an accelerated t-PA regimen, TNK 30 mg bolus or TNK 50 mg bolus, followed by 90-min angiogram. After substitution of 40 mg dose of TNK for the higher dose owing to the high rate of intracranial hemorrhage in the 50 mg arm, nearly identical rates of TIMI 3 flow at 90 min. There was no difference in the rate of ICH between the groups. In addition, this trial emphasized that weight-adjusting TNK appears to be important in achieving optimal reperfusion and that reduced heparin dosing improved safety for both agents. Coupled with safety data from a large trial of TNK [57], the stage was set to assess the relative clinical efficacy of TNK.

The ASSENT-2 trial compared TNK with t-PA [58] in 16,949 STEMI patients presenting within 6 h of symptom onset [58]. Patients were randomized to weight-adjusted accelerated t-PA (maximum 100 mg) over 90 min (8488 patients) or weight-adjusted TNK (30–50 mg) as a bolus over 5–10 seconds (8461 patients). All patients received aspirin 150–325 mg and weight-adjusted heparin 4000–5000 U bolus followed by an infusion of 800–1000 U/h adjusted to maintain the aPTT at 50–75 sec, for 48–72 h. The primary endpoint, 30-day all-cause mortality, occurred in 6.18% and 6.15% of the TNK and t-PA groups, fulfilling the criteria for equivalency. Multiple univariate analyses for death at 30 days were performed with respect to age, gender, time-to-treatment, infarct location, Killip class, diabetes, hypertension and previous CABG or MI. Only patients randomized more than 4 h from symptom onset demonstrated a lower (unadjusted) mortality for TNK compared with t-PA (7.0% vs 9.2%, *p*-value = 0.018). These data regarding the efficacy of TNK coupled with its enhanced safety and ease of administration have led to its approval by the FDA for treatment of patients with STEMI.

FIBRINOLYTIC RESISTANCE

Rupture of an atherosclerotic plaque with the resultant adhesion of circulating platelets, elaboration of coagulants such as thrombin, and the generation of cross-linked fibrin can culminate in occlusion of the coronary artery clinically represented by acute STEMI. The three integral components of an occlusive thrombus – platelets, thrombin and fibrin – may all need to be adequately targeted in order to achieve optimal reperfusion. Fibrinolytic therapy, however, targets only one of these components, fibrin, in part contributing to their noted reperfusion rates. Through their actions on fibrin, these agents release clot-bound thrombin, accentuating the prothrombotic milieu via platelet activation and the resultant generation of vasoactive amines and activation of the coagulation cascade [59, 60]. Given this prothrombotic milieu, adjunctive therapies targeting both thrombin and platelets seem essential.

Platelets play a significant role in promoting the incomplete efficacy achieved with fibrinolytic therapy. The pivotal role of platelets in acute STEMI was established in the ISIS-2 trial. Compared to placebo, aspirin reduced mortality following MI by 23%, a risk reduction similar to that of SK alone [4]. In addition the combination of aspirin and SK appeared to have an additive benefit on mortality. Furthermore, aspirin has been shown to decrease the risk of reocclusion following fibrinolytic therapy [61]. Despite these beneficial effects, aspirin's incomplete inhibition of platelet activation and the existence of aspirin resistance [62], have prompted the search for more potent antiplatelet therapies.

At the site of arterial injury, platelets adhere to exposed collagen, vWF and fibrinogen. Adherent platelets are then activated by several mechanisms including collagen, thrombin, serotonin and ADP. Activated platelets degranulate, prompting secretion of vasoactive amines, clotting factors and chemotaxins, promoting more thrombin generation and additional platelet accumulation: a cycle of thrombosis. With activation, the final common pathway of platelet aggregation, the GP IIb/IIIa receptor undergoes a conformational change and becomes receptive to ligand binding [63]. Platelet aggregation culminates in a large platelet core at the site of vascular injury: an ideal milieu for thrombus formation as well as a mechanism of resistance.

'ENHANCED' FIBRINOLYTIC REGIMENS

The benefit of fibrinolytic therapy for STEMI is limited by inadequate reperfusion or reocclusion of the IRA in a considerable proportion of patients. Initial reperfusion fails to occur in approximately 20% of patients and is associated with a doubling of mortality rates [43]. Furthermore, reinfarction secondary to reocclusion of the IRA occurs in an additional 4–5% of patients during their index hospitalization, and this event is associated with 3.5-fold increase in mortality rates [64]. An understanding of the underlying pathophysiology of this limitation of fibrinolytic therapy is essential in order to comprehend the development of 'enhanced' fibrinolytic regimens.

Fibrinolysis plus GP IIb/IIIa inhibition

Observations in several trials suggested that the use of GP IIb/IIIa inhibitors alone would result in TIMI 3 flow rates in up to 32% of patients [12, 65–67]. While these rates are dwarfed by the rate of TIMI 3 flow achieved with fibrinolytics, 50–60%, the use of GP IIb/IIIa inhibitors is not hindered by the paradoxical prothrombotic effects seen with fibrinolysis. In addition, several early phase II trials revealed improved angiographic and electrocardiographic evidence of reperfusion when combining GP IIb/IIIa inhibitors with full-dose fibrinolytics (Table 8.3). However, the increased bleeding complications associated with this therapy prompted further evaluation with the combination of half-dose fibrinolytics with GP IIb/IIIa antagonism. The encouraging results, revealing improved IRA patency without increased bleeding risks, set the stage for assessing the clinical benefit of combination therapy.

Despite the encouraging data from phase II trials, two large-scale clinical trials failed to show a survival benefit with combination therapy compared to conventional therapy, with evidence of increased bleeding, especially in elderly patients [14, 15]. The GUSTO-V trial randomized 16,588 patients in an open-label fashion to either a reduced-dose of the fibrinolytic r-PA combined with a full dose of the platelet GP IIb/IIIa inhibitor abciximab or to full-dose r-PA alone in patients with STEMI. The primary endpoint, 30-day mortality, was essentially the same in both groups. However there was evidence of more stable reperfusion with this approach as manifest by reductions in the incidences of reinfarction, recurrent ischemia, the need for urgent 'bailout' mechanical revascularization and other ischemic complications. This benefit was achieved at the cost of an increase in non-intracranial bleeding complications.

Given that LMWH and platelet GP IIb/IIIa inhibitors have shown the potential to improve pharmacological reperfusion therapy, a randomized, open-label trial was performed to compare the efficacy and safety of TNK plus enoxaparin or abciximab, with that of TNK plus weight-adjusted UH in 6095 patients with acute STEMI presenting within 6 h of symptom onset [14]. Patients were randomly assigned one of three regimens: full-dose TNK and enoxaparin for a maximum of 7 days, half-dose TNK with weight-adjusted low-dose UH and a 12-h infusion of abciximab, or full-dose TNK with weight-adjusted UH for 48 h. The primary endpoints, the composites of 30-day mortality, in-hospital reinfarction, or in-hospital refractory ischemia (efficacy endpoint), and the above endpoint plus in-hospital intracranial hemorrhage or in-hospital major bleeding complications (efficacy plus safety endpoint) were significantly improved with either abciximab or enoxaparin in combination with TNK. Coupled with the GUSTO-V data, these data suggest that combination therapy may be a viable alternative to full-dose fibrinolytics with the caveat being to not administer this therapy to elderly ($\geq$75 years) patients as a result of increased bleeding complications. However, in keeping with the 2004 ACC/AHA guidelines for the management of patients with STEMI, combined half-dose fibrinolytics with GP IIb/IIIa inhibitors can not be recommended at the current time [68].

Fibrinolysis plus clopidogrel

Similar to the impetus to assess GP IIb/IIIa inhibitors combined with reduced-dose fibrinolysis – that incomplete reperfusion and/or reocclusion of the IRA occur in substantial proportions of patients treated with fibrinolysis – prompted the evaluation of clopidogrel

Table 8.3 Phase II trials of GP IIb/IIIa inhibitors combined with fibrinolytics for STEMI

Trial	N	GP IIb/IIIa inhibitor	Fibrinolytic	UH	ASA given	TIMI 3 flow at 90 min (%)	Major hemorrhage (%)	Major findings
TAMI-8 [129]	70	m7E3 FAB	Full dose t-PA	+	+	–	25	Increased patency at coronary angiography. Combination therapy deemed safe
IMPACT-AMI [130]	132	Eptifibatide	Full dose t-PA, accelerated regimen	40 U/kg bolus; then 15 U/kg per h	+	66	4	The highest Integrilin dose groups had more complete reperfusion (TIMI grade 3 flow, 66% vs 39% for t-PA alone; p-value = 0.006) and a shorter median time to ST-segment recovery (65 vs 116 min for t-PA alone; p-value = 0.05)
PARADIGM [11]	345	Lamifiban	Full dose t-PA or SK	5000 U bolus; then 1000 U/h	+	–	16.1	Increased bleeding at highest doses but also increased ST-segment resolution vs fibrinolytic alone
TIMI-14 [65]	888	Abciximab	½ dose t-PA	60 U/kg bolus; then 7 U/kg per h	+	77	7	Abciximab produced early, marked increases in TIMI 3 flow when combined with half the usual dose of alteplase. This improvement in reperfusion with alteplase occurred without an increase in the risk of major bleeding
		Abciximab	½ dose t-PA	30 U/kg bolus; then 4 U/kg per h		69	1	
		Placebo	Full dose t-PA	70 U/kg bolus; then 15 U/kg per h		62	6	

SPEED [12]	528	Abciximab	½ dose r-PA	60 U/kg boluses	+	61	6.3	Combination therapy improved early patency in patients with STEMI
		Abciximab	½ dose r-PA	40 U/kg boluses		51	10.5	
		Placebo	Full dose r-PA	70 U/kg boluses		47	3.7	
INTRO-AMI [67]	649	Eptifibatide	½ dose t-PA	60 U/kg bolus; then 7 U/kg per h	+	56	11	Eptifibatide plus ½ dose t-PA improved early TIMI 3 flow and exhibited a similar safety profile to other combination regimens
		Placebo	Full dose t-PA	60 U/kg bolus; then 7 U/kg per h		40	6	
INTEGRITI [21]	438	Eptifibatide	½ dose TNK	60 U/kg bolus; then 7 U/kg per h	+	59	7.6	Double-bolus eptifibatide (180/2/180) plus half-dose TNK tended to improve angiographic flow and ST-segment resolution compared with TNK monotherapy, but was associated with more transfusions and non-cerebral bleeding
		Placebo	Full dose TNK	60 U/kg bolus; then 12 U/kg per h		49	2.5	

ASA = aspirin; h = hour; IMPACT-AMI = Integrillin to Minimise Platelet Aggregation and Thrombosis-Acute Myocardial Infarction; INTEGRITI = Integrillin and Tenecteplase in acute myocardial infarction; INTRO-AMI = Integrillin and low-dose Thrombolysis in Acute Myocardial Infarction; PARADIGM = Platelet Aggregation Receptor Antagonist Dose Investigation and Reperfusion Gain in Myocardial Infarction; SPEED = Strategies for Patency Enhancement in the Emergency Department; TAMI = Thrombolysis and Angioplasty in Myocardial Infarction combined with standard full-dose fibrinolytics (Chapter 3). Clopidogrel use in this setting significantly improved the rate of a patent IRA at angiography and reduced ischemic endpoints with a similar risk of hemorrhagic complications to fibrinolysis alone. If expanded upon by future trials, the P2Y12 receptor antagonists as a class may provide a seamless transition from the pharmacologic to the mechanical worlds of reperfusion. That there were no increased risks of bleeding including in patients who underwent cardiac surgical procedures early after presentation further emphasizes the promise of this therapeutic pathway.

PRE-HOSPITAL FIBRINOLYSIS

Given that time to reperfusion is paramount to enjoying the maximal benefits, it seems logical to hypothesize that administration of fibrinolytic therapy in the pre-hospital setting would improve mortality in patients with STEMI. Prehospital fibrinolysis in several studies has been found to reduce time to treatment [19, 69] but this did not translate into a reduction in mortality. However, a meta-analysis of pre-hospital fibrinolytic trials did find a 17% reduction of in-hospital mortality [70]. When compared to primary angioplasty, pre-hospital fibrinolysis resulted in similar outcomes to primary angioplasty in patients presenting with early STEMI [71]. Furthermore, if administered within the first 2 h, pre-hospital fibrinolysis may be associated with better outcomes than primary PCI in eligible patients [72]. Nevertheless, it remains to be seen whether this strategy can improve long-term outcomes in clinical practice.

FIBRINOLYTICS IN ELDERLY PATIENTS

The optimal reperfusion strategy in elderly patients with STEMI remains a topic of debate. This lack of consensus stems from the exclusion or perceived under-representation of elderly people in clinical trials. While some observational studies have raised concerns about the lack of short-term benefit or possibility of harm with fibrinolysis [73, 74], most observational studies demonstrate improved intermediate-term survival with fibrinolysis [75, 76]. In addition, a meta-analysis of nine randomized placebo-controlled trials, including a total of 5754 patients >75 years of age, revealed that while the relative risk reduction was less for patients >75 years of age, the absolute risk reduction was 10 lives saved per 1000 patients treated (odds ratio 0.94, 95% CI 0.84 to 1.07) [9]. Similarly, the effects of age on outcomes was examined in patients enrolled in the GUSTO-I trial, which found that the greatest absolute reduction in mortality with fibrinolysis occurred in patients 65 to 85 years of age [77]. Therefore, evidence from randomized trials suggests a decreasing relative benefit with fibrinolysis in elderly people, but there remains an absolute gain in lives saved. In contrast, clinical trials and observational studies indicate improved survival and low risk of stroke with primary PCI compared with fibrinolysis in elderly patients with STEMI [78]. Thus, the current 'best' treatment of acute STEMI in elderly patients appears to be primary PCI. Nevertheless, continued evaluation is necessary to evaluate the relative merits of available reperfusion strategies as well as newer antithrombotic adjunctive therapies in elderly patients with STEMI.

LATE ADMINISTRATION OF FIBRINOLYTICS

Although fibrinolytic therapy is optimal when given within 70 min, there may be benefit in patients presenting 12 h after symptom onset and possibly up to 24 h if the patient has on-going or stuttering chest pain [79, 80]. Although most myocardial necrosis occurs early (within the first 90–180 min), the advantages of late reperfusion are presumably related to the presence of a patent infarct-related vessel, leading to improved ventricular healing, reduced infarct expansion and greater electrical stability.

A 2004 task force of the American College of Cardiology (ACC) and the American Heart Association (AHA) recommended fibrinolytic therapy for patients without contraindications presenting within 12 h of onset of symptoms [68]. They also concluded that it is reasonable to administer fibrinolytic therapy to patients presenting 12 to 24 h after the onset of symptoms if they have continuing symptoms and persistent ST segment elevation on the ECG. In all cases, it was recommended that the time from presentation to drug administration should be less than 30 min.

COMPLICATIONS OF FIBRINOLYSIS

Through experience and extensive literature a list of absolute and relative contraindications to fibrinolytic therapy has accrued with the purpose of assisting in the identification of patients at maximal risk of adverse events (Table 8.4).

Table 8.4 Contraindications to fibrinolytic therapy

Absolute contraindications

- Any prior ICH
- Known structural cerebrovascular lesion (i.e. AVM)
- Known malignant intracranial neoplasm (primary or metastatic)
- Ischemic stroke within 3 months EXCEPT acute ischemic stroke within 3 h
- Suspected aortic dissection
- Active bleeding or bleeding diathesis (except menses)
- Significant closed-head or facial trauma within 3 months

Relative Contraindications

- History of chronic, severe, poorly controlled hypertension
- Severe uncontrolled hypertension upon presentation (SBP >160 mmHg or DBP >110 mmHg)
- History of prior ischemic stroke more than 3 months previously, dementia, or known intracranial pathology not covered in absolute contraindications
- Traumatic or prolonged (>10 minutes) CPR
- Major surgery (within 3 weeks)
- Recent (within 2–4 weeks) internal bleeding
- Noncompressible vascular punctures
- Pregnancy
- Active peptic ulcer disease
- Current anticoagulant use: the higher the INR the higher the risk
- For SK/APSAC: prior exposure (>5 days previously) or prior allergic reaction

APSAC = Anisoylated streptokinase plasminogen activator complex; AVM = arteri-venous malformation: CPR = cardiopulmonary resuscitation; DBP = diastolic blood pressure; ICH = intracranial hemorrhage; mmHg = millimeters of mercury; SBP = systolic blood pressure

Bleeding

Unfortunately, the benefits of the currently available fibrinolytic agents remain limited by two complications, bleeding and their 'Achilles' heel,' stroke associated with ICH. These two complications are the most common reasons cited by physicians when the decision is made not to administer this life-saving therapy. Although severe bleeding occurs in approximately 2% of cases, the majority of bleeding complications occur without associated hemodynamic compromise or need for intervention [81]. In clinical trials, bleeding was most often procedure related, occurring with CAPG in 3.6%, and at the groin site of a PCI in 2%. The presence of severe bleeding, however, has been associated with longer hospitalization and higher mortality at 30 days, as well as other adverse clinical outcomes such as recurrent ischemia, left ventricular dysfunction, arrhythmia and stroke.

When assessing the risk of non-cerebral hemorrhage, it appears there are differences between the various fibrin-specific fibrinolytic agents. Although no difference in the overall rate of ICH is seen between TNK and t-PA, the rate of non-cerebral bleeding complications (26.4% vs 29%) and need for transfusion (4.3% vs 5.5%) were significantly lower with TNK [58]. The improved safety profile of TNK may reflect only minimal depletion of fibrinogen and weight-adjusted dosing. That the benefit of bolus fibrinolytics in their associated risk of bleeding complications is related to a lower risk of dosing errors must also be considered.

Stroke/ICH

Although the risk of stroke and ICH are low with the use of fibrinolytic therapy, the risk is not trivial. In a pooled analysis of over 200,000 patients receiving fibrinolytic therapy with or without UH, the risks of stroke and ICH were 1.34 and 0.59, respectively [68]. Comparable rates (1.2% and 0.7%) were also noted in a non-trial community registry of 12,739 patients [82].

Fortunately, a body of literature has accrued that permits identification of clinical and pharmacologic risk factors for the development of stroke or ICH after fibrinolysis. The increased risk with fibrin-specific agents vs SK [68] and the association with dose of concomitant AT therapy has been described [8]. The history of a previous stroke or TIA places patients at particularly high risk (6.9% and 5.5%, respectively) [83]. Other notable risk factors have included greater age, female sex, systolic blood pressure >160 mmHg, diastolic blood pressure >110 mmHg, lower body weight and t-PA dose above 1.5 mg/kg [82–86].

In order to facilitate the determination of risk of ICH in patients receiving fibrinolytic therapy, the Cooperative Cardiovascular Project analyzed clinical data from 31,732 patients who received fibrinolytic therapy and developed a prediction model [87]. The risk of ICH in this model ranged from 0.69% for patients with zero or one risk factors to 4.11% for patients with five risk factors (Table 8.5). Coupled with data that immediate administration of beta blockers may protect against ICH [85], these data may assist in allaying the fear of fibrinolytic therapy sufficiently to provide the best chance of improved mortality for the large proportion of eligible patients who have been shielded from the benefits of pharmacologic reperfusion.

Table 8.5 Risk model for intracranial hemorrhage with fibrinolytic therapy. Data from Brass *et al.* [87]

Independent predictors*	
• Age ≥75 years	
• Black race	
• Female gender	
• Prior history of stroke	
• Systolic blood pressure ≥160 mmHg	
• Weight ≤65 kg for women or ≤80 kg for men	
• INR >4 or PT >24	
• Use of t-PA (vs other fibrinolytic)	
Risk Score	**Rate of ICH (%)**
0 or 1	0.69
2	1.02
3	1.63
4	2.49
≥5	4.11

*Each independent predictor is worth 1 point if present, 0 points if absent ICH = intracranial hemorrhage; PT = prothrombin time

8.3 FIBRINOLYTICS FOR VTE

DVT

The use of fibrinolytic therapy for the treatment of DVT remains controversial. Although an improvement in the rate of clot dissolution and of normal follow-up venography compared with UH is seen with these agents, the major benefit of fibrinolytic therapy rests with its ability to decrease the risk of complications of proximal occlusive DVT (i.e. phlegmasia cerulea dolens) and of post-phlebitic syndrome [88–91]. However, given the increased risk of bleeding with fibrinolytic therapy in these patients, and the suggestion that most patients would prefer to live with the post-phlebitic syndrome rather than accept the small increased risk of death or disability due to bleeding [92], these agents are reserved for patients with limb-threatening DVT or DVT associated with severe symptoms.

PE

Three fibrinolytic agents with specific regimens have been approved by the FDA for use in patients with an acute PE (Table 8.6). Key issues relating to the use of fibrinolytics for the treatment of PE will be briefly discussed. For a more in-depth discussion of the use of these agents, the reader is referred elsewhere [93–96].

Fibrinolytics versus UH

Whereas a clear role of fibrinolytics for patients with DVT remains to be more optimally defined, the role of fibrinolytics in the management of massive PE appears to be somewhat

Table 8.6 FDA-approved fibrinolytic regimens for the treatment of PE

Agent	Regimen
SK	250,000 U over 30 min followed by 100,000 U/h for 24 h
Urokinase	4400 U/kg over 10 min followed by 4400 U/kg per h for 24 h
rt-PA	100 mg over 2 h

clearer. Several randomized clinical trials comparing various fibrinolytic agents with UH have demonstrated improvements in angiographic and hemodynamic abnormalities early after treatment [97–104]. However, this advantage appears to be short-lived. Although significant differences in echocardiographic parameters of right ventricular pressure overload were evident within 12 h in patients treated with fibrinolysis compared with those treated with UH, these differences were no longer evident at 1 week of follow-up [97]. In addition, a recent meta-analysis suggested that, compared with UH, fibrinolytic therapy does not appear to have therapeutic benefit in unselected patients, but is associated with an increased risk of major hemorrhage [95]. Thus, these data mandate the identification of specific patient populations with acute PE in whom the benefits of fibrinolytic therapy clearly outweigh the risks.

Comparative fibrinolytic trials

Several randomized comparative trials have been performed comparing urokinase (UK) with SK [105], UK with recombinant tissue plasminogen activator (rt-PA) [106–108], SK with rt-PA [109] and rt-PA with r-PA [110] in patients with PE. These trials again demonstrated resolution of angiographic, radiographic and echocardiographic abnormalities and a reduction in pulmonary arterial pressures with fibrinolysis. However, no significant differences between the various protocols and regimens were noted.

Characteristics of patients with PE who may benefit from fibrinolysis

Currently, there is consensus that patients with massive PE presenting with overt right ventricular failure (clinical instability and cardiogenic shock) should promptly be treated with fibrinolytic agents, since they are at a particularly high risk of death or life-threatening complications during the acute phase [104, 111]. At the other end of the clinical spectrum, fibrinolysis for PE is not indicated in the absence of right ventricular dysfunction. In fact, the prognosis of patients with small pulmonary emboli (not affecting pulmonary artery pressure and right ventricular afterload), is excellent and, as a result, the bleeding risks of fibrinolysis may outweigh the potential benefits of this treatment. Where the divergence of opinion occurs is with patients presenting with submassive PE (i.e. presenting with signs of impending right heart failure). While these patients may be difficult to identify, echocardiographic [112, 113], and biomarker abnormalities [114, 115] coupled with clinical factors such as age over 70 years, cancer, congestive heart failure, chronic obstructive lung disease, hypotension and tachypnea [113] may facilitate the recognition of patients with submassive PE who would benefit from fibrinolytic therapy. In a randomized, double-blind study of 256 patients presenting with submassive PE, pulmonary hypertension or right ventricular dysfunction without arterial hypotension or shock, a significant decrease in the primary endpoint of in-hospital death or clinical deterioration requiring an escalation of treatment was noted in patients randomized to receive t-PA (100 mg over 2 h) plus UH compared with those who received UH alone (p-value = 0.006) [116]. Despite these encouraging data, the controversy will continue until data from well-designed prospective clinical trials are available.

Timing of fibrinolysis

Several trials of PE fibrinolysis indicated that the duration of symptoms did not affect lung scan reperfusion or angiographic clot lysis [104, 107, 117–119]. However, a pooled analysis composed of 308 patients from these trials demonstrated an inverse relationship between duration of symptoms and improvement on post-treatment lung scan reperfusion scores [120]. For each additional day of symptoms before PE fibrinolysis, there was a decrement of 0.8% of lung tissue reperfusion on lung scanning (95% CI 0.2% to 1.4%, p-value = 0.008). Similarly, on angiography, less clot lysis immediately following fibrinolysis was observed in the group of patients with the longest duration of symptoms compared with those with the shortest symptom duration. Although fibrinolysis is still useful in patients who have had symptoms for 6–14 days, this inverse relationship between the duration of symptoms and the response to fibrinolysis indicates that fibrinolytic treatment should begin as soon as possible after PE is diagnosed in the appropriate clinical situation.

Novel methods of fibrinolytic delivery

Rapid Infusion of Fibrinolysis

Although demonstrated to be effective when given in a rapid fashion (i.e. t-PA 0.6 mg/kg over 2 min) [98], the administration of fibrinolytic therapy for the management of PE is a more prolonged endeavor than that for an STEMI (Table 8.6). Theoretically, more rapid infusion regimens should maintain efficacy while decreasing hemorrhagic risk, a clinically significant advantage that remains to be proven.

Catheter-directed Fibrinolysis

While the intravenous route has been the primary method of delivery, local pulmonary arterial fibrinolytic therapy has been utilized in the setting of massive PE when surgical embolectomy might otherwise have been considered. A number of investigators have employed standard or low-dose intrapulmonary arterial fibrinolytic infusions in order to deliver a high concentration of drug in close proximity to the clot [121–127]. While theoretically this approach should result in less systemic anticoagulation, the presence of systemic effects of these locally delivered agents has been well documented [98, 123]. In one study of 34 patients with acute massive PE receiving IV heparin the efficacy of intrapulmonary vs IV t-Pa was assessed [127]. Pulmonary arteriography after treatment revealed that the severity of embolism decreased by 38% in both the intrapulmonary arterial and IV groups. The results of this randomized trial suggest that intrapulmonary arterial delivery of fibrinolytic agents offers no advantage over the IV route. Although the clinical implications remain poorly defined, a plausible explanation for the apparent lack of benefit is the fact that the fibrinolytic agent was not delivered directly into massive emboli. While direct, intra-embolic delivery of fibrinolytic utilizes a fraction, 10–20%, of the usual dose and may broaden the patient populations eligible for fibrinolysis, no trial has demonstrated improved efficacy over the IV route. Thus, this should not be the delivery method of choice except in extenuating circumstances.

8.4 CONCLUSIONS

Fibrinolytic therapy has provided those caring for patients with acute thrombotic disorders ammunition against an adverse prognosis especially when administered in a timely fashion. For both arterial and venous thrombotic disorders, IV administration appears to be the safest and most efficacious route of delivery. Despite the benefits of fibrinolysis, this therapeutic modality is plagued by the risk of severe hemorrhagic complications of which intracranial hemorrhage remains the most ominous. Nevertheless, with careful patient selection and close attention to the patient's clinical condition, these agents can be safely used and associated with improved clinical outcomes across a spectrum of CV disease states.

REFERENCES

[1] Fletcher, A.P., *et al.*, (1958) The treatment of patients suffering from early myocardial infarction with massive and prolonged streptokinase therapy. *Trans Assoc Am Physicians*, 71:287–96.

[2] Yusuf, S., *et al.*, (1985) Intravenous and intracoronary fibrinolytic therapy in acute myocardial infarction: overview of results on mortality, reinfarction and side-effects from 33 randomized controlled trials. *Eur Heart J*, 6(7):556–85.

[3] Gruppo Italiano per lo Studio della Streptochinasi nell'Infarto Miocardico (GISSI), (1986) Effectiveness of intravenous thrombolytic treatment in acute myocardial infarction. *Lancet*, 1(8478):397–402.

[4] ISIS-2 (Second International Study of Infarct Survival) collaborative group, (1988) Randomised trial of intravenous streptokinase, oral aspirin, both, or neither among 17,187 cases of suspected acute myocardial infarction: ISIS-2. *Lancet*, 2(8607):349–60.

[5] Gruppo Italiano per lo Studio della Sopravvivenza nell'Infarto Miocardico, (1990) GISSI-2: a factorial randomised trial of alteplase versus streptokinase and heparin versus no heparin among 12,490 patients with acute myocardial infarction. *Lancet*, 336(8707):65–71.

[6] The international study group, (1990) In-hospital mortality and clinical course of 20,891 patients with suspected acute myocardial infarction randomised between alteplase and streptokinase with or without heparin. *Lancet*, 336(8707):71–5.

[7] ISIS-3 (Third International Study of Infarct Survival) collaborative group, (1992) ISIS-3: a randomised comparison of streptokinase vs tissue plasminogen activator vs anistreplase and of aspirin plus heparin vs aspirin alone among 41,299 cases of suspected acute myocardial infarction. *Lancet*, 339(8796):753–70.

[8] The GUSTO investigators, (1993) An international randomized trial comparing four thrombolytic strategies for acute myocardial infarction. *N Eng J Med*, 329(10):673–82.

[9] Fibrinolytic Therapy Trialists' (FTT) collaborative group, (1994) Indications for fibrinolytic therapy in suspected acute myocardial infarction: collaborative overview of early mortality and major morbidity results from all randomised trials of more than 1000 patients. *Lancet*, 343(8893):311–22.

[10] The GUSTO III investigators, (1997) A comparison of reteplase with alteplase for acute myocardial infarction. *N Eng J Med*, 337(16):1118–23.

[11] The PARADIGM investigators, (1998) Combining thrombolysis with the platelet glycoprotein IIb/IIIa inhibitor lamifiban: results of the Platelet Aggregation Receptor Antagonist Dose Investigation and Reperfusion Gain in Myocardial Infarction (PARADIGM) trial. *J Am Coll Cardiol*, 32(7):2003–10.

[12] The SPEED group, (2000) Trial of abciximab with and without low-dose reteplase for acute myocardial infarction. Strategies for Patency Enhancement in the Emergency Department (SPEED). *Circulation*, 101(24):2788–94.

[13] In TIME-II investigators, (2000) Intravenous NPA for the treatment of infarcting myocardium early; InTIME-II, a double-blind comparison of single-bolus lanoteplase vs accelerated alteplase for the treatment of patients with acute myocardial infarction. *Eur Heart J*, 21(24): 2005–13.

[14] The ASSENT 3 investigators, (2001) Efficacy and safety of tenecteplase in combination with enoxaparin, abciximab, or unfractionated heparin: the ASSENT-3 randomised trial in acute myocardial infarction. *Lancet*, 358(9282):605–13.

[15] The GUSTO V Investigators, (2001) Reperfusion therapy for acute myocardial infarction with fibrinolytic therapy or combination reduced fibrinolytic therapy and platelet glycoprotein IIb/IIIa inhibition: the GUSTO V randomized trial. *Lancet*, 357:1905–1914.

[16] Coussement, P.K., *et al.*, (2001) A synthetic factor-Xa inhibitor (ORG31540/SR9017A) as an adjunct to fibrinolysis in acute myocardial infarction. The PENTALYSE study. *Eur Heart J*, 22(18):1716–24.

[17] Ross, A.M., *et al.*, (2001) Randomized comparison of enoxaparin, a low-molecular-weight heparin, with unfractionated heparin adjunctive to recombinant tissue plasminogen activator thrombolysis and aspirin: second trial of Heparin and Aspirin Reperfusion Therapy (HART II). *Circulation*, 104(6):648–52.

[18] White, H., (2001) Thrombin-specific anticoagulation with bivalirudin versus heparin in patients receiving fibrinolytic therapy for acute myocardial infarction: the HERO-2 randomised trial. *Lancet*, 358(9296):1855–63.

[19] Morrow, D.A., *et al.*, (2002) Evaluation of the time saved by prehospital initiation of reteplase for ST-elevation myocardial infarction: results of The Early Retavase-Thrombolysis in Myocardial Infarction (ER-TIMI) 19 trial. *J Am Coll Cardiol*, 40(1):71–7.

[20] Wallentin, L., *et al.*, (2003) Efficacy and safety of tenecteplase in combination with the low-molecular-weight heparin enoxaparin or unfractionated heparin in the prehospital setting: the Assessment of the Safety and Efficacy of a New Thrombolytic Regimen (ASSENT)-3 PLUS randomized trial in acute myocardial infarction. *Circulation*, 108(2): 135–42.

[21] Giugliano, R.P., *et al.*, (2003) Combination reperfusion therapy with eptifibatide and reduced-dose tenecteplase for ST-elevation myocardial infarction: results of the integrilin and tenecteplase in acute myocardial infarction (INTEGRITI) Phase II Angiographic Trial. *J Am Coll Cardiol*, 41(8):1251–60.

[22] Roe, M.T., *et al.*, (2004) Improved speed and stability of ST-segment recovery with reduced-dose tenecteplase and eptifibatide compared with full-dose tenecteplase for acute ST-segment elevation myocardial infarction. *J Am Coll Cardiol*, 43(4):549–56.

[23] Sabatine, M.S., *et al.*, (2005) Addition of clopidogrel to aspirin and fibrinolytic therapy for myocardial infarction with ST-segment elevation. *N Eng J Med*, 352(12):1179–89.

[24] Kastrati, A., *et al.*, (2004) Early administration of reteplase plus abciximab vs abciximab alone in patients with acute myocardial infarction referred for percutaneous coronary intervention: a randomized controlled trial. *JAMA*, 291(8):947–54.

[25] Pino, R., *et al.*, (2004) Invasive strategy following fibrinolysis in ST-elevation acute myocardial infarction. *Ital Heart J*, 5(9):688–92.

[26] Di Mario, C., *et al.*, (2004) Combined Abciximab REteplase Stent Study in acute myocardial infarction (CARESS in AMI). *Am Heart J*, 148(3):378–85.

[27] Cutlip, D.E., *et al.*, (2003) Effect of tirofiban before primary angioplasty on initial coronary flow and early ST-segment resolution in patients with acute myocardial infarction. *Am J Cardiol*, 92(8):977–80.

[28] Scheller, B., *et al.*, (2003) Beneficial effects of immediate stenting after thrombolysis in acute myocardial infarction. *J Am Coll Cardiol*, 42(4):634–41.

[29] Fernandez-Aviles, F., *et al.*, (2004) Routine invasive strategy within 24 h of thrombolysis versus ischaemia-guided conservative approach for acute myocardial infarction with ST-segment elevation (GRACIA-1): a randomised controlled trial. *Lancet*, 364(9439):1045–53.

[30] de Lemos, J.A., *et al.*, (2000) ST-segment resolution and infarct-related artery patency and flow after thrombolytic therapy. Thrombolysis in Myocardial Infarction (TIMI) 14 investigators. *Am J Cardiol*, 85(3):299–304.

[31] French, J.K., *et al.*, (2002) Early ST-segment recovery, infarct artery blood flow, and long-term outcome after acute myocardial infarction. *Am Heart J*, 143(2):265–71.

[32] Gibson, C.M., *et al.*, (2004) Angiographic perfusion score: an angiographic variable that integrates both epicardial and tissue level perfusion before and after facilitated percutaneous coronary intervention in acute myocardial infarction. *Am Heart J*, 148(2):336–40.

[33] Tillet, W.S., Garner, R.I., (1933) The fibrinolytic activity of hemolytic streptococci. *J Expl Med*, 58:485–502.

[34] Rentrop, K.P., *et al.*, (1979) Acute myocardial infarction: intracoronary application of nitroglycerin and streptokinase. *Clin Cardiol*, 2(5):354–63.

[35] Anderson, J.L., *et al.*, (1983) A randomized trial of intracoronary streptokinase in the treatment of acute myocardial infarction. *N Eng J Med*, 308(22):1312–18.

[36] Simoons, M.L., *et al.*, (1986) Early thrombolysis in acute myocardial infarction: limitation of infarct size and improved survival. *J Am Coll Cardiol*, 7:717–28.

[37] The EMERAS (Estudio Multicentrico Estreptoquinasa Republicas de America del Sur) collaborative group, (1993) Randomised trial of late thrombolysis in patients with suspected acute myocardial infarction. *Lancet*, 342(8874):767–72.

[38] Franzosi, M.G., *et al.*, (1998) Ten-year follow-up of the first megatrial testing thrombolytic therapy in patients with acute myocardial infarction: results of the Gruppo Italiano per lo Studio della Sopravvivenza nell'Infarto-1 study. The GISSI Investigators. *Circulation*, 98(24): 2659–65.

[39] Neuhaus, K.L., *et al.*, (1989) Improved thrombolysis with a modified dose regimen of recombinant tissue-type plasminogen activator. *J Am Coll Cardiol*, 14(6):1566–9.

[40] Carney, R.J., *et al.*, (1992) Randomized angiographic trial of recombinant tissue-type plasminogen activator (alteplase) in myocardial infarction. RAAMI Study Investigators. *J Am Coll Cardiol*, 20(1):17–23.

[41] Neuhaus, K.L., *et al.*, (1992) Improved thrombolysis in acute myocardial infarction with front-loaded administration of alteplase: results of the rt-PA-APSAC patency study (TAPS). *J Am Coll Cardiol*, 19(5):885–91.

[42] Cannon, C.P., *et al.*, (1994) Comparison of front-loaded recombinant tissue-type plasminogen activator, anistreplase and combination thrombolytic therapy for acute myocardial infarction: results of the Thrombolysis in Myocardial Infarction (TIMI) 4 trial. *J Am Coll Cardiol*, 24(7):1602–10.

[43] The GUSTO Angiographic Investigators, (1993) The effects of tissue plasminogen activator, streptokinase, or both on coronary-artery patency, ventricular function, and survival after acute myocardial infarction. *N Eng J Med*, 329(22):1615–22.

[44] Simes, R.J., *et al.*, (1995) Link between the angiographic substudy and mortality outcomes in a large randomized trial of myocardial reperfusion. Importance of early and complete infarct artery reperfusion. GUSTO-I Investigators. *Circulation*, 91(7):1923–8.

[45] Llevadot, J., Giugliano, R.P., Antman, E.M., (2001) Bolus fibrinolytic therapy in acute myocardial infarction. *JAMA*, 286(4):442–9.

[46] Hu, C.K., *et al.*, (1994) Tissue-type plasminogen activator domain-deletion mutant BM 06.022: modular stability, inhibitor binding, and activation cleavage. *Biochemistry*, 33(39): 11760–6.

[47] Martin, U., Sponer, G., Strein, K., (1992) Evaluation of thrombolytic and systemic effects of the novel recombinant plasminogen activator BM 06.022 compared with alteplase, anistreplase, streptokinase and urokinase in a canine model of coronary artery thrombosis. *J Am Coll Cardiol*, 19(2):433–40.

[48] Randomised, double-blind comparison of reteplase double-bolus administration with streptokinase in acute myocardial infarction (INJECT): trial to investigate equivalence. International Joint Efficacy Comparison of Thrombolytics, (1995) *Lancet*, 346(8971):329–36.

[49] Smalling, R.W., *et al.*, (1995) More rapid, complete, and stable coronary thrombolysis with bolus administration of reteplase compared with alteplase infusion in acute myocardial infarction. RAPID Investigators. *Circulation*, 91(11):2725–32.

[50] Bode, C., *et al.*, (1996) Randomized comparison of coronary thrombolysis achieved with double-bolus reteplase (recombinant plasminogen activator) and front-loaded, accelerated alteplase (recombinant tissue plasminogen activator) in patients with acute myocardial infarction. The RAPID II Investigators. *Circulation*, 94(5):891–8.

[51] Gurbel, P.A., *et al.*, (1998) Effects of reteplase and alteplase on platelet aggregation and major receptor expression during the first 24 h of acute myocardial infarction treatment. GUSTO-III Investigators. Global Use of Strategies to Open Occluded Coronary Arteries. *J Am Coll Cardiol*, 31(7):1466–73.

[52] Gurbel, P.A., *et al.*, (2005) The platelet-related effects of tenecteplase versus alteplase versus reteplase. *Blood Coagul Fibrinolysis*, 16(1):1–7.

[53] Paoni, N.F., *et al.*, A slow clearing, fibrin-specific, PAI-1 resistant variant of t-PA (T103N, KHRR 296-299 AAAA). *Thromb Haemost*, 70(2):307–12.

[54] Collen, D., *et al.*, (1994) Comparative thrombolytic properties of tissue-type plasminogen activator and of a plasminogen activator inhibitor-1-resistant glycosylation variant, in a combined arterial and venous thrombosis model in the dog. *Thromb Haemost*, 72(1):98–104.

[55] Cannon, C.P., *et al.*, (1997) TNK-tissue plasminogen activator in acute myocardial infarction. Results of the Thrombolysis in Myocardial Infarction (TIMI) 10A dose-ranging trial. *Circulation*, 95(2):351–6.

[56] Cannon, C.P., *et al.*, (1998) TNK-tissue plasminogen activator compared with front-loaded alteplase in acute myocardial infarction: results of the TIMI 10B trial. Thrombolysis in Myocardial Infarction (TIMI) 10B Investigators. *Circulation*, 98(25):2805–14.

[57] Van de Werf, F., *et al.*, (1999) Safety assessment of single-bolus administration of TNK tissue-plasminogen activator in acute myocardial infarction: the ASSENT-1 trial. The ASSENT-1 Investigators. *Am Heart J*, 137(5):786–91.

[58] The ASSENT-2 investigators, (1999) Single-bolus tenecteplase compared with front-loaded alteplase in acute myocardial infarction: the ASSENT-2 double-blind randomised trial. Assessment of the Safety and Efficacy of a New Thrombolytic Investigators. *Lancet*, 354(9180):716–22.

[59] Merlini, P.A., *et al.*, (1995) Thrombin generation and activity during thrombolysis and concomitant heparin therapy in patients with acute myocardial infarction. *J Am Coll Cardiol*, 25(1):203–9.

[60] Coulter, S.A., *et al.*, (2000) High levels of platelet inhibition with abciximab despite heightened platelet activation and aggregation during thrombolysis for acute myocardial infarction: results from TIMI (thrombolysis in myocardial infarction) 14. *Circulation*, 101(23):2690–5.

[61] Roux, S., S. Christeller, E. Ludin, (1992) Effects of aspirin on coronary reocclusion and recurrent ischemia after thrombolysis: a meta-analysis. *J Am Coll Cardiol*, 19(3):671–7.

[62] Gum, P.A., *et al.*, (2003) A prospective, blinded determination of the natural history of aspirin resistance among stable patients with cardiovascular disease. *J Am Coll Cardiol*, 41(6):961–5.

[63] Lefkovits, J., Plow, E.F., Topol, E.J., (1995) Platelet glycoprotein IIb/IIIa receptors in cardiovascular medicine. *N Eng J Med*, 332(23):1553–9.

[64] Hudson, M.P., *et al.*, (2001) Early reinfarction after fibrinolysis: experience from the global utilization of streptokinase and tissue plasminogen activator (alteplase) for occluded coronary arteries (GUSTO I) and global use of strategies to open occluded coronary arteries (GUSTO III) trials. *Circulation*, 104(11):1229–35.

[65] Antman, E.M., *et al.*, (1999) Abciximab facilitates the rate and extent of thrombolysis: results of the thrombolysis in myocardial infarction (TIMI) 14 trial. The TIMI 14 Investigators. *Circulation*, 99(21):2720–32.

[66] Gold, H.K., *et al.*, (1997) Restoration of coronary flow in myocardial infarction by intravenous chimeric 7E3 antibody without exogenous plasminogen activators. Observations in animals and humans. *Circulation*, 95(7):1755–9.

[67] Brener, S.J., *et al.*, (2002) Eptifibatide and low-dose tissue plasminogen activator in acute myocardial infarction: the integrilin and low-dose thrombolysis in acute myocardial infarction (INTRO AMI) trial. *J Am Coll Cardiol*, 39(3):377–86.

[68] Antman, E.M., *et al.*, (2004) ACC/AHA guidelines for the management of patients with ST-elevation myocardial infarction—executive summary: a report of the American College of Cardiology/American Heart Association Task Force on Practice Guidelines (Writing Committee to Revise the 1999 Guidelines for the Management of Patients With Acute Myocardial Infarction). *Circulation*, 110(5):588–636.

[69] Weaver, W.D., *et al.*, (2003) Prehospital-initiated vs hospital-initiated thrombolytic therapy. *JAMA*, 270:1211–16.

[70] Morrison, L.J., *et al.*, (2000) Mortality and prehospital thrombolysis for acute myocardial infarction: A meta-analysis. *JAMA*, 283(20):2686–92.

[71] Bonnefoy, E., *et al.*, (2002) Primary angioplasty versus prehospital fibrinolysis in acute myocardial infarction: a randomised study. *Lancet*, 360(9336):825–9.

[72] Steg, P.G., *et al.*, (2003) Impact of time to treatment on mortality after prehospital fibrinolysis or primary angioplasty: data from the CAPTIM randomized clinical trial. *Circulation*, 108(23):2851–6.

[73] Thiemann, D.R., *et al.*, (2000) Lack of benefit for intravenous thrombolysis in patients with myocardial infarction who are older than 75 years. *Circulation*, 101(19):2239–46.

[74] Soumerai, S.B., *et al.*, (2002) Effectiveness of thrombolytic therapy for acute myocardial infarction in the elderly: cause for concern in the old-old. *Arch Intern Med*, 162(5):561–8.

[75] Berger, A.K., *et al.*, (2000) Thrombolytic therapy in older patients. *J Am Coll Cardiol*, 36(2): 366–74.

[76] Stenestrand, U., Wallentin, L., (2003) Fibrinolytic therapy in patients 75 years and older with ST-segment-elevation myocardial infarction: one-year follow-up of a large prospective cohort. *Arch Intern Med*, 163(8):965–71.

[77] White, H.D., *et al.*, (1996) Age and outcome with contemporary thrombolytic therapy. Results from the GUSTO-I trial. Global Utilization of Streptokinase and TPA for Occluded coronary arteries trial. *Circulation*, 94(8):1826–33.

[78] de Boer, M.J., *et al.*, (2002) Reperfusion therapy in elderly patients with acute myocardial infarction: a randomized comparison of primary angioplasty and thrombolytic therapy. *J Am Coll Cardiol*, 39(11):1723–8.

[79] Late Assessment of Thrombolytic Efficacy (LATE) study group, (1993) Late Assessment of Thrombolytic Efficacy (LATE) study with alteplase 6–24 h after onset of acute myocardial infarction. *Lancet*, 342(8874):759–66.

[80] Steinberg, J.S., *et al.*, (1994) Effects of thrombolytic therapy administered 6 to 24 h after myocardial infarction on the signal-averaged ECG. Results of a multicenter randomized trial. LATE Ancillary Study Investigators. Late Assessment of Thrombolytic Efficacy. *Circulation*, 90(2):746–52.

[81] Berkowitz, S.D., *et al.*, (1997) Incidence and predictors of bleeding after contemporary thrombolytic therapy for myocardial infarction. The Global Utilization of Streptokinase and Tissue Plasminogen activator for Occluded coronary arteries (GUSTO) I Investigators. *Circulation*, 95(11):2508–16.

[82] Huynh, T., *et al.*, (2004) Predictors of intracranial hemorrhage with fibrinolytic therapy in unselected community patients: a report from the FASTRAK II project. *Am Heart J*, 148(1): 86–91.

[83] Gore, J.M., *et al.*, (1995) Stroke after thrombolysis. Mortality and functional outcomes in the GUSTO-I trial. Global Use of Strategies to Open Occluded Coronary Arteries. *Circulation*, 92(10):2811–18.

[84] Aylward, P.E., *et al.*, (1996) Relation of increased arterial blood pressure to mortality and stroke in the context of contemporary thrombolytic therapy for acute myocardial infarction. A randomized trial. GUSTO-I Investigators. *Ann Intern Med*, 125(11):891–900.

[85] Barron, H.V., *et al.*, (2000) Intracranial hemorrhage rates and effect of immediate beta-blocker use in patients with acute myocardial infarction treated with tissue plasminogen activator. Participants in the National Registry of Myocardial Infarction-2. *Am J Cardiol*, 85(3): 294–8.

[86] Gurwitz, J.H., *et al.*, (1998) Risk for intracranial hemorrhage after tissue plasminogen activator treatment for acute myocardial infarction. Participants in the National Registry of Myocardial Infarction 2. *Ann Intern Med*, 129(8):597–604.

[87] Brass, L.M., *et al.*, (2000) Intracranial hemorrhage associated with thrombolytic therapy for elderly patients with acute myocardial infarction: results from the Cooperative Cardiovascular Project. *Stroke*, 31(8):1802–11.

[88] Turpie, A.G., *et al.*, (1990) Tissue plasminogen activator (rt-PA) vs heparin in deep vein thrombosis. Results of a randomized trial. *Chest*, 97(4 Suppl):172S–175S.

[89] Rogers, L.Q., Lutcher, C.L., (1990) Streptokinase therapy for deep vein thrombosis: a comprehensive review of the English literature. *Am J Med*, 88(4):389–95.

[90] Goldhaber, S.Z., (1990) Thrombolytic therapy for venous thromboembolism. *Baillieres Clin Haematol*, 3(3):693–704.

[91] Mohr, D.N., *et al.*, (2000) The venous stasis syndrome after deep venous thrombosis or pulmonary embolism: a population-based study. *Mayo Clin Proc*, 75(12):1249–56.

[92] O'Meara, J.J., 3rd, *et al.*, (1994) A decision analysis of streptokinase plus heparin as compared with heparin alone for deep-vein thrombosis. *N Eng J Med*, 330(26):1864–9.

[93] Wan, S., *et al.*, (2004) Thrombolysis compared with heparin for the initial treatment of pulmonary embolism: a meta-analysis of the randomized controlled trials. *Circulation*, 110(6):744–9.

[94] Buller, H.R., *et al.*, (2004) Antithrombotic therapy for venous thromboembolic disease: the Seventh ACCP Conference on Antithrombotic and Thrombolytic Therapy. *Chest*, 126(3 Suppl):401S–428S.

[95] Thabut, G., *et al.*, (2002) Thrombolytic therapy of pulmonary embolism: a meta-analysis. *J Am Coll Cardiol*, 40(9):1660–7.

[96] Goldhaber, S.Z., (2002) Thrombolysis for pulmonary embolism. *N Eng J Med*, 347(15):1131–2.

[97] Konstantinides, S., *et al.*, (1998) Comparison of alteplase versus heparin for resolution of major pulmonary embolism. *Am J Cardiol*, 82(8):966–70.

[98] Levine, M., *et al.*,(1990) A randomized trial of a single bolus dosage regimen of recombinant tissue plasminogen activator in patients with acute pulmonary embolism. *Chest*, 98(6):1473–9.

[99] Tibbutt, D.A., *et al.*, (1974) Comparison by controlled clinical trial of streptokinase and heparin in treatment of life-threatening pulmonay embolism. *Br Med J*, 1(904):343–7.

[100] Dalla-Volta, S., *et al.*, (1992) PAIMS 2: alteplase combined with heparin versus heparin in the treatment of acute pulmonary embolism. Plasminogen activator Italian multicenter study 2. *J Am Coll Cardiol*, 20(3):520–6.

[101] Ly, B., *et al.*, (1978) A controlled clinical trial of streptokinase and heparin in the treatment of major pulmonary embolism. *Acta Med Scand*, 203(6):465–70.

[102] The PIOPED investigators, (1990) Tissue plasminogen activator for the treatment of acute pulmonary embolism. A collaborative study by the PIOPED Investigators. *Chest*, 97(3):528–33.

[103] The urokinase pulmonary embolism trial. A national cooperative study. *Circulation*, 1973. 47(Suppl 2):1–108.

[104] Goldhaber, S.Z., *et al.*, (1993) Alteplase versus heparin in acute pulmonary embolism: randomised trial assessing right-ventricular function and pulmonary perfusion. *Lancet*, 341(8844):507–11.

[105] Urokinase-streptokinase embolism trial. Phase 2 results. A cooperative study. *JAMA*, 1974. 229(12):1606–13.

[106] Goldhaber, S.Z., *et al.*, (1988) Randomised controlled trial of recombinant tissue plasminogen activator versus urokinase in the treatment of acute pulmonary embolism. *Lancet*, 2(8606):293–8.

[107] Goldhaber, S.Z., *et al.*, (1992) Recombinant tissue-type plasminogen activator versus a novel dosing regimen of urokinase in acute pulmonary embolism: a randomized controlled multicenter trial. *J Am Coll Cardiol*, 20(1):24–30.

[108] Meyer, G., *et al.*, (1992) Effects of intravenous urokinase versus alteplase on total pulmonary resistance in acute massive pulmonary embolism: a European multicenter double-blind trial. The European Cooperative Study Group for Pulmonary Embolism. *J Am Coll Cardiol*, 19(2):239–45.

[109] Meneveau, N., *et al.*, (1998) Comparative efficacy of a two-hour regimen of streptokinase versus alteplase in acute massive pulmonary embolism: immediate clinical and hemodynamic outcome and one-year follow-up. *J Am Coll Cardiol*, 31(5):1057–63.

[110] Tebbe, U., *et al.*, (1999) Hemodynamic effects of double bolus reteplase versus alteplase infusion in massive pulmonary embolism. *Am Heart J*, 138(1 Pt 1):39–44.

[111] Kasper, W., *et al.*, (1997) Management strategies and determinants of outcome in acute major pulmonary embolism: results of a multicenter registry. *J Am Coll Cardiol*, 30(5):1165–71.

[112] Goldhaber, S.Z., (2002) Echocardiography in the management of pulmonary embolism. *Ann Intern Med*, 136(9):691–700.
[113] Goldhaber, S.Z., Visani, L., De Rosa, M., (1999) Acute pulmonary embolism: clinical outcomes in the International Cooperative Pulmonary Embolism Registry (ICOPER). *Lancet*, 353(9162):1386–9.
[114] Pruszczyk, P., *et al.*, (2003) Cardiac troponin T monitoring identifies high-risk group of normotensive patients with acute pulmonary embolism. *Chest*, 123(6):1947–52.
[115] Kucher, N., Printzen, G., Goldhaber, S.Z., (2003) Prognostic role of brain natriuretic peptide in acute pulmonary embolism. *Circulation*, 107(20):2545–7.
[116] Konstantinides, S., *et al.*, (2002) Heparin plus alteplase compared with heparin alone in patients with submassive pulmonary embolism. *N Eng J Med*, 347(15):1143–50.
[117] Goldhaber, S.Z., Loscalzo, J., (1988) Urokinase versus tissue plasminogen activator in pulmonary embolism. *Lancet*, 2(8616):915.
[118] Goldhaber, S.Z., *et al.*, (1986) Acute pulmonary embolism treated with tissue plasminogen activator. *Lancet*, 2(8512):886–9.
[119] Goldhaber, S.Z., Agnelli, G., Levine, M.N., (1994) Reduced dose bolus alteplase vs conventional alteplase infusion for pulmonary embolism thrombolysis. An international multicenter randomized trial. The Bolus Alteplase Pulmonary Embolism Group. *Chest*, 106(3):718–24.
[120] Daniels, L.B., *et al.*, (1997) Relation of duration of symptoms with response to thrombolytic therapy in pulmonary embolism. *Am J Cardiol*, 80(2):184–8.
[121] Leeper, K.V. Jr., *et al.*, (1988) Treatment of massive acute pulmonary embolism. The use of low doses of intrapulmonary arterial streptokinase combined with full doses of systemic heparin. *Chest*, 93(2):234–40.
[122] Vujic, I., *et al.*, (1983) Massive pulmonary embolism: treatment with full heparinization and topical low-dose streptokinase. *Radiology*, 148(3):671–5.
[123] Rubenfire, M., *et al.*, (1984) The systemic fibrinolytic effect of low-dose intraarterial streptokinase: observations in 12 patients. Work in progress. *Radiology*, 152(1):41–3.
[124] Barberena, J., (1983) Intraarterial infusion of urokinase in the treatment of acute pulmonary thromboembolism: preliminary observations. *AJR Am J Roentgenol*, 140(5):883–6.
[125] The UKEP study research group, (1987) The UKEP study: multicentre clinical trial on two local regimens of urokinase in massive pulmonary embolism. *Eur Heart J*, 8(1):2–10.
[126] Tapson, V.F., *et al.*, (1994) Pharmacomechanical thrombolysis of experimental pulmonary emboli. Rapid low-dose intraembolic therapy. *Chest*, 106(5):1558–62.
[127] Verstraete, M., *et al.*, (1988) Intravenous and intrapulmonary recombinant tissue-type plasminogen activator in the treatment of acute massive pulmonary embolism. *Circulation*, 77(2):353–60.
[128] Schroder, R., *et al.*, (1987) A prospective placebo-controlled double-blind multicenter trial of intravenous streptokinase in acute myocardial infarction (ISAM): long-term mortality and morbidity. *J Am Coll Cardiol*, 9(1):197–203.
[129] Kleiman, N.S., *et al.*, (1993) Profound inhibition of platelet aggregation with monoclonal antibody 7E3 Fab after thrombolytic therapy. Results of the Thrombolysis and Angioplasty in Myocardial Infarction (TAMI) 8 Pilot Study. *J Am Coll Cardiol*, 22(2):381–9.
[130] Ohman, E.M., *et al.*, (1997) Combined accelerated tissue-plasminogen activator and platelet glycoprotein IIb/IIIa integrin receptor blockade with Integrilin in acute myocardial infarction. Results of a randomized, placebo-controlled, dose-ranging trial. IMPACT-AMI Investigators. *Circulation*, 95(4):846–54.

9 Acute ST-Segment-Elevation Myocardial Infarction

9.1 INTRODUCTION

Acute STEMI remains a leading cause of morbidity and mortality. Although the optimal therapy for this clinical presentation in patients with coronary artery disease remains a process in evolution, the central paradigm mandates prompt and complete reperfusion in the setting of acute STEMI in order to reduce mortality and morbidity [1–6]. The improved outcomes enjoyed by patients with acute STEMI have arisen out of improved pharmacologic and mechanical revascularization approaches along with an expanding repertoire of adjunctive therapies including beta blockers, angiotensin-converting enzyme inhibitors, aldosterone antagonists, HMG CoA reductase inhibitors and the continued evolution of the repertoire of anti-platelet and antithrombin therapy.

Despite the improved outcome in patients with acute MI treated with reperfusion therapy, a substantial mortality and morbidity persists [7]. The benefits imparted by this treatment modality are, in part, determined by time to therapy, and transcends various patient characteristics including age, gender and the presence of diabetes mellitus, as well as the location of MI [8–12]. A substantial contributor to the improved mortality is the decreased myocardial necrosis and preserved left ventricular function achieved with successful reperfusion [13]. However, only 50–60% of patients receiving fibrinolytic therapy achieve complete angiographic reperfusion defined as TIMI grade 3 flow [14]. In addition, a substantial proportion of patients who do achieve TIMI 3 flow fail to achieve microvascular, or tissue-level, reperfusion, manifested by persistent ST-segment elevation [15]. This weakness of pharmacologic reperfusion therapy has clearly been shown to contribute to suboptimal outcomes [16–18].

Recent clinical trials of acute MI testing 'enhanced' reperfusion strategies have failed to demonstrate a significant improvement in mortality through an inability to break through this 'ceiling' of reperfusion [19–21]. In addition, no significant progress has been made on encouraging patients to present earlier with their symptoms, since the time to presentation for patients enrolled in clinical trials, nearly 3 h after symptom onset, has not changed over the past decade. As a result, IHD remains the leading cause of heart failure (HF), the prevalence of which is substantial and expected to increase to astronomical proportions by the third decade of this century [22].

Primary PCI has addressed some of the important limitations of fibrinolytic therapy including the 'ceiling' of benefit, the time dependence of benefit and the risks of ICH but remains limited in its own right. Several obstacles to instituting primary PCI as the universal treatment of STEMI include:

Management Strategies in Antithrombotic Therapy Arman T. Askari, Adrian W. Messerli and A. Michael Lincoff

- the lack of timely availability
- the dependence on the technical expertise of center and operator
- the need to address patient subgroups that are not studied in randomized trials
- comparisons of primary PCI to newer pharmacologic regimens.

In addition it appears that, at least in some form, the future treatment of STEMI may actually be one of a pharmaco-invasive morphology.

This chapter will review the currently available antithrombotic treatment strategies for STEMI including the benefits and limitations of the available fibrinolytic regimens, adjunctive therapies including AT and antiplatelet agents, a brief review of the advantages and disadvantages of mechanical reperfusion techniques and the possibility of a pharmaco-invasive approach to STEMI, and will address specific clinical considerations relevant to this patient population.

9.2 DEFINITIVE THERAPY

It has been well established that a key to myocardial salvage and improved outcomes in patients with STEMI is the time to restoration of antegrade coronary perfusion within the IRA. What remains controversial is how best to achieve complete reperfusion. Despite dramatic strides in the area of percutaneous intervention, fibrinolysis remains the most used form of reperfusion treatment worldwide. The interest in fibrinolytic therapy as a key player in the field of reperfusion rests with several advantages, including its widespread availability, its ease of use and its ability to be administered rapidly. On the other hand, fibrinolytic therapy has been limited by the lack of uniform efficacy, the risk of major hemorrhagic complications, and the figurative 'ceiling' of benefit. Coupled with the advantages of primary mechanical reperfusion techniques, these limitations of fibrinolytic therapy have prompted the search for 'enhanced' regimens that address the limitations and may potentially bridge the worlds of pharmacologic and mechanical reperfusion in order to improve outcomes for these patients.

PHARMACOLOGIC REPERFUSION

Fibrinolytic therapy

Although the use of fibrinolytic therapy was first described in 1958 [23], its utility in improving mortality in the setting of an STEMI was not formally suggested until the mid-1980s [24]. Since then a burgeoning body of literature has confirmed fibrinolytic therapy as a therapy that revolutionized treatment of these patients. Observations from the initial trials helped define the therapeutic window, the limitations and complications of fibrinolysis, and the role of adjunctive medications [4–6, 25–28]. Since the mid-1990s, attention has been focused on methods to further improve the outcomes while minimizing the adverse effects of fibrinolysis. The administration of potent antiplatelet and AT agents with fibrinolytic agents have been assessed in an attempt to break through the 'ceiling' of benefit associated with fibrinolysis [14, 19–21, 29–37]. The use of fibrinolysis in the setting of STEMI is continuing to evolve with a suggestion of improved outcomes when used in a 'facilitated' approach in combination with PCI [38–43]. Although primary PCI has demonstrated superior outcomes compared with fibrinolysis, associated delays in transfer of patients for primary

PCI may essentially eliminate its benefits in the United States. Combined with the improved mortality achieved with fibrinolysis, this further supports the role of pharmacologic reperfusion strategies in the current era. The central theme to treatment of STEMI remains early and complete restoration of antegrade blood. As to what method to use, that remains a process in evolution.

Fibrinolytic agents

Since the initial benefits of fibrinolytic therapy were demonstrated in the mid-1980s the specific fibrinolytic agents and treatment regimens have continued to evolve. Importantly, fibrinolytic therapy has been shown to restore IRA patency, reduce infarct size, preserve LV function and reduce mortality in patients with STEMI. Furthermore, the current generation of bolus fibrinolytics has been associated with simplified dosing regimens, reduced door-to-needle time and reduced potential for dosing errors. This has culminated in the lowest mortality rate to date achieved with pharmacologic reperfusion [21, 44]. In addition, irrespective of the fibrinolytic agent used for reperfusion strategies, the efficacy of the fibrinolytic is strongly dependent on the time to therapy and to the degree of both epicardial and tissue-level reperfusion obtained [11, 15, 45]. An in-depth view of the pharmacology of the various fibrinolytics is available in Chapter 8. Characteristics of the most commonly used fibrinolytic agents are summarized in Table 9.1.

Complications of fibrinolysis

Through experience and extensive literature a list of absolute and relative contraindications to fibrinolytic therapy has accrued with the purpose of assisting in the identification of the patients at maximal risk of adverse events (Table 9.2).

Bleeding

Unfortunately, the benefit of the currently available fibrinolytic agents remains limited by two complications, bleeding and their 'Achilles' heel,' stroke associated with ICH. These two complications are the most common reasons cited by physicians when the decision is made not to administer this life-saving therapy. Although severe bleeding occurs in approximately 2% of cases, the majority of bleeding complications occurs without associated hemodynamic compromise or need for intervention [46]. In clinical trials, bleeding was most often procedure related, occurring with CAPG in 3.6%, and at the groin site of a PCI in 2%. The presence of severe bleeding, however, has been associated with longer hospitalization and higher mortality at 30 days, as well as other adverse clinical outcomes such as recurrent ischemia, left ventricular dysfunction, arrhythmia and stroke.

When assessing the risk of non-cerebral hemorrhage, it appears there are differences between the various fibrin-specific fibrinolytic agents. Although no difference in the overall rate of ICH is seen between TNK and t-PA, the rate of non-cerebral bleeding complications (26.4% vs 29%) and need for transfusion (4.3% vs 5.5%) were significantly lower with TNK [29]. The improved safety profile of TNK may reflect only minimal depletion of fibrinogen and weight-adjusted dosing. That the benefit of bolus fibrinolytics in their associated risk of bleeding complications is related to a lower risk of dosing errors must also be considered.

Table 9.1 Characteristics of fibrinolytic agents

Agent	Source	Fibrin specificity	Systemic fibrinogen depletion	Antigenic	Effect on plasminogen	Plasma $T_{1/2}$ (min)	Metabolism	Dosing	Heparin therapy	90-min TIMI 3 flow rates (%)	Cost per dose (US$)
SK	Group A streptococci	–	Marked	Yes	Via activator complex	18–23	Hepatic	1.5 million IU IV over 1 h	SC or IV UH	30–35	613
t-PA	Recombinant, human	++	Mild	No	Direct	4–8	Hepatic	15 mg bolus, then 0.75 mg/kg (max 50 mg) over 30 min, then 0.5 mg/kg (max 35 mg) over 60 min	IV UH	54–60	2974
r-PA	Recombinant, human. Single chain deletion of t-PA.	+	Moderate	No	Direct	13–16	Renal	Double bolus (10 U IV over 2 min) 30 min apart.	IV UH	∼60	2750
TNK	Recombinant plus point substitutions of t-PA	+++	Minimal	No	Direct	20–24	Hepatic	Single bolus IV. For wt <60 kg:30 mg For wt 60–69 kg:35 mg For wt 70–79 kg:40 mg For wt 80–89 kg:45 mg For wt >90 kg:50 mg	IV UH or LMWH	∼60	2833

Table 9.2 Contraindications to fibrinolytic therapy

Absolute contraindications

- Any prior ICH
- Known structural cerebrovascular lesion (i.e. AVM)
- Known malignant intracranial neoplasm (primary or metastatic)
- Ischemic stroke within 3 months EXCEPT acute ischemic stroke within 3 h
- Suspected aortic dissection
- Active bleeding or bleeding diathesis (except menses)
- Significant closed-head or facial trauma within 3 months

Relative contraindications

- History of chronic, severe, poorly controlled hypertension
- Severe uncontrolled hypertension upon presentation (SBP >180 mmHg or DBP >110 mmHg)
- History of prior ischemic stroke more than 3 months previously, dementia, or known intracranial pathology not covered in absolute contraindications
- Traumatic or prolonged (>10 min) CPR
- Major surgery (within 3 weeks)
- Recent (within 2–4 weeks) internal bleeding
- Noncompressible vascular punctures
- Pregnancy
- Active peptic ulcer disease
- Current anticoagulant use: the higher the INR the higher the risk
- For SK/APSAC: prior exposure (>5 days previously) or prior allergic reaction

APSAC = Anisoylated streptokinase plasminogen activator complex; AVM = arteri-venous malformation: CPR = cardiopulmonary resuscitation; DBP = diastolic blood pressure; ICH = intracranial hemorrhage; SBP = systolic blood pressure

Stroke/ICH

Although the risk of stroke and ICH are low with the use of fibrinolytic therapy, the risk is not trivial. In a pooled analysis of over 200,000 patients receiving fibrinolytic therapy with or without UH, the risks of stroke and ICH were 1.34 and 0.59, respectively [47]. Comparable rates (1.2% and 0.7%) were also noted in a non-trial community registry of 12,739 patients [48].

Fortunately, a body of literature has accrued that permits identification of clinical and pharmacologic risk factors for the development of stroke or ICH after fibrinolysis. The increased risk with fibrin-specific agents vs SK [47] and the association with dose of concomitant AT therapy has been described [5]. The history of a previous stroke or TIA places patients at particularly high risk (6.9% and 5.5%, respectively) [49]. Other notable risk factors have included greater age, female sex, systolic blood pressure 140 mmHg, diastolic blood pressure 100 mmHg, lower body weight, and t-PA dose above 1.5 mg/kg [48–52].

In order to facilitate the determination of risk of ICH in patients receiving fibrinolytic therapy, the Cooperative Cardiovascular Project analyzed clinical data from 31,732 patients who received fibrinolytic therapy and developed a prediction model [53]. The risk of ICH in this model ranged from 0.69% for patients with zero or one risk factors to 4.11% for patients with five risk factors (Table 9.3). Coupled with data that immediate administration of beta blockers may protect against ICH [51], these data may assist in allaying the fear of

Table 9.3 Risk model for intracranial hemorrhage with fibrinolytic therapy. Data from Brass *et al.* [53].

Independent predictors *

- Age ≥75 years
- Black race
- Female gender
- Prior history of stroke
- Systolic blood pressure ≥160 mmHg
- Weight ≤65 kg for women or ≤80 kg for men
- INR >4 or PT >24
- Use of t-PA (vs other fibrinolytic)

Risk Score	**Rate of ICH (%)**
0 or 1	0.69
2	1.02
3	1.63
4	2.49
≥5	4.11

* Each independent predictor is worth 1 point if present, 0 points if absent
ICH = intracranial hemorrhage; PT = prothrombin time

fibrinolytic therapy sufficiently to provide the best chance of improved mortality for the large proportion of eligible patients who have been shielded from the benefits of pharmacologic reperfusion.

MECHANICAL REPERFUSION

Fibrinolytic therapy has been an important means of establishing reperfusion for decades. However, limitations to the use of fibrinolytic therapy include perceived or definite contraindications, intracranial bleeding, inability to establish TIMI 3 flow in many patients and high rates of recurrent ischemia and reocclusion. Compared to fibrinolysis, primary PCI achieves a higher rate of TIMI 3 flow (more than 90%), does not carry the risk of ICH and is associated with improved outcomes. Thus, primary PCI has emerged as the preferred reperfusion strategy.

Primary angioplasty versus fibrinolysis

Knowledge of coronary anatomy allows immediate triage to surgery, medical therapy or primary PCI, when appropriate, and results in earlier hospital discharge compared to fibrinolytic therapy. Primary PCI establishes TIMI 3 flow in 90% of patients and is associated with reduced rates of recurrent ischemia and reocclusion [54]. With the addition of stenting, reocclusion has been further reduced to 5% at routine 6-month angiography. Small studies have suggested that pharmacological adjuncts to PCI such as abciximab may improve myocardial perfusion and limit infarct size without the risk of bleeding observed with fibrinolytic therapy. Finally, new technologies such as coronary thrombectomy and distal protection are increasingly being employed in the catheterization laboratory and may further improve myocardial perfusion and infarct size.

To date, 23 published randomized controlled trials (RCT) have compared primary PCI with fibrinolytic therapy. These trials differ in many respects, including patient sample size, type of fibrinolytic therapy and whether stents, with or without platelet GP IIb/IIIa inhibitors, were used. A recent meta-analysis of these trials compared short-term and long-term outcomes in 7739 patients presenting with STEMI randomized to either primary PCI or to fibrinolytic therapy [55]. Primary PCI was better than fibrinolytic therapy at reducing overall short-term death (7% vs 9%, p-value = 0.0002), non-fatal reinfarction (3% vs 7%, p-value <0.0001), stroke (1% vs 2%, p-value = 0.0004), and the combined endpoint of death, non-fatal reinfarction, and stroke (8% vs 14%, p-value <0.0001). The results seen with primary PCI remained better than those seen with fibrinolytic therapy during long-term follow-up, and were independent of both the type of fibrinolytic agent used and whether or not the patient was transferred for primary PCI.

Primary PCI appears to address an important limitation of fibrinolysis, that of time dependence. Although mortality is associated with to door-to-balloon time [56, 57], a number of reports suggest that mortality with PCI is less time dependent than the mortality benefits of early fibrinolysis [58–60]. As a result, a greater number of patients may derive benefit from an initial PCI approach.

Despite the data supporting primary PCI as the reperfusion strategy of choice, this technique for restoring IRA perfusion is associated with several limitations of its own. Primary PCI remains less widely available than fibrinolytics. This often results in 'real-world' delays in reperfusion and can make this therapy quite inconvenient for patients who are eligible for fibrinolysis. In addition, outcomes of primary PCI are clearly dependent on the expertise of the primary operator and center performing the primary PCI, with high-volume operators enjoying the best outcomes for these patients [61]. Thus, because of its widespread availability, ease of administration and favorable outcomes in patients with an STEMI, fibrinolysis will continue to have a pivotal role in reperfusion therapy.

Transfer for primary PCI versus on-site fibrinolysis

Several recent trials including DANAMI-2 [62], AIR-PAMI [63] and PRAGUE [64] have investigated the benefit of on-site fibrinolysis in comparison to transfer to tertiary centers for direct PCI. These studies have found improved outcomes in patients randomized to a transfer strategy and direct PCI, even after taking into account the increased time for patient transfer. For example, patients in DANAMI-2 randomized to transfer PCI had a significantly lower 30-day incidence of death, MI or stroke (8.5% vs 14.3%, p-value = 0.002). In addition, a recent meta-analysis also demonstrated that primary PCI was associated with a significant reduction in the incidence of the combined end point of death, reinfarction or stroke compared to fibrinolysis (relative risk 0.58, 95% CI 0.47–0.71) [65]. Although interhospital transfer with direct PCI appears to be an attractive therapeutic option for acute MI based on clinical trial data, where the difference in time to reperfusion is routinely less than 60 min with balloon angioplasty compared with fibrinolysis, it remains to be seen whether such dramatic results can be obtained in the 'real world,' where transfer times are much longer.

Facilitated PCI

Facilitated PCI refers to pharmacologic therapy just prior to planned primary PCI for STEMI in an attempt to achieve an open IRA before arrival in the catheterization laboratory. Observations from PCI trials have suggested that patients undergoing primary PCI in whom TIMI 3 flow is present before intervention show greater clinical and angiographic evidence of myocardial salvage, are less likely to develop complications related to left ventricular failure and have improved early and late survival [66]. These data helped forge the hypothesis that the administration of fibrinolytics and other adjunctive therapies such as GP IIb/IIIa inhibitors before mechanical revascularization could enhance pre-procedural TIMI 3 flow rates which, in turn, could better prepare patients for primary PCI. A combined pharmacologic and mechanical approach for STEMI, therefore, has an inherent appeal, as it blends the benefits of both strategies. On the one hand, mechanical reperfusion offers more complete and sustained IRA patency with less ICH but is not widely available and is often associated with prohibitive time delays. On the other hand, fibrinolytics are associated with less intrinsic time delay and are universally available. Thus, combining these reperfusion strategies could 'facilitate' primary PCI and lead to superior clinical outcomes. Chapter 11 discusses this topic in more detail.

Although not formally tested in a large prospective randomized fashion, the facilitated approach to reperfusion has been suggested by observations from recent clinical studies. The results of the ADVANCE MI trial demonstrated no improvement in clinical outcomes with facilitated PCI in a small sample of patients from this prematurely terminated randomized trial [67]. Thus, the impact of facilitated PCI with GpIIb/IIIa inhibitors plus reduced-dose fibrinolytics before primary PCI on clinical outcomes remains uncertain, as a result of the small numbers of patients studied to date in dedicated randomized trials. This technique could potentially become appropriate for the management of patients with acute MI who present to hospitals without 24-hour catheterization laboratories. The FINESSE trial will study the feasibility and efficacy of facilitated PCI strategies.

Angiography after fibrinolysis

An important issue that remains unresolved is the role of elective coronary angiography and revascularization in patients who receive fibrinolytic therapy. While initial older trials showed no improvement in outcomes, more recent trials using major therapeutic advances, such as low-profile catheters, stents, GP IIb/IIIa inhibitors, thienopyridines and fibrin-specific fibrinolytic agents, have suggested a benefit from PCI performed within hours (adjunctive PCI) or a few days (early elective PCI) after fibrinolysis [68]. Two relatively small randomized trials (SIAM III and GRACIA) have demonstrated a reduction in subsequent ischemic events, but no reduction in mortality, with adjunctive PCI [42, 43], while a significant mortality benefit after early elective PCI was noted in a retrospective review of 20,100 patients from the TIMI and InTIME-II trials (2.6 vs 6.3% compared to no PCI among patients who had not had a recurrent MI) [69]. Although these data are relatively new, a report from the Second National Registry of Myocardial Infarction of 61,232 patients with an uncomplicated MI who were treated with fibrinolytic therapy between 1994 and 1998 previously underwent a high frequency (78%) of routine cardiac catheterization following fibrinolysis; for those below age 50 the frequency was 85% [70].

Rescue PCI

Rescue percutaneous revascularization is defined as the use of PCI when fibrinolytic therapy has proven unsuccessful. Despite the proven mortality benefit, >30% of patients who receive fibrinolytic therapy have essentially occluded infarct arteries at 90 min [71]. If reperfusion is not clearly evident 90 min after initiation of fibrinolytic therapy, particularly among patients with large acute MI, the decision to perform emergency angiography and mechanical reperfusion should be made promptly. Patients in cardiogenic shock after fibrinolytic therapy should undergo immediate coronary angiography and should not await clinical assessment of reperfusion.

It can be difficult to determine clinically whether a patient has successfully reperfused with fibrinolytic therapy. Resolution of chest pain is an inaccurate measure of reperfusion, because the pain may be blunted by narcotic analgesia or the partial denervation that is known to occur among some patients with MI. Serial assessment of 12-lead ECGs is a more reliable indicator of reperfusion, although it also is suboptimal. An accelerated idioventricular rhythm (AIVR) is fairly specific for reperfusion, but arrhythmias other than AIVR are not reliable indicators because a variety of ventricular and supraventricular arrhythmias may be observed in patients with a non-reperfused IRA. The complete resolution of chest pain and ECG changes (defined as >70% resolution of ST-segment elevation), accompanied by a run of AIVR, is highly specific for successful reperfusion, but it occurs among less than 10% of patients receiving lytic therapy. Resolution of ST-segment elevation by >70% is correlated with effective tissue level reperfusion and this finding has been correlated with better clinical outcome and angiographic reperfusion.

The patients who are known to derive definite benefit from rescue angioplasty are patients with anterior MI who have undergone unsuccessful fibrinolysis (TIMI 0 or 1 flow). These data were originally from the RESCUE trial, in which patients with TIMI 2 or 3 flow did not undergo revascularization [72]. More recently, a multicenter trial assessed the efficacy of repeat fibrinolysis, conservative therapy or rescue PCI on the combined endpoint of death, reinfarction, stroke or severe heart failure within 6 months in 427 patients presenting with an STEMI in whom fibrinolysis failed to achieve reperfusion [73]. Event-free survival after failed fibrinolytic therapy was significantly higher with rescue PCI (84.6%) than with repeated fibrinolysis (68.7%) or conservative treatment (70.1%) (overall p-value = 0.004). With the available evidence, rescue PCI should be considered for patients in whom reperfusion fails to occur after fibrinolytic therapy.

9.3 ADJUNCTIVE THERAPY

ANTIPLATELET THERAPY

The recognition of the central role of the platelet, in addition to fibrin and thrombin in arterial thrombosis, has provided a potential means for further improving the benefits of fibrinolytic therapy. It is hypothesized that in order to achieve more rapid and complete coronary and tissue reperfusion, and ultimately improve survival following acute STEMI, a combination of agents targeted to these key components of thrombosis may be necessary. The hope is that combination chemotherapy for acute STEMI would improve early patency and, ultimately, survival.

Aspirin

The benefits of aspirin in the treatment of STEMI are unequivocal (Chapter 2). Aspirin should be administered immediately to all patients with acute STEMI, unless there is a clear history of true aspirin allergy (not intolerance). Aspirin therapy conveys as much mortality benefit as SK, and the combination provides additive benefit [4]. The dose should be either four chewable 80 mg tablets (for more rapid absorption) or one 325 mg non-chewable tablet. If oral administration is not possible, a rectal suppository can be given. Alternatively, aspirin may be administered via the IV route at equipotent doses. Treatment with 75–162 mg/day of aspirin should be continued indefinitely. If true aspirin allergy is present, alternative antiplatelet agents can be utilized.

Clopidogrel

Once thought of simply as an alternative to aspirin in the treatment of STEMI, the use of clopidogrel in addition to aspirin has been associated with improved outcomes in patients with STEMI when administered as a 300 mg loading dose followed by 75 mg daily in addition to fibrinolysis within 12 h of symptom onset [37] and when administered as a 75 mg daily dose to patients as an adjunct to 'usual' therapy when administered within 24 h of symptom onset [74]. Based on these data, patients with STEMI treated with fibrinolysis should also receive a 300 mg loading dose of clopidogrel followed by 75 mg daily. Caution is advised in patients who are deemed at high risk of requiring CABG surgery [37], as prior data have suggested an increase in peri-operative bleeding complications in patients requiring CABG within 5–7 days of clopidogrel administration [75–77].

GP IIb/IIIa Inhibitors

Given the lack of a mortality benefit and increased risk of bleeding demonstrated with the combination of half-dose fibrinolytics and GP IIb/IIIa inhibitors (Chapter 8), the use of GP IIb/IIIa inhibitors as an adjunct to fibrinolysis cannot be recommended currently.

On the other hand, several clinical trials have documented the benefits of GP IIb/IIIa inhibitors in improving clinical outcomes after direct PCI with or without stenting in patients with acute MI [78–81]. Furthermore, a recent meta-analysis demonstrated that, when compared with the control group, adjunctive abciximab for STEMI is associated with a significant reduction in 30-day (2.4% vs 3.4%, p-value = 0.047) and long-term (4.4% vs 6.2%, p-value = 0.01) mortality in patients treated with primary angioplasty [81]. Thus, abciximab (0.25 mg/kg bolus intravenously followed by 0.125 mg/kg per min infusion over 12 h) should be considered in the care of all patients undergoing direct PCI for acute MI.

ANTITHROMBIN THERAPY

UH

The rationale for administering UH in patients with STEMI includes preventing ventricular thrombus formation, VTE and cerebral thromboembolism in addition to maintaining patency of the IRA.

UH Without Fibrinolytics in STEMI

Prior to the fibrinolytic era, AT therapy with UH and oral anticoagulation served to limit ischemic complications and prevent peripheral, cerebral or pulmonary embolization. Whereas the combination of aspirin and UH resulted in improved outcomes in patients with ACS, the benefit of combining these agents in patients with STEMI has been more difficult to establish. Observational data from clinical trials of fibrinolytic therapy have revealed conflicting results. Both a lack of a survival benefit [4] and improved survival [82] have been suggested. However, the clinical applicability of these data to present day management of STEMI is ambiguous, given that the vast majority of patients remain eligible for either fibrinolysis or primary PCI.

UH with Fibrinolytics in STEMI

Clinically relevant data assessing the utility of UH added to a regimen of fibrinolytics and aspirin remain limited. The majority of the benefit of UH therapy in these patients arises from a decreased incidence of ischemic and thrombotic complications rather than from a mortality benefit. The added benefit of UH to aspirin in patients receiving fibrinolysis was assessed in the GISSI-2 [27] and ISIS-3 [28] trials. Important considerations for UH therapy also addressed by these trials included the timing and route of administration. In the combined data set of GISSI-2 and ISIS-3 (totaling over 62,000 patients), the 35-day mortality was 10.0% in the patients receiving IV UH vs 10.2% in the patients not receiving any IV UH. Similar outcomes were seen in the GUSTO study, where no difference was seen in the 35-day mortality rate in patients receiving SK plus IV UH (7.2%) or IV UH (7.4%) [5]. Thus, the available information suggests that IV UH is probably of no benefit in patients receiving SK plus aspirin.

On the other hand, IV UH has found an adjunctive role with the fibrin-specific agents. After being associated with an improved patency combined with accelerated t-PA, studies of the newer fibrinolytic agents all uniformly used IV UH (Table 9.4). Although IV UH is commonly used after fibrinolytic therapy, this therapy appears to have a narrow therapeutic window with the optimal benefit and minimal risk of bleeding complications occurring at an aPTT between 50 and 70 sec [83]. The relationship between aPTT and clinical outcome may be confounded to some degree by the influence of baseline prognostic characteristics, aPTTs higher than 70 sec have been associated with higher likelihood of mortality, stroke, bleeding and reinfarction. The use of an early 3-h aPTT in the InTIME-II trial resulted in an observed ICH rate of 0.62%. A 60 U/kg bolus (with a maximum dose of 4000 U) followed by a maintenance infusion of 12 U/kg per h (maximum of 1000 U/h) is adequate with fibrin-specific agents [47]. These clinical trials involving UFH have used universal therapeutic aPTT ranges – typically 50 to 70 sec – regardless of the responsiveness of the thromboplastin reagent in use at the participating institutions. It is important to remember that the aPTT should be normalized to correspond to a 0.2 to 0.5 U/mL anti-factor Xa activity, given the variability responsiveness of thromboplastin reagents [84].

UH in Primary PCI

When primary PCI is chosen as the route of reperfusion, weight-adjusted boluses of heparin of 70 to 100 U/kg are recommended. This recommendation comes from general observations

Table 9.4 ICH rate in selected trials assessing t-PA plus heparin

Trial	*N*	Fibrinolytic arm	UH dose	Target aPTT	ICH rate (%)	Comment
ISG [25]	5,170	t-PA	12,500 SC bid	–	0.4	SC heparin was associated with an excess of major bleeds (1.0% with heparin vs 0.5% without heparin) but did not affect the incidence of stroke or reinfarction
GUSTO-1 [5]	10,268	Accelerated t-PA	5000 U bolus then 1000 U/h (1200 U/h if >80 kg)	60–85	0.72	Significant excess of ICH noted with the use of the accelerated t-PA regimen although absolute risk was still low
GUSTO IIA [97]	436	t-PA	5000 U bolus then 1000 U/h (1300 U/h if >80 kg)	60–90	0.90	Heparin, at a slightly higher dose than previously used in a large-scale trial (approximately 20% increase) was accompanied by a twofold risk of hemorrhagic stroke in patients receiving fibrinolytic therapy
GUSTO IIB [103]	1,163	t-PA	5000 U bolus then 1000 U/h	60–85	0.77	No difference in outcomes with t-PA combined with heparin or with the DTI hiudin

TIMI 9A [98]	368	t-PA	5000 U bolus then 1000 U/h (1300 U/h if >80 kg)	60–90	1.90	UH associated with extremely high rate of ICH
TIMI 9B [99]	1,456	Accelerated t-PA	5000 U bolus then 1000 U/h	50–85	0.90	UH was administered for 96 h
GUSTO III [14]	4,921	Accelerated t-PA	5000 U bolus then 1000 U/h (800 U/h if <80 kg)	50–70	0.87	No significant difference in hemorrhagic stroke between the t-PA and reteplase regimens
ASSENT II [29]	8,488	Accelerated t-PA	5000 U bolus then 1000 U/h (>67 kg); 4000 U bolus; then 800 U/h (<67 kg)	50–75	0.94	Rates of intracranial hemorrhage were similar with TNK (0.93%) and t-PA (0.94%)
TIMI 10B [105]	316	Accelerated t-PA	5000 U bolus then 1000 U/h (800 U/h if <67 kg)	55–80	1.9	Significantly lower rates were observed for both tPA after the heparin doses were lowered and titration of the heparin was started at 6 h
IN-TIME-II [106]	5,027	Accelerated t-PA	70 U/kg (max 4000 U) bolus; then 15 U/kg per h (max 1000 U/h)	50–70	0.64	Heparin titration started 6 h after initial bolus. Adjustment to aPTT titration at 3 h had no effect on ICH rates

ASSENT = Assessment of the Safety and Efficacy of a New Thrombolytic; GUSTO = The Global Use of Strategies to Open Occluded Coronary Arteries; ICH = intracranial hemorrhage; IN-TIME = Intravenous NPA for the treatment of infarcting myocardium early; ISG = International Study Group in the setting of angioplasty without GP IIb/IIIa blockade that an activated clotting time of at least 250 to 350 sec with the HemoTec device and 300 to 350 sec with the Hemochron device is associated with a lower rate of complications than lower activated clotting times [85–87]

When GP IIb/IIIa antagonists are used the UH bolus should be reduced to 50–70 U/kg to achieve a target activated clotting time of 200 sec with either the HemoTec or Hemochron device [88]. UH doses used during PCI for failed fibrinolysis should be similarly reduced and further lowered if used with GP IIb/IIIa antagonists as well.

LMWH

The safety and efficacy of two LMWHs, dalteparin and enoxaparin, as an adjunct to fibrinolysis in the setting of an STEMI has been evaluated in several trials to date focusing on such endpoints as left ventricular thrombus formation and subsequent thromboembolism [89], IRA patency [31, 90–93] and clinical outcomes [20, 34, 94]. In general, these trials have demonstrated improved late coronary artery patency and lower rates of late ischemic events with LMWH compared to UH as an adjunct to fibrinolytic therapy (Table 9.5).

Three trials have assessed the efficacy of enoxaparin combined with fibrinolysis with respect to IRA patency and have revealed absolute increases in IRA patency between 1% and 12%. In each trial, the addition of enoxaparin (30 mg IV bolus followed by 1 mg/kg subcutaneously twice daily) to either t-PA [31], SK [91] or TNK [90], improved IRA patency without an increase in major bleeding. These trials also suggested that less reocclusion, enhanced tissue level reperfusion and combination with a GP IIb/IIIa inhibitor could be achieved with enoxaparin. The addition of enoxaparin to half-dose TNK and abciximab did result, however, in more hemorrhagic complications.

Several additional trials have also assessed the clinical efficacy of enoxaparin as an adjunct to fibrinolysis using SK, TNK or either SK, antistreplase or t-PA [93–95]. The use of enoxaparin combined with each of these fibrinolytics resulted in an absolute reduction in clinical events ranging between 1.1% and 10%. However, the use of enoxaparin in this setting has also been associated with increased hemorrhagic risk.

The ASSENT-3 trial compared the fibrinolytic agent TNK combined with enoxaparin or abciximab, with TNK plus UH in 6095 patients randomized within 6 h of the onset of an acute MI to single-bolus TNK plus IV enoxaparin, TNK plus UH (48-h infusion, aPTT 50–70 sec), or half-dose TNK plus IV UH and IV abciximab [20]. The combined end point of 30-day mortality, in-hospital reinfarction, or refractory ischemia was significantly lower in the enoxaparin and abciximab groups (11.4% and 11.1%, respectively, p-value = 0.0001) than in the UFH group (15.4%). Although not powered to assess mortality, this traditional endpoint of fibrinolytic trials was not affected by combining TNK with either enoxaparin or abciximab. Despite a slight increase hemorrhagic complications with enoxaparin, the incidence of ICH was similar (0.9%) in each group. The results of this trial suggest that the combination of full-dose TNK and up to 7 days of enoxaparin may be the optimal pharmacologic treatment for patients with acute MI presenting within 6 h of symptom onset.

DTIs

Despite the beneficial effects on coronary reperfusion seen with hirudin combined with t-PA in animal models [96], several large trials failed to show a significant benefit of hirudin over

Table 9.5 LMWH trials in STEMI

LMWH	Dose	Control arm	*N*	Duration	Fibrinolytic regimen	Primary endpoint	Timing of outcome	LMWH (%)	Control (%)	Absolute difference (%)
Dalteparin										
FRAMI [89]	150 IU/kg SC	Placebo	517	Hospitalization	SK	Reduction in LV thrombus and arterial TE	9 days	14.2	21.9	−7.7 *p*-value = 0.02
BIOMACS II [92]	100 IU/kg before SK; 120 IU/kg 12 h after SK SC	Placebo	101	24 h	SK	TIMI 3 flow	20–28 h	68	51	17 *p*-value = 0.10
ASSENT-PLUS [93]	30 IU/kg IV then 120 IU/kg bid	UH	439	4–7 days	t-PA	TIMI 3 flow	4–7 days	69.3	62.5	6.8 *p*-value = 0.163
Enoxaparin										
ASENOX [94]	40 mg IV then 1 mg/kg SC bid	UH	412	2–3 days	SK	D Reperfusion	30 days Not defined	7.1 79.8	8.2 75.9	−1.1 3.9
Baird *et al.* [95]	40 mg IV then 40 mg SC tid	UH	300	4 days	SK, antistreplase, t-PA	D/MI/RH	3 months	26	36	−10 *p*-value = 0.04

Table 9.5 *(Continued)*

LMWH	Dose	Control arm	*N*	Duration	Fibrinolytic regimen	Primary endpoint	Timing of outcome	LMWH (%)	Control (%)	Absolute difference (%)
AMI-SK [91]	30 mg IV then 1 mg/kg SC bid	Placebo	496	3–8 days	SK	TIMI 3 flow	5–10 days	70	58	12 *p*-value = 0.01
HART-II [31]	30 mg IV then 1 mg/kg SC bid	UH	400	≥3 days	t-PA	IRA patency	90 min	80.1	75.1	5
ENTIRE-TIMI 23 [90]	±30 mg IV then 1 mg/kg SC bid	UH	483	Max 8 days	TNK, 1/2 TNK with abciximab	TIMI 3 flow-angiographic	60 min	51	50	1 *p*-value = NS
						D/MI – clinical	30 days	4.9	11.3	−6.4 *p*-value = 0.01
ASSENT-3 [20]	30 mg IV then 1 mg/kg SC bid	UH	4075	Max 7 days	TNK	In-hospital D/MI/RI	30 days	11.4	15.4	−4 *p*-value <0.001
ASSENT-3 PLUS [34]	Pre-hospital 30 mg IV then 1 mg/kg SC bid	UH	1639	Max 7 days	TNK	In-hospital D/MI/RI	30 days	14.2	17.4	−3.2

bid = twice daily; D = death; RI = recurrent ischemia; TE = thrombo-embolism; tid = three times a day

UH during fibrinolysis in acute STEMI [97–100]. A similar trend has also been noted with the newer DTIs studied in recent trials. The HERO-2 trial found no mortality difference at 30 days in patients with acute STEMI treated with SK and adjunctive bivalirudin in comparison to SK and UH [32]. The bivalirudin arm had significantly fewer reinfarctions, but significantly higher rates of bleeding. Additional study is needed before DTIs can be routinely recommended in acute MI.

A clear indication for these agents is HIT. A form of hirudin, lepuridin (0.4 mg/kg bolus up to 44 mg, followed by an infusion of 0.15 mg/kg for 2–10 days) has been approved. Argatroban (2 μg/kg per min infusion) is also approved for this indication.

Fondaparinux

The synthetic heparin pentasaccharide fondaparinux as an adjunctive AT agent has been compared to both placebo and UH in patients with STEMI [101]. The use of fondaparinux (2.5 mg once daily for up to 8 days or to hospital discharge) was associated with a significant reduction in the primary endpoint of death or MI at 30 days compared to control (9.7% vs 11.2%, respectively, p-value = 0.008). Whereas this benefit was seen compared to placebo (11.2% vs 14.0%, HR 0.79) and UH in patients not undergoing primary PCI (11.5% vs 13.8%, HR 0.82), a trend towards increased event rates was seen compared to UH in those undergoing primary PCI (more frequent guide catheter thromboses (1.2% vs 0%, p-value <0.001) and 'coronary complications' (14.3% vs 11.9%, p-value = 0.04)). Fondaparinux was also associated with a trend towards fewer bleeding complications. There is clinical promise for the use of this AT agent as an adjunct in the management of STEMI. However, further studies are necessary to better elucidate the mechanism of benefit (Is it due to the longer duration of therapy?) and whether the increased event rate in those undergoing primary PCI can be eliminated.

9.4 RECOMMENDATIONS

The optimal management of patients with STEMI continues to evolve. Although patients with STEMI have enjoyed the lowest mortality rate to date with currently available therapies, the search for even better outcomes continues. General recommendations are listed in Figure 9.1; however, these recommendations need to be individualized to each patient and their specific circumstances.

REPERFUSION STRATEGY

That the IRA should be reperfused as quickly as possible should be the goal of reperfusion therapy for STEMI (Figure 9.2). Given the benefits of primary PCI, this should be the preferred strategy if it can be performed within 90 min of first medical contact. The 2004 ACC/AHA guidelines recommend the use of fibrinolytic therapy for any patient with an acute STEMI who presents within 12 h of symptom onset, has no contraindications for fibrinolysis and presents to a facility without the capability for expert, prompt intervention with primary PCI within 90 min of first medical contact. Fibrinolytic therapy is also recommended if the relative delay necessary to perform primary PCI (the expected door-to-balloon time minus the expected door-to-needle time) is greater than 1 h. Transfer for direct PCI may not be

Step 1: Assess Time and Risk

- *Time since symptom onset*
- *Time to transfer to a facility with PCI*
- *Risk of STEMI*
- *Risk of fibrinolysis*

Step 2: Determine Strategy of Choice: Fibrinolysis versus Primary PCI

- *Either strategy acceptable if: presentation within 3 hours and no delay to invasive strategy*

Fibrinolytics preferred if:

- *Early presentation (<3 hours)*
- *Invasive strategy not an option*
- *Delay to invasive strategy*

Primary PCI preferred if:

- *Late presentation (>3 hours)*
- *Contraindications to fibrinolysis present*
- *High risk from STEMI*
- *Skilled PCI laboratory available with surgical backup*

Figure 9.1 Assessment of reperfusion options for patients with STEMI. ICH = intracranial hemorrhage; skilled PCI laboratory = Operator experience greater than a total of 75 primary PCI cases per year and team experience greater than a total of 36 primary PCI cases per year; high risk from STEMI = Killip Class 3 or 4

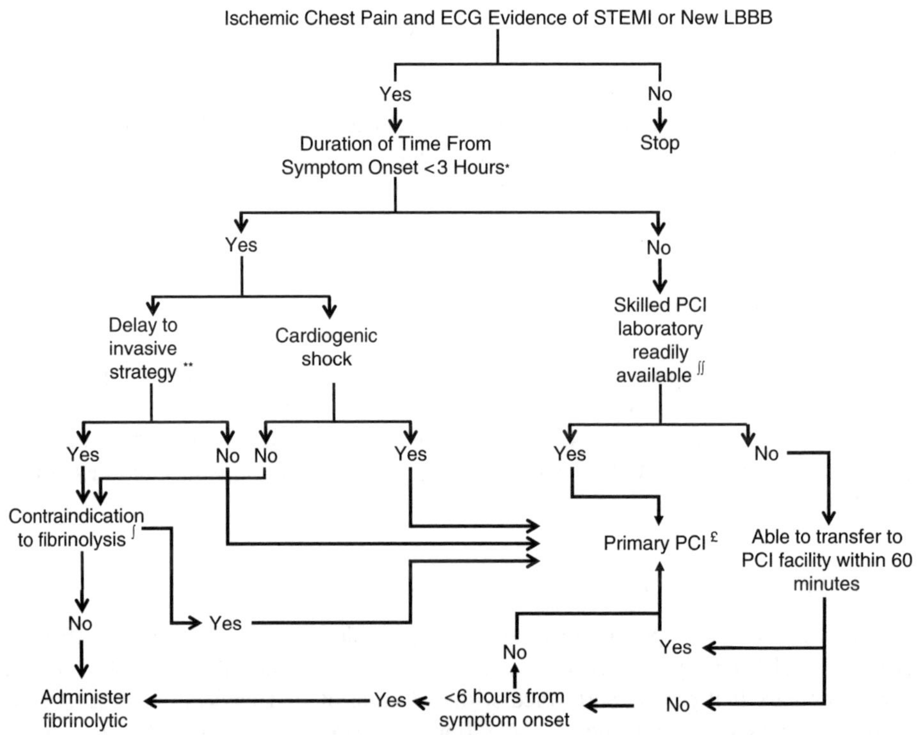

Figure 9.2 Proposed reperfusion selection strategy. * = If presentation is within 3 h of symptom onset and there is no delay for an invasive strategy, either reperfusion technique is acceptable in eligible patients. ** = prolonged transport time (>60 min) or prolonged medical contact-to-balloon time (>90 min). $\int$ = Contraindications to fibrinolysis, see Table 9.2). $\int\int$ = Door-to-balloon time <60 min. £ = primary PCI imparts a significant benefit up to at least 12 h following symptom onset

feasible in the current state of affairs with regards to inter-institution patient transport times. Hence the enduring importance of fibrinolysis.

The choice of fibrinolytic will depend on the setting, prehospital or hospital, whether the patients have been previously exposed to SK, patient age, time from symptom onset and intent to transfer for routine 'facilitated' PCI. Of the four commonly used fibrinolytics (Table 9.1) TNK is easiest to administer (single bolus), while t-PA requires an initial bolus followed by an infusion over 1.5 h and r-PA requires two boluses 30 min apart. Coronary recanalization may occur more rapidly with TNK than with t-PA (mean 32 min vs 49 min from initiation of treatment in one report) [101], although any such difference has not translated into an advantage with regard to mortality. TNK also appears to be safer than t-PA. In ASSENT-2, TNK was associated with a lower rate of non-cerebral bleeding (26.4% vs 29.0%) and a less-frequent requirement for blood transfusion (4.3% vs 5.5%) [29]. The improved safety profile of TNK may reflect only minimal depletion of fibrinogen and weight-adjusted dosing. These advantages have made TNK the fibrinolytic agent of choice in many hospitals in the United States.

Whether or not one is to initiate prehospital fibrinolysis depends on several issues. Prehospital fibrinolysis is reasonable in those settings in which physicians are present in the ambulance or prehospital transport times are more than 60 min in high-volume (more than 25,000 runs per year) EMS systems. In addition, other considerations for implementing a prehospital fibrinolytic service include the ability to transmit ECGs, paramedic initial and ongoing training in ECG interpretation and MI treatment, a medical director with experience in the management of STEMI and full-time paramedics. Unless these key issues are addressed, one can not advocate a prehospital fibrinolytic program.

ADJUNCTIVE THERAPY

Whether primary PCI or fibrinolysis is employed as the reperfusion strategy, concomitant AT and antiplatelet therapies improve the outcomes and are essential components of management strategies for STEMI (Figure 9.3).

With respect to antiplatelet therapies, aspirin remains a cornerstone. Irrespective of fibrinolysis or PCI, aspirin should be given at a dose of 162–325 mg at initial evaluation and 75–162 mg/day indefinitely thereafter unless contraindications exist. Clopidogrel should be added to patients less than 75 years of age at the 300 mg load and 75 mg daily doses thereafter. This dosing regimen may also be used as an alternative to aspirin in allergic patients. In patients older than 75 years of age, clopidogrel at 75 mg daily without a loading bolus should be employed. Although useful as an adjunct to primary PCI, the use of GP IIb/IIIa inhibitors in addition to fibrinolysis can not be advocated at the present time.

Despite inconclusive evidence, UH has remained an integral component of standard therapy for STEMI (Chapter 5). Current guidelines for adjunctive UH in patients receiving fibrin-specific fibrinolytics recommend UH at a 60 U/kg bolus (maximum 4000 U), followed by a 12 U/kg per h IV infusion (maximum 1000 U/h). The aPTT should be measured at 6 h and the infusion dose adjusted to maintain the aPTT between 50 and 70 sec (1.5 to 2 × control). This level of anticoagulation should be maintained for 48 h unless the presence of additional indications for more prolonged UH use exist (e.g. atrial fibrillation, history of pulmonary embolus, LV apical thrombus, etc.).

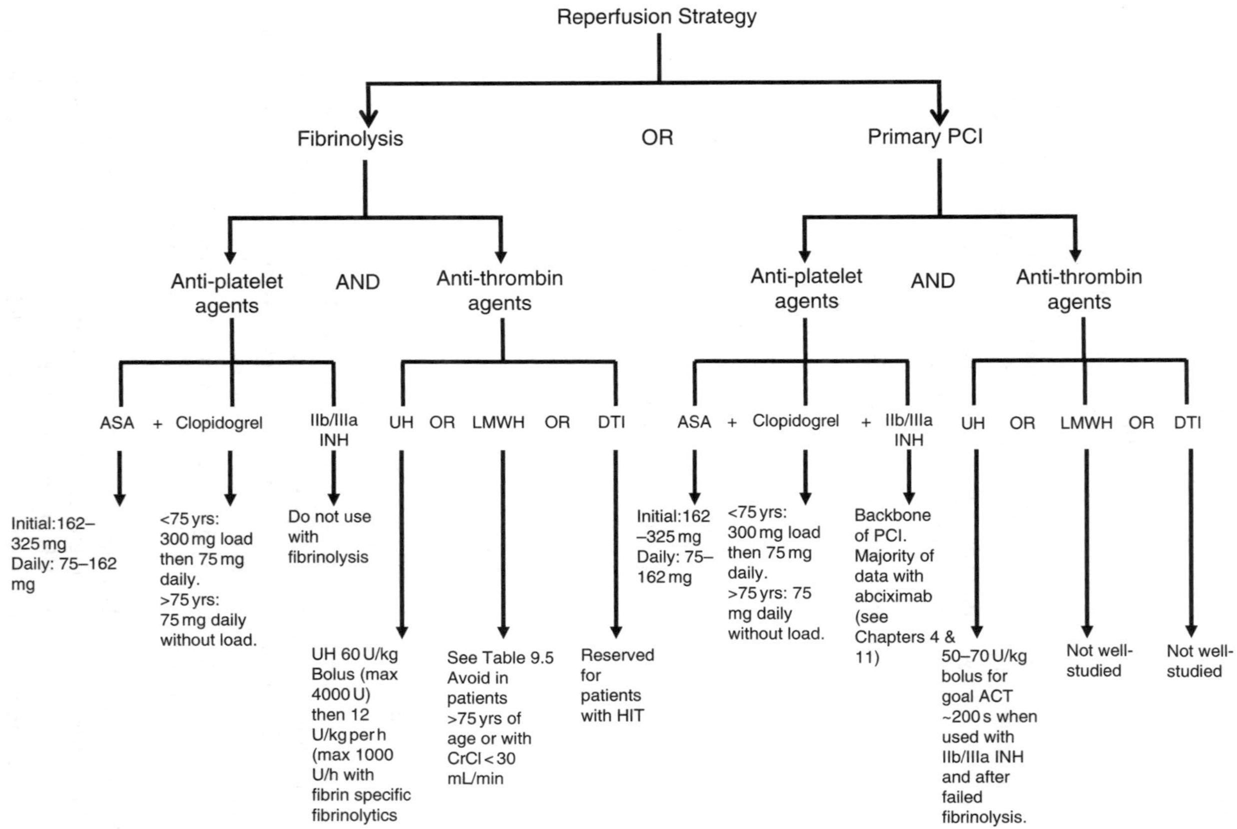

Figure 9.3 Recommendations for adjunctive antithrombotic agents in the setting of reperfusion therapy for STEMI. Aspirin should be universally administered unless a true allergy exists. Clopidogrel may also be used irrespective of reperfusion strategy. Combining IIb/IIIa inhibitors with fibrinolysis should be avoided, although these agents remain beneficial in the primary PCI setting. UH remains the mainstay of adjunctive antithrombin therapy for STEMI. UH should be dosed to achieve an aPTT of 50–70 sec when combined with fibrin-specific fibrinolytics. An ACT of ~200 sec should be the goal when UH and IIb/IIIa inhibitors are employed for primary PCI or for rescue PCI following failed fibrinolysis. LMWH may be used in selected populations receiving fibrinolysis but should be avoided in the primary PCI setting. DTIs remain reserved for patients with HIT in the STEMI setting

With respect to primary PCI, IV UH should be given to all patients undergoing primary PCI during the procedure to prevent acute vessel closure due to thrombosis. Heparin monitoring is usually performed via the ACT with a common target being an ACT of 250 to 350 sec. Postprocedural heparin is not recommended in patients with an uncomplicated procedure.

The use of LMWH as an adjunct to fibrinolysis requires careful patient selection. Although enoxaparin has been associated with clinical benefit when combined with TNK, the increased risk of ICH in patients older than 75 years precludes its use in STEMI for this population [20, 90]. Enoxaparin can be considered as an adjunctive therapy in patients younger than 75 years who have relatively well preserved renal function. It is worth noting that a recent trial of a different LMWH, reviparin, suggested that in patients with acute ST-segment elevation or new left bundle-branch block MI, reviparin could reduce mortality and reinfarction, without a substantive increase in overall stroke rates [102]. However, even though the benefits outweighed the risks of a small absolute excess of life-threatening bleeding in that trial, these data should be corroborated before this agent can be accepted as a routine adjunctive therapy.

Data regarding the DTIs dictate that, at the present time, they be reserved for patients with STEMI who have a history of HIT.

9.5 CONCLUSIONS

Somewhat unique to the treatment of STEMI is the ability to substantially and readily improve outcomes for these patients. Remarkable progress has been made, initially in the field of fibrinolytics and subsequently with advances in PCI techniques and adjunct therapies. However, a substantial burden of this disease continues to persist. One approach has been the suggestion that combining pharmacologic and mechanical reperfusion techniques, so-called 'facilitated PCI,' will achieve further improvement in outcomes. However, this has yet to be determined decisively. Furthermore, the possibility exists that immunomodulatory and cellular adjuncts to various antithrombotic regimens may improve the chances of breaking through the current 'ceiling' of benefit. A rigorous search for methods to continue to 'push the envelope' will be required to achieve the hoped for optimal outcomes in this population.

REFERENCES

[1] Machecourt, J., *et al.*, (2005) Primary angioplasty is cost-minimizing compared with pre-hospital thrombolysis for patients within 60 min of a percutaneous coronary intervention center: the Comparison of Angioplasty and Pre-hospital Thrombolysis in Acute Myocardial Infarction (CAPTIM) cost-efficacy sub-study. *J Am Coll Cardiol*, 45(4):515–24.

[2] Schroder, R., *et al.*, (1995) Extent of early ST segment elevation resolution: a strong predictor of outcome in patients with acute myocardial infarction and a sensitive measure to compare thrombolytic regimens. A substudy of the International Joint Efficacy Comparison of Thrombolytics (INJECT) trial. *J Am Coll Cardiol*, 26(7):1657–64.

[3] Steg, P.G., *et al.*, (2003) Impact of time to treatment on mortality after prehospital fibrinolysis or primary angioplasty: data from the CAPTIM randomized clinical trial. *Circulation*, 108(23):2851–6.

[4] The ISIS-2 collaborative group, (1988) Randomised trial of intravenous streptokinase, oral aspirin, both, or neither among 17,187 cases of suspected acute myocardial infarction: ISIS-2. *Lancet*, 2(8607):349–60.

[5] The GUSTO investigators, (1993) An international randomized trial comparing four thrombolytic strategies for acute myocardial infarction. *N Eng J Med*, 329(10):673–82.

[6] Fibrinolytic Therapy Trialists' (FTT) collaborative group, (1994) Indications for fibrinolytic therapy in suspected acute myocardial infarction: collaborative overview of early mortality and major morbidity results from all randomised trials of more than 1000 patients. *Lancet*, 343(8893):311–22.

[7] Gibson, C.M., (2004) NRMI and current treatment patterns for ST-elevation myocardial infarction. *Am Heart J*, 148(5 Suppl):S29–33.

[8] De Luca, G., *et al.*, (2004) Time delay to treatment and mortality in primary angioplasty for acute myocardial infarction: every minute of delay counts. *Circulation*, 109(10):1223–5.

[9] Gurm, H.S., *et al.*, (2004) Outcome of acute ST-segment elevation myocardial infarction in diabetics treated with fibrinolytic or combination reduced fibrinolytic therapy and platelet glycoprotein IIb/IIIa inhibition: lessons from the GUSTO V trial. *J Am Coll Cardiol*, 43(4):542–8.

[10] Griffith, D., *et al.*, (2005) Early and late mortality after myocardial infarction in men and women: prospective observational study. *Heart*, 91(3):305–7.

[11] French, J.K., *et al.*, (2002) Early ST-segment recovery, infarct artery blood flow, and long-term outcome after acute myocardial infarction. *Am Heart J*, 143(2):265–71.

[12] Woodfield, S.L., *et al.*, (1997) Gender and acute myocardial infarction: is there a different response to thrombolysis? *J Am Coll Cardiol*, 29(1):35–42.

[13] Simoons, M.L., *et al.*, (1986) Early thrombolysis in acute myocardial infarction: limitation of infarct size and improved survival. *J Am Coll Cardiol*, 7:717–28.

[14] The GUSTO III investigators, (1997) A comparison of reteplase with alteplase for acute myocardial infarction. *N Eng J Med*, 337(16):1118–23.

[15] de Lemos, J.A., *et al.*, (2000) ST-segment resolution and infarct-related artery patency and flow after thrombolytic therapy. Thrombolysis in Myocardial Infarction (TIMI) 14 investigators. *Am J Cardiol*, 85(3):299–304.

[16] Ito, H., *et al.*, (1992) Lack of myocardial perfusion immediately after successful thrombolysis. A predictor of poor recovery of left ventricular function in anterior myocardial infarction. *Circulation*, 85(5):1699–705.

[17] Lincoff, A.M., Topol, E.J., (1993) Illusion of reperfusion. Does anyone achieve optimal reperfusion during acute myocardial infarction? *Circulation*, 88(3):1361–74.

[18] Fu, Y., *et al.*, (2001) Time to treatment influences the impact of ST-segment resolution on one-year prognosis: insights from the assessment of the safety and efficacy of a new thrombolytic (ASSENT-2) trial. *Circulation*, 104(22):2653–9.

[19] The SPEED group, (2000) Trial of abciximab with and without low-dose reteplase for acute myocardial infarction. Strategies for Patency Enhancement in the Emergency Department (SPEED). *Circulation*, 101(24):2788–94.

[20] Efficacy and safety of tenecteplase in combination with enoxaparin, abciximab, or unfractionated heparin: the ASSENT-3 randomised trial in acute myocardial infarction, (2001) *Lancet*, 358(9282):605–13.

[21] The GUSTO V investigators, (2001) Reperfusion therapy for acute myocardial infarction with fibrinolytic therapy or combination reduced fibrinolytic therapy and platelet glycoprotein IIb/IIIa inhibition: the GUSTO V randomized trial. *Lancet*, 357:1905–1914.

[22] Robbins, M.A., O'Connell, J.B., (1998) Economic impact of heart failure, in *Management of End-Stage Heart Disease*, (eds E.A. Rose, L.W. Stevenson), Lippincott-Raven: Philadelphia, PA, pp. 3–13.

[23] Fletcher, A.P., *et al.*, (1958) The treatment of patients suffering from early myocardial infarction with massive and prolonged streptokinase therapy. *Trans Assoc Am Physicians*, 71: 287–96.

[24] Yusuf, S., *et al.*, (1985) Intravenous and intracoronary fibrinolytic therapy in acute myocardial infarction: overview of results on mortality, reinfarction and side-effects from 33 randomized controlled trials. *Eur Heart J*, 6(7):556–85.

[25] The international study group, (1990) In-hospital mortality and clinical course of 20,891 patients with suspected acute myocardial infarction randomised between alteplase and streptokinase with or without heparin. *Lancet*, 336(8707):71–5.

[26] Gruppo Italiano per lo Studio della Streptochinasi nell'Infarto Miocardico (GISSI), (1986) Effectiveness of intravenous thrombolytic treatment in acute myocardial infarction. *Lancet*, 1(8478):397–402.

[27] Gruppo Italiano per lo Studio della Streptochinasi nell'Infarto Miocardico (GISSI), (1990) GISSI-2: a factorial randomised trial of alteplase versus streptokinase and heparin versus no heparin among 12,490 patients with acute myocardial infarction. *Lancet*, 336(8707):65–71.

[28] The ISIS-3 collaborative group, (1992) ISIS-3: a randomised comparison of streptokinase vs tissue plasminogen activator vs anistreplase and of aspirin plus heparin vs aspirin alone among 41,299 cases of suspected acute myocardial infarction. *Lancet*, 339(8796):753–70.

[29] The ASSENT-2 investigators, (1999) Single-bolus tenecteplase compared with front-loaded alteplase in acute myocardial infarction: the ASSENT-2 double-blind randomised trial. *Lancet*, 354(9180):716–22.

[30] Coussement, P.K., *et al.*, (2001) A synthetic factor-Xa inhibitor (ORG31540/SR9017A) as an adjunct to fibrinolysis in acute myocardial infarction. The PENTALYSE study. *Eur Heart J*, 22(18):1716–24.

[31] Ross, A.M., *et al.*, (2001) Randomized comparison of enoxaparin, a low-molecular-weight heparin, with unfractionated heparin adjunctive to recombinant tissue plasminogen activator thrombolysis and aspirin: second trial of Heparin and Aspirin Reperfusion Therapy (HART II). *Circulation*, 104(6):648–52.

[32] White, H., (2001) Thrombin-specific anticoagulation with bivalirudin versus heparin in patients receiving fibrinolytic therapy for acute myocardial infarction: the HERO-2 randomised trial. *Lancet*, 358(9296):1855–63.

[33] Morrow, D.A., *et al.*, (2002) Evaluation of the time saved by prehospital initiation of reteplase for ST-elevation myocardial infarction: results of The Early Retavase-Thrombolysis in Myocardial Infarction (ER-TIMI) 19 trial. *J Am Coll Cardiol*, 40(1):71–7.

[34] Wallentin, L., *et al.*, (2003) Efficacy and safety of tenecteplase in combination with the low-molecular-weight heparin enoxaparin or unfractionated heparin in the prehospital setting: the Assessment of the Safety and Efficacy of a New Thrombolytic Regimen (ASSENT)-3 PLUS randomized trial in acute myocardial infarction. *Circulation*, 108(2):135–42.

[35] Giugliano, R.P., *et al.*, (2003) Combination reperfusion therapy with eptifibatide and reduced-dose tenecteplase for ST-elevation myocardial infarction: results of the integrilin and tenecteplase in acute myocardial infarction (INTEGRITI) Phase II Angiographic Trial. *J Am Coll Cardiol*, 41(8):1251–60.

[36] Roe, M.T., *et al.*, (2004) Improved speed and stability of ST-segment recovery with reduced-dose tenecteplase and eptifibatide compared with full-dose tenecteplase for acute ST-segment elevation myocardial infarction. *J Am Coll Cardiol*, 43(4):549–56.

[37] Sabatine, M.S., *et al.*, (2005) Addition of clopidogrel to aspirin and fibrinolytic therapy for myocardial infarction with ST-segment elevation. *N Eng J Med*, 352(12):1179–89.

[38] Kastrati, A., *et al.*, (2004) Early administration of reteplase plus abciximab vs abciximab alone in patients with acute myocardial infarction referred for percutaneous coronary intervention: a randomized controlled trial. *JAMA*, 291(8):947–54.

[39] Pino, R., *et al.*, (2004) Invasive strategy following fibrinolysis in ST-elevation acute myocardial infarction. *Ital Heart J*, 5(9):688–92.

[40] Di Mario, C., *et al.*, Combined Abciximab REteplase Stent Study in acute myocardial infarction (CARESS in AMI). *Am Heart J*, 148(3):378–85.

[41] Cutlip, D.E., *et al.*, (2003) Effect of tirofiban before primary angioplasty on initial coronary flow and early ST-segment resolution in patients with acute myocardial infarction. *Am J Cardiol*, 92(8):977–80.

[42] Scheller, B., *et al.*, (2003) Beneficial effects of immediate stenting after thrombolysis in acute myocardial infarction. *J Am Coll Cardiol*, 42(4):634–41.

[43] Fernandez-Aviles, F., *et al.*, (2004) Routine invasive strategy within 24 h of thrombolysis versus ischaemia-guided conservative approach for acute myocardial infarction with ST-segment elevation (GRACIA-1): a randomised controlled trial. *Lancet*, 364(9439):1045–53.

[44] The MAGIC trial investigators, (2002) Early administration of intravenous magnesium to high-risk patients with acute myocardial infarction in the Magnesium in Coronaries (MAGIC) Trial: a randomised controlled trial. *Lancet*, 360(9341):1189–96.

[45] Gibson, C.M., *et al.*, (2004) Angiographic perfusion score: an angiographic variable that integrates both epicardial and tissue level perfusion before and after facilitated percutaneous coronary intervention in acute myocardial infarction. *Am Heart J*, 148(2):336–40.

[46] Berkowitz, S.D., *et al.*, (1997) Incidence and predictors of bleeding after contemporary thrombolytic therapy for myocardial infarction. The Global Utilization of Streptokinase and Tissue Plasminogen activator for Occluded coronary arteries (GUSTO) I Investigators. *Circulation*, 95(11):2508–16.

[47] Antman, E.M., *et al.*, (2004) ACC/AHA guidelines for the management of patients with ST-elevation myocardial infarction—executive summary: a report of the American College of Cardiology/American Heart Association Task Force on Practice Guidelines (Writing Committee to Revise the 1999 Guidelines for the Management of Patients With Acute Myocardial Infarction). *Circulation*, 110(5):588–636.

[48] Huynh, T., *et al.*, (2004) Predictors of intracranial hemorrhage with fibrinolytic therapy in unselected community patients: a report from the FASTRAK II project. *Am Heart J*, 148(1): 86–91.

[49] Gore, J.M., *et al.*, (1995) Stroke after thrombolysis. Mortality and functional outcomes in the GUSTO-I trial. Global Use of Strategies to Open Occluded Coronary Arteries. *Circulation*, 92(10):2811–8.

[50] Aylward, P.E., *et al.*, (1996) Relation of increased arterial blood pressure to mortality and stroke in the context of contemporary thrombolytic therapy for acute myocardial infarction. A randomized trial. GUSTO-I Investigators. *Ann Intern Med*, 125(11):891–900.

[51] Barron, H.V., *et al.*, (2000) Intracranial hemorrhage rates and effect of immediate beta-blocker use in patients with acute myocardial infarction treated with tissue plasminogen activator. Participants in the National Registry of Myocardial Infarction-2. *Am J Cardiol*, 85(3):294–8.

[52] Gurwitz, J.H., *et al.*, (1998) Risk for intracranial hemorrhage after tissue plasminogen activator treatment for acute myocardial infarction. Participants in the National Registry of Myocardial Infarction 2. *Ann Intern Med*, 129(8):597–604.

[53] Brass, L.M., *et al.*, (2000) Intracranial hemorrhage associated with thrombolytic therapy for elderly patients with acute myocardial infarction: results from the Cooperative Cardiovascular Project. *Stroke*, 31(8):1802–11.

[54] Zeymer, U., *et al.*, (2001) The Na(+)/H(+) exchange inhibitor eniporide as an adjunct to early reperfusion therapy for acute myocardial infarction. Results of the evaluation of the safety and cardioprotective effects of eniporide in acute myocardial infarction (ESCAMI) trial. *J Am Coll Cardiol*, 38(6):1644–50.

[55] Keeley, E.C., Boura, J.A., Grines, C.L., (2003) Primary angioplasty versus intravenous thrombolytic therapy for acute myocardial infarction: a quantitative review of 23 randomised trials. *Lancet*, 361(9351):13–20.

[56] Cannon, C.P., *et al.*, (2000) Relationship of symptom-onset-to-balloon time and door-to-balloon time with mortality in patients undergoing angioplasty for acute myocardial infarction. *JAMA*, 283(22):2941–7.

[57] Berger, P.B., *et al.*, (1999) Relationship between delay in performing direct coronary angioplasty and early clinical outcome in patients with acute myocardial infarction: results from the global use of strategies to open occluded arteries in Acute Coronary Syndromes (GUSTO-IIb) trial. *Circulation*, 100(1):14–20.

[58] Brodie, B.R., *et al.*, (2001) Importance of time to reperfusion on outcomes with primary coronary angioplasty for acute myocardial infarction (results from the Stent Primary Angioplasty in Myocardial Infarction Trial). *Am J Cardiol*, 88(10):1085–90.

[59] van't Hof, A.W., *et al.*, (1998) Clinical presentation and outcome of patients with early, intermediate and late reperfusion therapy by primary coronary angioplasty for acute myocardial infarction. *Eur Heart J*, 19(1):118–23.

[60] Zijlstra, F., *et al.*, (2002) Clinical characteristics and outcome of patients with early (<2h), intermediate (2–4 h) and late (>4 h) presentation treated by primary coronary angioplasty or thrombolytic therapy for acute myocardial infarction. *Eur Heart J*, 23(7):550–7.

[61] Vakili, B.A., Kaplan, R., Brown, D.L., (2001) Volume-outcome relation for physicians and hospitals performing angioplasty for acute myocardial infarction in New York state. *Circulation*, 104(18):2171–6.

[62] Andersen, H.R., *et al.*, (2003) A comparison of coronary angioplasty with fibrinolytic therapy in acute myocardial infarction. *N Eng J Med*, 349(8):733–42.

[63] Grines, C.L., *et al.*, (2002) A randomized trial of transfer for primary angioplasty versus on-site thrombolysis in patients with high-risk myocardial infarction: the Air Primary Angioplasty in Myocardial Infarction study. *J Am Coll Cardiol*, 39(11):1713–9.

[64] Widimsky, P., *et al.*, (2000) Multicentre randomized trial comparing transport to primary angioplasty vs immediate thrombolysis vs combined strategy for patients with acute myocardial infarction presenting to a community hospital without a catheterization laboratory. The PRAGUE study. *Eur Heart J*, 21(10):823–31.

[65] Dalby, M., *et al.*, (2003) Transfer for primary angioplasty versus immediate thrombolysis in acute myocardial infarction: a meta-analysis. *Circulation*, 108(15):1809–14.

[66] Stone, G.W., *et al.*, (2001) Normal flow (TIMI-3) before mechanical reperfusion therapy is an independent determinant of survival in acute myocardial infarction: analysis from the primary angioplasty in myocardial infarction trials. *Circulation*, 104(6):636–41.

[67] The ADVANCE MI investigators, (2005) Facilitated percutaneous coronary intervention for acute ST-segment elevation myocardial infarction: results from the prematurely terminated ADdressing the Value of facilitated ANgioplasty after Combination therapy or Eptifibatide monotherapy in acute Myocardial Infarction (ADVANCE MI) trial. *Am Heart J*, 150(1):116–22.

[68] O'Neill, W.W., (2003) 'Watchful waiting' after thrombolysis: it's time for a re-evaluation. *J Am Coll Cardiol*, 42(1):17–9.

[69] Gibson, C.M., *et al.*, (2003) Early and long-term clinical outcomes associated with reinfarction following fibrinolytic administration in the Thrombolysis in Myocardial Infarction trials. *J Am Coll Cardiol*, 42(1):7–16.

[70] Spencer, F.A., *et al.*, (2001) Age and the utilization of cardiac catheterization following uncomplicated first acute myocardial infarction treated with thrombolytic therapy (The Second National Registry of Myocardial Infarction [NRMI-2]). *Am J Cardiol*, 88(2):107–11.

[71] The GUSTO angiographic investigators, (1993) The effects of tissue plasminogen activator, streptokinase, or both on coronary-artery patency, ventricular function, and survival after acute myocardial infarction. *N Eng J Med*, 329(22):1615–22.

[72] Ellis, S.G., *et al.*, (1994) Randomized comparison of rescue angioplasty with conservative management of patients with early failure of thrombolysis for acute anterior myocardial infarction. *Circulation*, 90:2280–2284.

[73] Gershlick, A.H., *et al.*, (2005) Rescue angioplasty after failed thrombolytic therapy for acute myocardial infarction. *N Eng J Med*, 353(26):2758–68.

[74] Chen, Z., (2005) Clopidogrel Metoprolol Myocardial Infarction (COMMIT) trial in *American College of Cardiology Scientific Sessions*. Orlando, FL.

[75] Englberger, L., *et al.*, (2004) Impact of clopidogrel in coronary artery bypass grafting. *Eur J Cardiothorac Surg*, 26(1):96–101.

[76] Chen, L., *et al.*, (2004) Clopidogrel and bleeding in patients undergoing elective coronary artery bypass grafting. *J Thorac Cardiovasc Surg*, 128(3):425–31.

[77] Kapetanakis, E.I., *et al.*, (2005) Clopidogrel administration prior to coronary artery bypass grafting surgery: the cardiologist's panacea or the surgeon's headache? *Eur Heart J*, 26(6):576–83.

[78] Brener, S.J., *et al.*, (1998) Randomized, placebo-controlled trial of platelet glycoprotein IIb/IIIa blockade with primary angioplasty for acute myocardial infarction. ReoPro and Primary PTCA Organization and Randomized Trial (RAPPORT) Investigators. *Circulation*, 98(8): 734–41.

[79] Montalescot, G., *et al.*, (2001) Platelet glycoprotein IIb/IIIa inhibition with coronary stenting for acute myocardial infarction. *N Eng J Med*, 344(25):1895–903.

[80] Kandzari, D.E., *et al.*, (2004) Improved clinical outcomes with abciximab therapy in acute myocardial infarction: a systematic overview of randomized clinical trials. *Am Heart J*, 147(3):457–62.

[81] De Luca, G., *et al.*, (2005) Abciximab as adjunctive therapy to reperfusion in acute ST-segment elevation myocardial infarction: a meta-analysis of randomized trials. *JAMA*, 293(14):1759–65.

[82] Late Assessment of Thrombolytic Efficacy (LATE) study with alteplase 6–24 hours after onset of acute myocardial infarction. *Lancet*, 1993. 342(8874):759–66.

[83] Granger, C., *et al.*, (1996) Activated partial thromboplastin time and outcome after thrombolytic therapy for acute myocardial infarction. *Circulation*, 93:870–8.

[84] Hirsh, J., Raschke, R., (2004) Heparin and low-molecular-weight heparin: the Seventh ACCP Conference on Antithrombotic and Thrombolytic Therapy. *Chest*, 126(3 Suppl):188S–203S.

[85] Narins, C.R., *et al.*, (1996) Relation between activated clotting time during angioplasty and abrupt closure. *Circulation*, 93:667–71.

[86] Chew, D.P., *et al.*, (2001) Defining the optimal activated clotting time during percutaneous coronary intervention: aggregate results from 6 randomized, controlled trials. *Circulation*, 103(7):961–6.

[87] Ferguson, J.J., *et al.*, (1994) Relation between procedural activated coagulation time and outcome after percutaneous transluminal coronary angioplasty. *J Am Coll Cardiol*, 23(5):1061–5.

[88] Tolleson, T.R., *et al.*, (2003) Relationship between heparin anticoagulation and clinical outcomes in coronary stent intervention: observations from the ESPRIT trial. *J Am Coll Cardiol*, 41(3): 386–93.

[89] Kontny, F., *et al.*, (1997) Randomized trial of low molecular weight heparin (dalteparin) in prevention of left ventricular thrombus formation and arterial embolism after acute anterior myocardial infarction: the Fragmin in Acute Myocardial Infarction (FRAMI) Study. *J Am Coll Cardiol*, 30(4):962–9.

[90] Antman, E.M., *et al.*, (2002) Enoxaparin as adjunctive antithrombin therapy for ST-elevation myocardial infarction: results of the ENTIRE-Thrombolysis in Myocardial Infarction (TIMI) 23 Trial. *Circulation*, 105(14):1642–9.

[91] Simoons, M., *et al.*, (2002) Improved reperfusion and clinical outcome with enoxaparin as an adjunct to streptokinase thrombolysis in acute myocardial infarction. The AMI-SK study. *Eur Heart J*, 23(16):1282–90.

[92] Frostfeldt, G., *et al.*, (1999) Low molecular weight heparin (dalteparin) as adjuvant treatment of thrombolysis in acute myocardial infarction–a pilot study: biochemical markers in acute coronary syndromes (BIOMACS II). *J Am Coll Cardiol*, 33(3):627–33.

[93] Wallentin, L., *et al.*, (2003) Low molecular weight heparin (dalteparin) compared to unfractionated heparin as an adjunct to rt-PA (alteplase) for improvement of coronary artery patency in acute myocardial infarction-the ASSENT Plus study. *Eur Heart J*, 24(10):897–908.

[94] Tatu-Chitoiu, G., *et al.*, (2003) Efficacy and safety of a new streptokinase regimen with enoxaparin in acute myocardial infarction. *J Thromb Thrombolysis*, 15(3):171–9.

[95] Baird, S.H., *et al.*, (2002) Randomized comparison of enoxaparin with unfractionated heparin following fibrinolytic therapy for acute myocardial infarction. *Eur Heart J*, 23(8): 627–32.

[96] Kaiser, B., Simon, A., Markwardt, F., (1990) Antithrombotic effects of recombinant hirudin in experimental angioplasty and intravascular thrombolysis. *Thromb Haemost*, 63(1):44–7.

[97] The GUSTO IIa investigators, (1994) Randomized trial of intravenous heparin versus recombinant hirudin for acute coronary syndromes. *Circulation*, 90(4):1631–7.

[98] Antman, E.M., (1994) Hirudin in acute myocardial infarction. Safety report from the Thrombolysis and Thrombin Inhibition in Myocardial Infarction (TIMI) 9A Trial. *Circulation*, 90(4):1624–30.

[99] Antman, E.M., (1996) Hirudin in acute myocardial infarction. Thrombolysis and Thrombin Inhibition in Myocardial Infarction (TIMI) 9B trial. *Circulation*, 94(5):911–21.

[100] The GUSTO IIb angioplasty substudy investigators, (1997) A clinical trial comparing primary coronary angioplasty with tissue plasminogen activator for acute myocardial infarction. *N Eng J Med*, 336(23):1621–8.

[101] Yusuf, S., *et al.*, (2006) Effects of fondaparinux on mortality and reinfarction in patients with acute ST-segment elevation myocardial infarction: the OASIS-6 randomized trial. *JAMA*, 295(13):1519–30.

[102] Binbrek, A.S., *et al.*, (2004) Comparison of rapidity of coronary recanalization in men with tenecteplase versus alteplase in acute myocardial infarction. *Am J Cardiol*, 93(12): 1465–8.

[103] Yusuf, S., *et al.*, (2005) Effects of reviparin, a low-molecular-weight heparin, on mortality, reinfarction, and strokes in patients with acute myocardial infarction presenting with ST-segment elevation. *JAMA*, 293(4):427–35.

[104] Metz, B.K., *et al.*, (1998) Randomized comparison of direct thrombin inhibition versus heparin in conjunction with fibrinolytic therapy for acute myocardial infarction: results from the GUSTO-IIb Trial. Global Use of Strategies to Open Occluded Coronary Arteries in Acute Coronary Syndromes (GUSTO-IIb) Investigators. *J Am Coll Cardiol*, 31(7):1493–8.
[105] Cannon, C.P., *et al.*, (1998) TNK-tissue plasminogen activator compared with front-loaded alteplase in acute myocardial infarction: results of the TIMI 10B trial. Thrombolysis in Myocardial Infarction (TIMI) 10B Investigators. *Circulation*, 98(25):2805–14.
[106] Intravenous NPA for the treatment of infarcting myocardium early; InTIME-II, a double-blind comparison of single-bolus lanoteplase vs accelerated alteplase for the treatment of patients with acute myocardial infarction. *Eur Heart J*, 21(24):2005–13.

10 Acute Coronary Syndromes: Unstable Angina / Non-ST-Segment-Elevation Myocardial Infarction (NSTE ACS)

10.1 INTRODUCTION

UA and NSTEMI remain leading causes of morbidity and mortality in the United States, accounting for approximately 700,000 hospital admissions per year. These conditions are part of a continuum of ACS that ranges from UA and NSTEMI to STEMI. Whereas the treatment paradigm for the readily identifiable patients that present with an STEMI (ST-segment elevations, new left bundle branch block or true posterior MI) remains complete and rapid restoration of antegrade coronary perfusion, the treatment paradigm for the much larger group of patients that present with UA or a NSTEMI remains one in evolution. An explanation for the discrepancy rests with the fact that the latter groups of patients require further risk stratification to distinguish where they fall on the continuum from non-cardiac chest pain to UA and NSTEMI, as the need for and response to the potpourri of available therapies differ between these groups. Nevertheless, it has become increasingly clear that early identification of patients with UA or NSTEMI (referred to as NSTE ACS) and treatment with various permutations of antiplatelet and AT therapies coupled with PCI has contributed to the improved outcomes experienced by a substantial proportion of patients.

IDENTIFICATION OF HIGH-RISK PATIENTS

Risk assessment: utility of risk scores

Given the heterogeneous nature of NSTE ACS and the associated varying risk, accurate yet simple risk assessment tools have been developed in order to facilitate appropriate delivery of care to this patient population [1, 2]. While risk calculation tools focus on both clinical and biochemical information, only the TIMI risk score has been validated in several trial datasets [3–8] (Figure 10.1). Importantly, a progressively greater benefit from newer therapies such as LMWH, platelet GP IIb/IIIa receptor antagonists and an early invasive strategy with increasing risk score has been reported.

Risk assessment: utility of biomarkers

The cardiac troponins have proven useful not only in identifying patients presenting with NSTE ACS who have had myocardial damage but also in risk stratification. A ‘positive’

Management Strategies in Antithrombotic Therapy Arman T. Askari, Adrian W. Messerli and A. Michael Lincoff

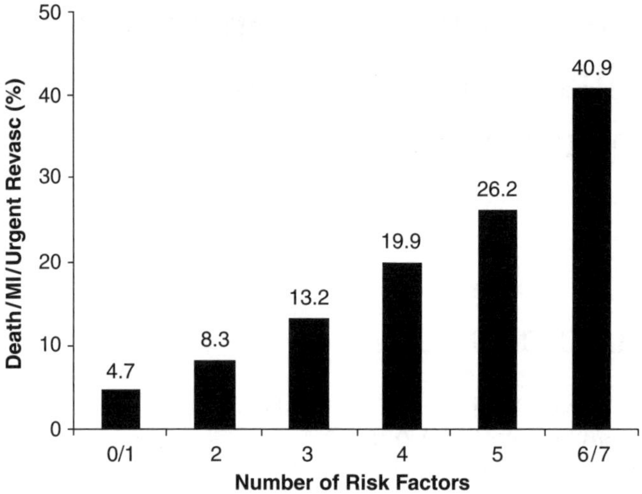

Figure 10.1 The TIMI risk score elements and associated prognostic ability. Risk factors included in the risk score include age ≥65 years, three or more CAD risk factors, prior CAD, aspirin within the previous 7 days, two or more anginal events within 24 h, ST-segment deviations, and elevated cardiac biomarkers (CK-MB or troponin). Adapted from Antman *et al.*[1]

troponin identifies patients at an increased risk for future adverse events, with the future risk being directly proportional to the level of troponin elevation [9]. Furthermore, the utility of troponin elevations primarily resides with the identification of patients who derive the greatest benefit from more aggressive antithrombotic and revascularization approaches to their therapy.

Although the cardiac troponins are specific for identifying myocardial necrosis, the elevation of this marker is not always secondary to atherosclerotic coronary artery disease. Any systemic condition that increases myocardial oxygen demand (e.g. fever, thyrotoxicosis), decreases overall coronary blood flow (e.g. systemic hypotension), or decreases oxygen delivery (e.g. profound anemia) can cause myocardial ischemia, necrosis and increases in the circulating levels of cardiac troponins. Although these may be considered instances of NSTEMI, they should be distinguished on clinical grounds from the more common form of NSTEMI secondary to coronary atherosclerosis. Therefore, in establishing the diagnosis of NSTEMI, cardiac troponins should be used in conjunction with appropriate clinical features and electrocardiographic changes. This chapter will serve to review the myriad of AT therapies available, and to frame recommendations for the management of patients with this diverse clinical syndrome.

10.2 ANTITHROMBOTIC APPROACH TO PATIENTS WITH ACS/NSTEMI

Rupture of a vulnerable atherosclerotic plaque followed by local thrombosis resulting in varying levels of occlusion of the culprit artery is the usual inciting event in an ACS. Ultimately, the goals of therapy for an ACS are to prevent progression of intracoronary thrombus, to promote atherosclerotic plaque stabilization and to decrease the risk of subsequent ischemic events.

ANTIPLATELET THERAPY

Given the central role of platelet activation and aggregation in thrombus formation, it is reasonable to expect that antiplatelet therapy would be at the core of NSTE ACS management. Recommended agents include aspirin, which inhibits platelet aggregation and activation primarily by inhibiting thromboxane A_2 synthesis, clopidogrel, which inhibits platelet activation by blocking the adenosine diphosphate receptor, and the Gp IIb/IIIa inhibitors.

Aspirin

Despite the pursuit and development of alternative antiplatelet agents, aspirin remains a pillar of strength in the management of patients with NSTE ACS (Chapter 2). The use of aspirin in this setting has been shown to be safe and, when combined with antithrombin therapy such as UH, to provide a readily evident, durable and additive benefit [10–13].

The optimal dose of aspirin for the treatment of UA/NSTEMI remains incompletely defined. While the risk of side effects, particularly GI bleeding, appears to increase with increasing dose, the relationship between efficacy and aspirin dose is less certain. However, based on the available data, an initial loading dose of 162–325 mg should be given as soon as possible to these patients [14]. Thereafter, a dose of 7–150 mg daily may provide optimal efficacy with limited toxicity [15].

Clopidogrel

While proven to be efficacious in the secondary prevention of patients with IHD when used as the sole antiplatelet agent [16], clopidogrel has demonstrated an additive effect when combined with aspirin in patients presenting with ACS [17] as well as in those undergoing PCI [18]. Given the beneficial effects and the improved safety profile compared with ticlopidine, clopidogrel should be the additional or alternative oral antiplatelet therapy of choice.

Given the need for an antithrombotic regimen that provides a seamless beneficial effect on both the short- and long-term outcomes in those patients who initially present with ACS, who undergo an early invasive strategy and who receive definitive therapy, the markedly enhanced efficacy of combining a thienopyridine with aspirin on reducing stent thrombosis provided the backdrop for investigating the utility of clopidogrel for the management of ACS. Clopidogrel's role in ACS was assessed in the CURE trial [17]. This trial of 12,562 patients presenting within 24 h of symptom onset demonstrated a significant impact on clinical outcomes that were associated with clopidogrel use in addition to usual therapy (including aspirin in all patients). That the addition of clopidogrel to standard care provided an avenue for the seamless transition between the pharmacologic and percutaneous management of patients with ACS was further suggested by the CURE trial, wherein clopidogrel was shown to be effective regardless of treatment strategy received, invasive or conservative, and regardless of baseline risk profile [19]. Coupled with the consistent benefit of clopidogrel amongst trials regardless of patient population and setting [18], these data have strongly positioned clopidogrel as an integral component of the armamentarium available for these patients.

The beneficial effects of clopidogrel in patients with ACS have been limited by the associated increased hemorrhagic risk. This is particularly important in those patients presenting with ACS who are found to have surgical CAD, as treatment with clopidogrel within 5–7 days of cardiac surgery has been associated with more frequent reoperation for bleeding and blood product transfusions and greater peri-operative blood loss. However, it should be noted that very few NSTE ACS patients (~19% in the SYNERGY trial) go to CABG in the current era [20] and even fewer require CABG within 5–7 days. In addition, the benefit of thienopyridine use in these patients begins to accrue immediately. Thus, holding clopidogrel until after the coronary anatomy is defined in the catheterization laboratory does not seem prudent, as it would deprive the majority of patients of the benefit for the sake of the few who might need early surgery. Therefore, early clopidogrel use remains favored for patients with NSTE ACS unless the patient has a high pre-catheterization likelihood of needing surgery.

GP IIb/IIIa inhibitors

GP IIb/IIIa inhibitors target the final common pathway involved in platelet adhesion, activation and aggregation. Given the role of the platelet in forming and perpetuating the ischemic milieu in ACS, the development of these agents has provided additional armaments to battle the associated adverse outcomes. Three classes of these agents have been developed: murine–human chimeric antibodies (e.g. abciximab), synthetic peptides (e.g. eptifibatide) and synthetic non-peptide forms (e.g. tirofiban). Several trials with these agents, either as adjuncts to UH and aspirin in patients undergoing PCI [21–25] or as a multipronged approach to medical therapy [26–29] in patients with ACS, have demonstrated their worth (Chapter 4 and Table 10.1).

When used in conjunction with UH and aspirin for medical therapy of ACS, the small-molecule GP IIb/IIIa inhibitors have demonstrated an additive benefit [26–29]. In the largest study of these agents in ACS, the PURSUIT trial, the combination of eptifibatide, UH and aspirin significantly reduced the 30-day incidence of death or MI compared with UH plus aspirin (14.2% vs 15.7%, p-value = 0.04) in 10,948 patients [29]. However, patients in the combination group experienced a higher incidence of bleeding and need for transfusions; subsequent experience suggested that excess bleeding with GP IIb/IIIa blockade can be attenuated by reduced concomitant heparin dosing. A recent trial also suggested that the addition of abciximab to either UH or LMWH plus aspirin was not of benefit and was potentially harmful among patients managed conservatively (without revascularization) [30]. Combined with other trials of these agents in conjunction with antithrombin agents as stand-alone therapy for ACS, the majority of the benefit appears to be in patients at high risk as evidenced by positive serum cardiac biomarkers and/or dynamic ECG changes, those with chronic kidney disease or diabetes and in those undergoing PCI [31–35]. The utility of these agents combined with an early invasive approach is without question evident from the currently available data.

Based on the available data the following recommendations for the use of these agents can be made. In moderate- to high-risk patients presenting with NSTE ACS, the use of either eptifibatide or tirofiban for initial (early) treatment in addition to treatment with aspirin, heparin, and/or clopidogrel. No prospective, randomized trial has assessed GP IIb/IIIa inhibitors with clopidogrel in the medical phase of management of NSTE ACS, so some

Table 10.1 Selected trials of GP IIb/IIIa inhibitors for ACS

Trial	*N*	GP IIb/IIIa inhibitor	GP IIb/IIIa Inhibitor dose	Treatment groups	UH dose	Primary endpoint	Comment
GP IIb/IIIa as an Adjunct to UH in Patients Undergoing PCI							
EPIC [21]	2099	Abciximab	0.25 mg/kg bolus started 10 min before procedure then 10 μg/min × 12 h	Placebo Abciximab bolus Abciximab bolus + infusion	10,000–12,000 U bolus then targeted to ACT 300–350 s	30-d D/MI/CABG/PCI/stenting/IABP	Abciximab bolus plus infusion had 35% fewer endpoints compared with placebo (8.3% vs 12.8%, *p*-value = 0.008). Abciximab was associated with more bleeding (14% vs 7%, *p*-value = 0.001)
EPILOG [22]	2792	Abciximab	0.25 mg/kg bolus then 0.125 μg/kg per min × 12 h	Plabeo + UH (100 U/kg) Abciximab+UH (100 U/kg) Abciximab + UH (70 U/kg)	Standard dose = 100 U/kg Low dose = 70 U/kg	30-d D/MI/UR	Primary endpoint occurred in 5.2% abciximab + low dose UH. 5.4% abciximab + standard dose UH, 11.7% standard dose UH. No difference in major bleeding. Minor bleeding increased with abciximab + standard UH group
CAPTURE [23]	1265	Abciximab	0.25 mg/kg bolus then 10 μg/min × 18–24 h before and 1 h after PCI	Placebo Abciximab	Targeted to ACT 300 s	30-d D/MI/UR	Abciximab administered in this manner reduced recurrent ischemic events before, during, and after PTCA
IMPACT-II [24]	4010	Eptifibatide	135 μg/kg bolus 10–60 min before procedure then 0.5 or 0.75 μg/kg per min × 20–24 h	Placebo Eptifibatide 135 μg/kg, 0.5 μg/kg per min Eptifibatide 135 μg/kg, 0.75 μg/kg per min	100 U/kg then targeted to ACT 300–350 s	30-d D/MI/UR/stent	In the 135/0.5 group, treatment with eptifibatide during coronary intervention reduced rates of early abrupt closure and ischemic events at 30 days. Eptifibatide did not increase bleeding

Table 10.1 (*Continued*)

Trial	*N*	GP IIb/IIIa inhibitor	GP IIb/IIIa Inhibitor dose	Treatment groups	UH dose	Primary endpoint	Comment
RESTORE [25]	2139	Tirofiban	10 μg/kg bolus over 3 min then 0.15 μg/kg per min × 36 h	Placebo Tirofiban	UH max bolus 10,000 U or 150 U/kg if <70 kg, then targeted to ACT 300–400 s	30-d D/MI/CABG/ repeat PTCA/stenting	Tirofiban protects against early adverse cardiac events related to thrombotic closure. No increased bleeding with tirofiban
GP IIb/IIIa Inhibitors as an Adjunct to UH as Medical Therapy							
PRISM [26]	3232	Tirofiban	0.6 μg/kg per min × 30 min then 0.15 μg/kg per min × 47.5 h	UH + aspirin Tirofiban + aspirin	5000 U bolus then 1000 U/h titrated to aPTT	48 h D/MI/RI	Tirofiban was associated with a significant decrease in the primary endpoint. No increased bleeding was seen, but thrombocytopenia was seen more frequently with tirofiban
PRISM-PLUS [28]	1915	Tirofiban	0.6 μg/kg per min then 0.15 μg/kg per min 0.4 μg/kg per min bolus then 0.1 μg/kg per min	Tirofiban + aspirin UH + aspirin Tirofiban + UH + aspirin	5000 U bolus then 1000 U/h titrated to aPTT	7-d D/MI/RI	The trial was stopped early because the group receiving tirofiban alone experienced excess mortality at 7 days (4.6% vs 1.1% in the UH group)

PURSUIT [29]	10,948	Eptifibatide	180 μg/kg bolus then 1.3 μg/kg per min OR 180 μg/kg bolus then 2.0 μg/kg per min	Low dose eptifibatide + UH /aspirin High dose eptifibatide +UH/aspirin UH + aspirin + usual care	5000U bolus then 1000 U/h titrated to aPTT 50–70 s	30-d D/MI	Eptifibatide was associated with a 1.5% absolute reduction in the incidence of the primary end point (14.2%, vs 15.7% in the placebo group; *p*-value = 0.04). The benefit was apparent by 96 h and persisted through 30 days. Bleeding was more common in the eptifibatide group
GUSTO IV [30]	7800	Abciximab	0.25 mg/kg bolus then 0.125 μg/kg per min (max 10 mg/min) × 24 h OR 0.25 mg/kg bolus then 0.125 μg/kg per min (max 10 mg/min) × 48 h	Placebo Abciximab bolus + 24 h infusion Abciximab bolus + 48 h infusion	70 U/kg bolus (max 5000 U), then 10 U/kg per h (max 800 U/h) titrated to goal aPTT 50–70 s	30-d D/MI	Revealed that abciximab is not first line therapy for patients being treated medically for ACS. Bleeding increased with abciximab, especially when given for 48 h

D = death; IABP = intra-aortic balloon pump; PTCA = percutaneous transluminal coronary angioplasty; RI = refractory ischemia; UR = urgent revascularization caution may be warranted for the potential of with increased bleeding complications [36]. The use of abciximab as initial treatment outside of the coronary interventional laboratory can not be recommended except when the coronary anatomy is known and PCI is planned within 24 h [23].

AT THERAPY

That thrombin generation plays a pivotal role in the genesis of pathologic thrombosis across the spectrum of CVD ranging from ACS to venous thromboembolic disease has facilitated the expansion of the field of available antithrombotic agents. The emergence of several agents including LMWH and the DTIs have been born out of a need to address the limitations of UH (Chapter 5). Despite the assessment of these new agents in various drug combinations with antiplatelet agents, a benefit above and beyond that imparted by a regimen utilizing UH as the backbone of AT therapy has yet to be demonstrated.

UH

Intracoronary thrombus remains central to the pathogenesis of ACS. Although a large-scale randomized controlled trial assessing the efficacy of UH in ACS is lacking, several smaller studies have demonstrated the utility of UH in the management of these patients (Table 10.2). When used as the sole antithrombotic agent in ACS, UH has been associated with decreased recurrent angina or recurrent MI [13, 37, 38]. In addition, studies have suggested that combining UH and aspirin in ACS results in further benefit and, importantly, serves to reduce the rebound ischemia that occurs following cessation of UH therapy. Ultimately, irrespective of risk category, patients with NSTE ACS benefit from UH therapy compared with no UH therapy (Chapter 5). The available evidence supports a weight-adjusted dosing regimen with UH as a means to provide a more predictable and constant level of systemic anticoagulation (Table 10.3). An initial bolus of 60 to 70 U/kg (maximum, 5000 U) and initial infusion of 12 to 15 U/kg per h (maximum, 1000 U/h) titrated to a target aPTT of 50–75 sec is recommended.

Dosing of UH during PCI depends on several factors including the use of stents, the use of adjunctive antiplatelet agents (i.e. GP IIb/IIIa inhibitors) and the clinical scenario (elective PCI versus PCI in patients with ACS). However, in the setting of ACS, the routine use of ACTs to guide therapy remains clinically prudent. The concomitant use of UH with GP IIb/IIIa inhibitors dictates the use of lower, weight-adjusted dosing. In these cases, similar clinical outcomes can be achieved with fewer bleeding complications with ACTs in the range of >200 sec whether stents are used or not [39]. In addition, low-dose heparin (70 U of heparin per kilogram to a maximum of 7000 U), with additional boluses to maintain an ACT at approximately 200 seconds, has been associated with a reduced incidence of hemorrhagic complications without increasing coronary events [22].

In summary, the following empirical recommendations can be made with respect to anticoagulation during PCI. UH should be administered with either weight-adjusted (70–100 IU/kg) or gender-adjusted (7000 U for women and 8000 U for men) bolus doses to achieve an ACT of 250–350 sec. Weight-adjusted heparin can be used to avoid excessive levels of anticoagulation. When a GP IIb/IIIa inhibitor is used, the heparin bolus should be reduced to 50 to 70 IU/kg. In such patients, an ACT of 20–250 sec appears to be safe and effective.

Table 10.2 Trials of UH for the management of ACS

Trial	Type	*N*	Treatment	UH dose	Goal aPTT	ASA dose	Endpoint	Comment
Telford *et al.* [38]	RDBPCT	214	UH Atenolol Placebo UH + Atenolol	5000 U every 6 h		NA	Transmural MI	During the trial period, transmural MI developed in 17%, 13%, 2%, and 4% of patients in the placebo, atenolol, heparin, and heparin plus atenolol groups, respectively (p-value = 0.024)
Theroux *et al.* [13]	RDBPCT	479	Placebo UH ASA UH + ASA	1000 U/h Continuous IV infusion × 6 days	1.5–2 × normal	325 mg bid	RA/MI/D	The incidence of MI at a mean follow-up of 6 ±3 days was significantly reduced in heparin-treated patients (0.8% vs 3.3% with aspirin). The study was not powered to assess the effect of heparin vs aspirin on mortality. Aspirin blunted rebound of UA symptoms after discontinuation of heparin therapy
RISC [12]	RDBPCT	796	Placebo UH ASA UH + ASA	5000 U every 6 h × 5 days	Not stated	75 mg daily	D/MI	Aspirin reduced the event rate in non-Q-wave MI and UA, independently of ECG abnormalities or concurrent drug therapy. Heparin had no significant influence on event rate, although the group treated with aspirin and heparin had the lowest number of events during the initial 5 days

Table 10.2 (*Continued*)

Trial	Type	*N*	Treatment	UH dose	Goal aPTT	ASA dose	Endpoint	Comment
Neri Serneri *et al.* [37]	RDBT	97	UH–intermittent bolus UH–continuous IV ASA + alteplase	6000 U every 6 h 5000 U bolus f/b 1000 U/h IV				On the first days of treatment heparin infusion significantly decreased the frequency of angina (by 84–94%), episodes of silent ischemia (by 71–77%), and the overall duration of ischemia (by 81–86%). Heparin bolus and aspirin were not effective. Alteplase caused small (non-significant) reductions on the first day only
Cohen *et al.* [59]	Pilot	93	ASA f/b warfarin UH f/b warfarin ASA + UH f/b warfarin	Titrated to aPTT × 3–4 days	2 × normal	325 mg daily 80 mg daily	D/MI	
Theroux *et al.* [60]	RDBT	484	ASA UH	5000 U bolus then titrated to aPTT	1.5–2.5 × normal	325 mg bid	D/MI	UH was associated with significantly fewer MI than aspirin (0.8% vs 3.7%, respectively)
Cohen *et al.* [61]	PRT	214	ASA ASA + UH f/b ASA + warfarin	Titrated to aPTT × 3–4 days	2 × normal	162.5 mg daily	RA/MI/D	In nonprior aspirin users, combination antithrombotic therapy with aspirin plus anticoagulation significantly reduces recurrent ischemic events in the early phase of UA

Holdright *et al.* [62]	PRT	285	ASA ASA + UH	Titrated to aPTT × 2 days	1.5–2 × normal	150 mg daily		This study suggests that combined therapy with heparin and aspirin compared with aspirin alone makes no difference in the development of in hospital MI or death, nor does it reduce the development of transient myocardial ischemia
Gurfinkel *et al.* [63]	RDBT	219	ASA ASA + UH ASA + LMWH	400 IU/kg IV daily Titrated to aPTT × 5–7 days 214 UIC/kg SC bid	2 × normal	200 mg daily	RA/MI/UR/D and bleeding	Treatment with aspirin plus a high dose of LMWH during the acute phase of UA was significantly better than treatment with aspirin alone or aspirin plus regular heparin
Neri Serneri *et al.* [64]	PRT	108	IV UH SC UH ASA	Titrated to aPTT 5,000–75,000 q8h	1.5–2 × normal	325 mg daily	Reduced myocardial ischemia	Aspirin did not significantly affect the incidence of myocardial ischemia. On the first 3 days, infused and SC heparin significantly decreased the frequency of angina, episodes of silent ischemia, and the overall duration of ischemia vs run-in day and aspirin (*p*-value <0.001 for all variables). The favorable effects of heparin therapy remained evident during follow-up

bid = twice daily; D = death; ECG = electrocardiogram; f/b = followed by; NA = not applicable; PRT = prospective randomized trial; q8h = every 8 h; RA = recurrent angina. RDBPCT = randomized double blind placebo controlled trial; RDBT = randomized double blind trial; UR = urgent revascularization

Table 10.3 A weight-based UH dosing nomogram for ACS. Adapted from Becker *et al.* [65]

aPTT (s)	bolus	Infusion adjustment (U/kg per h)
<35	70 U/kg additional	+3
35–49	35 U/kg additional	+2
50–70	Therapeutic range *	0
71–90	0	−2
>100	Hold infusion for 30 min	−3

Initial dose: 60 U/kg bolus and 12 U/kg per h infusion

* The therapeutic range should be assessed at every institution by correlation with Anti-factor Xa levels between 0.3 and 0.7 U/mL

LMWH

Born out of the limitations of UH (Chapter 6), the LMWHs have emerged as potential viable alternative antithrombin agents for the treatment of NSTE ACS. Their safety and efficacy have been demonstrated in addition to aspirin when used alone, when combined with a thienopyridine, a GP IIb/IIIa inhibitor, or both and as a potential 'bridging' agent that may facilitate the transition from medical to percutaneous management of this patient population (Tables 10.4 and 10.5) (Chapter 6). Furthermore, the association of the use of the LMWH enoxaparin and improved outcomes in patients with NSTE ACS who were medically managed established a strong foothold for this class of AT agents [40–42]. When combined with additional trials comparing LMWH with UH in addition to aspirin it is evident that:

- dalteparin and nadroparin offer similar efficacy to UH in patients with ACS
- enoxaparin decreases the composite endpoint of death, MI and recurrent angina by 12–25% at varying time points (48 h to 43 days) following presentation of ACS among patients treated conservatively (without early revascularization)
- LMWH use in this patient population was safe, without an increase in major hemorrhagic events
- prolonged treatment with LMWH in this patient population does not provide any additional benefit.

While the data in those early trials suggested that LMWHs may afford some incremental benefit over that of UH, several limitations preclude the extrapolation of these data to contemporary practice patterns. These were studies primarily of medical management of patients with ACS. Based on clinical trials [43, 44], a substantial proportion of these patients would be treated with an early invasive approach. Furthermore, when these patients were taken to the catheterization laboratory, the majority had their AT therapy crossed over to UH, a practice that has been suggested to result in worse outcomes [20]. In addition, none of these trials assessed the added benefit of LMWH over UH in patients being treated with a GP IIb/IIIa inhibitor or a thienopyridine, two classes of adjunctive antiplatelet medications that confer additional benefit in these patients.

Whether combining enoxaparin with a GP IIb/IIIa inhibitor is as safe or as effective as the current standard combination of UH with GP IIb/IIIa inhibitors for the treatment of ACS was assessed in the A to Z trial [45]. This prospective, international, open-label, randomized non-inferiority trial of 3987 ACS patients receiving tirofiban compared enoxaparin (1 mg/kg twice

Table 10.4 Trials of LMWH in Patients Undergoing PCI

Trial	Study population	LMWH (Dose)	Control	*N*	Primary efficacy endpoint	Timing of outcome	LMWH(%)	Control(%)	Timing of PCI relative to last LMWH dose	Supplemental peri-procedural anticoagulant
Without GP IIb/IIIa inhibitors										
Rabah *et al.* [25]	Elective PCI	Enoxaparin (1 mg/kg IV × 1 dose)	UH	60	TIMI 3 Flow Ischemic complications	Post-PCI 30 days	97 0	93 10	Immediately	None
REDUCE [9]	Elective PCI	Reviparin (7000 U IV bolus + infusion)	UH	612	D/MI/R	30 weeks	33.3	32	Immediately	10,500 U IV over first 24 h then 3500 U SC QD × 28 days
PEPCI [53]	Elective PCI	Enoxaparin (1 mg/kg SC bid)	NA	40	D/MI/UR	30 days	5.4	NA	8–12 h	0.3 mg/kg IV
NICE 1 [26]	Elective or urgent PCI	Enoxaparin (1 mg/kg IV × 1 dose)	NA	828	D/MI/UR	30 days	7.7	NA	Immediately	None
Choussat *et al.* [27]	Elective PCI	Enoxaparin (0.5 mg/kg IV × 1 dose)	NA	242	D/MI/UR	30 days	2.5	NA	Immediately	None
ESSENCE/TIMI-11B [58]	UA/NSTEMI	Enoxaparin (1 mg/kg SC bid ± 30 mg IV bolus)	UH	924	D/MI	43 days	3.3	5.9	Physician discretion after 24 h	UH at discretion of investigator
Collet *et al.* [59]	UA/NSTEMI	Enoxaparin (1 mg/kg SC bid)	NA	132	D/MI	30 days	3.0	NA	4–8 h	None
FRISC II [48]	UA/NSTEMI	Dalteparin (120 IU/kg bid)	NA	1222	D/MI	6 months	9.4	NA	≤12 h pre-PCI	NA

Table 10.4 (*Continued*)

Trial	Study population	LMWH (Dose)	Control	*N*	Primary efficacy endpoint	Timing of outcome	LMWH(%)	Control(%)	Timing of PCI relative to last LMWH dose	Supplemental peri-procedural anticoagulant
With GP IIb/IIIa inhibitors										
SYNERGY [50]	UA/NSTEMI	Enoxaparin (1mg/kg SC bid)	UH	10,000	D/MI	30 days	14	14.5	6–8 h	0.3 mg/kg IV if >8 h from last SC dose
NICE 4 [30]	Elective or urgent PCI	Enoxaparin (0.75 mg/kg IV × 1 dose) (Abciximab)	NA	818	D/MI/UR	30 days	6.8	NA	Immediately	NA
Kereiakes *et al.* [29]	Elective or urgent PCI	Dalteparin (40 IU/kg IV × 1 dose; 60 IU/kg IV × 1 dose) (Abciximab)	NA	103	D/MI/UR	IH	11.1 17.1	NA NA	Immediately	NA
CRUISE [28]	Elective or urgent PCI	Enoxaparin (0.75 mg/kg IV × 1 dose) (Eptifibatide)	UH	261	D/MI/UR	48 h	8.5	7.6	Immediately	NA
NICE 3 [41]	UA/NSTEMI	Enoxaparin (1 mg/kg SC bid) (Tirofiban, Eptifibatide, or abciximab)	NA	283	D/MI/RI	30 days	11.3	NA	Physician discretion	NA

bid = twice daily; D = death; IH = in hospital; NA = not applicable; QD = once daily; UR = urgent revascularization

Table 10.5 LMWH without GP IIb/IIIa inhibitors in ACS: UA/NSTEMI

Trial	Duration of therapy	LMWH dose	Control	*N*	Primary endpoint	LMWH(%)	Control(%)	Absolute difference(%) (*p*-value)
Dalteparin								
FRIC [78]	6 days	120 IU/kg SC bid	UH 5000 IU bolus + 1000 IU/h (aPTT 1.5 × control)	1482	D/MI/RA	9.3	7.6	1.7 (NS)
	40 days	7500 IU SC qd	Placebo		D/MI/RA	12.3	12.3	–
FRISC [35]	6 days	120 IU/kg SC bid	Placebo	1506	D/MI	1.8	4.8	−3 (0.001)
	35–45 days	7500 IU SC qd	Placebo		D/MI/UR	18	23.7	−5.7 (0.005)
FRISC II [7]	3 months after ≥5 days open label dalteparin	120 IU/kg SC bid	Placebo	2267	D/MI (3 months)	10.0	11.2	−1.2 (NS)
Nadroparin								
Gurfinkel *et al.* [34]	5–7 days	214 ICU/kg SC bid	ASA	219	D/MI/UI/RA	22	ASA–59	−37 (0.00001)
			UH (titrated to aPTT)				UH–63	−41 (0.00001)

Table 10.5 *(Continued)*

Trial	Duration of therapy	LMWH dose	Control	N	Primary endpoint	LMWH(%)	Control(%)	Absolute difference(%) (*p*-value)
FRAXIS [38]	6 days	86 IU/kg SC bid (ST)	UH 5000 IU bolus + 1250 IU/h (ST)	3468	D/MI/RA (14D)	17.8	18.1	−0.3 (NS)
	14 days	86 IU SC bid (LT)	Placebo (LT)			20	18.1	1.9 (NS)
Enoxaparin								
ESSENCE [5]	2–8 days	1 mg/kg SC bid	UH 5000 U bolus plus infusion (aPTT 55–85 s)	3171	D/MI/RA(14D)	16.6	19.8	–3.2 (0.019)
TIMI 11B [6]	Max 8 days	1 mg/kg SC bid	UH 70 U/kg + 15 U/kg per h (aPTT 1.5–2.5 × control)	3910	D/MI/UR (8 days)	12.4	14.5	−2.1 (0.048)
	43 days		Placebo		D/MI/UR (43 days)	17.3	19.7	−2.4 (0.048)

bid = twice daily; D = death; LT = long term; MB = major bleed daily) with weight-adjusted IV UH. There were no differences in rates of death, recurrent MI or refractory ischemia at 7 days (8.4% with enoxaparin vs 9.4% with UH, p-value = NS), meeting the prespecified criterion for non-inferiority. In addition, the combination of enoxaparin and tirofiban did not impart an increased risk of bleeding (3.0% vs 2.2% UH, p-value = 0.13). Although approximately 60% of patients in each group underwent an 'early invasive' management strategy, this trial was not designed to address the key issue of efficacy and safety of enoxaparin for this purpose.

The safety and efficacy of combined enoxaparin and GP IIb/IIIa inhibitors was evaluated in the most relevant manner in the SYNERGY trial, the only definitively powered trial in the current era of early invasive management of patients with ACS [20]. This trial enrolled 10,000 high-risk ACS patients and randomized them to receive either enoxaparin (1 mg/kg subcutaneously twice daily) or UH (60 U/kg bolus then 12 U/kg per h adjusted to an aPTT of 50–70 sec). More than 90% of patients underwent an early invasive strategy (cardiac catheterization at a median of 21 h from randomization). Of these, patients 47% underwent PCI, 19% had coronary bypass surgery and 57% received a GP IIb/IIIa inhibitor. The primary endpoint of death or MI occurred at a similar rate in the two treatment arms (14.5% vs 14.0% in the UH and enoxaparin arms, respectively, p-value = 0.4), although patients tended to do worse when switched from enoxaparin to UH or vice versa. Major bleeding occurred more frequently among patients receiving enoxaparin (7.6% vs 9.1%, respectively, p-value = 0.008). Notably, enoxaparin provided an adequate level of anticoagulation for patients undergoing early PCI, as demonstrated by the similar proportion of patients experiencing untoward events during invasive management.

Thus, enoxaparin may be used either as the sole anticoagulant or in combination with GP IIb/IIIa inhibitors for patients undergoing PCI. Patients can safely undergo PCI while on SC enoxaparin 1 mg/kg twice daily if it is performed within 8 h following the last administered dose. If PCI is undertaken between 8–12 h after the last dose, an additional 0.3 mg/kg dose of enoxaparin should be administered. As recently suggested, switching from enoxaparin to UH in these patients should be avoided. Dalteparin may also be utilized in this setting, although the data supporting this remain limited. If used, dalteparin should be administered at a dose of 120 IU/kg subcutaneously twice daily if PCI is performed within 8 h of the last dose. If performed more than 8 h from the last SC dose, PCI should be preceded by an additional 60 IU/kg IV dose.

DTIs

The central role of thrombin in the initiation and propagation of intravascular thrombus provides a strong rationale for the use of DTIs in ACS. DTIs are theoretically likely to be more effective than indirect thrombin inhibitors, such as UH or LMWH, because the heparins block only circulating thrombin, whereas DTIs block both circulating and clot-bound thrombin. Nevertheless, the DTIs have not been widely accepted as a replacement for UH in the management of ACS, except in cases of HIT.

Several initial phase 3 trials did not demonstrate a convincing benefit of DTIs over UH. However, the Direct Thrombin Inhibitor Trialists' Collaboration meta-analysis suggested the superiority of DTIs, particularly hirudin and bivalirudin, over UH with respect to recurrent MI in patients presenting with NSTE ACS (odds ratio, 0.80, 95% CI, 0.70 to 0.91) [46]. The absolute risk reduction in the composite of death or MI at the end of treatment (0.8%) was similar at 30 days (0.7%), indicating no loss of benefit after cessation of therapy.

It should be noted that the trials included in the meta-analysis were heavily weighted to the use of hirudin, an agent associated with increased bleeding complications. Coupled with assessment of these agents at a time when an early conservative approach and PTCA dominated the treatment paradigm, the penetration of these agents into NSTE ACS management was thwarted. Encouraging results from a large-scale trial assessing the efficacy of bivalirudin in patients undergoing urgent or elective stenting has fostered interest in this agent as a potential enhancement to the currently available AT agents in the acute setting [47]. The definitive trial, the ACUITY trial, recently provided insight into the role of this antithrombin agent in the NSTE ACS setting (ACC 2006 Scientific Sessions). In this trial 13,819 patients with moderate- to high-risk ACS undergoing cardiac catheterization within 72 h were randomized to receive UH or enoxaparin plus routine GP IIb/IIIa inhibition, bivalirudin plus routine GP IIb/IIIa inhibition or bivalirudin alone. Although bivalirudin alone was associated with a non-significant increase in ischemic events, it was deemed non-inferior to heparin/enoxaparin plus a GP IIb/IIIa inhibitor. However, the bivalirudin group showed significantly fewer bleeding complications. The addition of a GP IIb/IIIa inhibitor to bivalirudin did not improve its efficacy but did negate its benefit with respect to bleeding complications.

Additional support for the use of bivalirudin in medium- to high-risk NSTE ACS patients comes from a study that compared this DTI with either UH or LMWH plus eptifibatide [48]. Bivalirudin was shown to be associated with greater coronary flow reserve, fewer minor bleeding and transfusion events and a similar rate of ischemic events when compared with the eptifibatide-utilizing groups. Thus the role of these agents in the management of NSTE ACS continues to evolve and it appears that bivalirudin can be considered an alternative to UH or enoxaparin plus a GP IIb/IIIa inhibitor for intermediate- and high-risk patients as well as the AT agent for those patients unable to take UH or LMWH (i.e. patients with HIT).

Fondaparinux

Fondaparinux is a synthetic molecule consisting of the essential pentasaccharide sequence of heparin which binds to and induces the conformational change in circulating antithrombin. Fondaparinux exclusively inhibits factor Xa, with no activity against thrombin. Based on an early suggestion that this agent possesses similar efficacy to enoxaparin in NSTE ACS [49], the OASIS-5 trial sought to compare the effects of fondaparinux (2.5 mg/day) with enoxaparin (1 mg/kg twice daily) for 6 days on death, MI or refractory ischemia at 9 days in 20,078 patients presenting with NSTE ACS [50]. Although a similar rate of the primary endpoint was demonstrated, fondaparinux was associated with reduced major bleeding and improved long-term morbidity and mortality. That there was a small but statistically significant increase in catheter-related thrombi (0.9% vs 0.4% with enoxaparin) in those undergoing PCI emphasizes the need for further investigation in patients with NSTE ACS undergoing early invasive therapy.

10.3 EARLY INVASIVE VERSUS EARLY CONSERVATIVE STRATEGIES

An early invasive approach to the management of patients with NSTE ACS, defined as coronary angiography with or without revascularization within 48 h of symptom onset, has

Table 10.6 Class I indications for an early invasive approach to patients with non-ST-segment elevation ACS. Data from Braunwald *et al.* [14]

High-risk characteristics*

- Recurrent angina/ischemia at rest or at low levels of activity despite intensive anti-ischemic therapy
- Elevated cardiac biomarkers (CKMB, cardiac troponin I or T)
- Dynamic ST-segment changes
- Recurrent angina/ischemia associated with HF symptoms or signs (S3 gallop, rales, new or worsening MR)
- Depressed LV systolic function (EF <40%)
- Hemodynamic instability associated with angina
- PCI within the previous 6 months
- Prior CABG
- Sustained ventricular tachycardia
- High-risk findings on non-invasive functional study

* In the absence of these features, either an early conservative or early invasive strategy in hospitalized patients without contraindications for revascularization is acceptable

CKMB = creatinine kinase MB fraction; EF = ejection fraction; HF = heart failure; MR = mitral regurgitation

become the standard of care especially for intermediate- and high-risk patients (Table 10.6). This approach reduces composite cardiac outcomes, largely by decreasing recurrent angina and the need for subsequent rehospitalizations and revascularizations [51]. Although the optimal timing between presentation and an early invasive strategy remains poorly defined, a recent meta-analysis of randomized contemporary clinical trials supports the implementation of this strategy within 48 h of presentation [52]. The decision to pursue an early invasive versus an early conservative approach may ultimately influence the antithrombotic regimen employed for a given patient. Irrespective of approach pursued, the use of both antiplatelet and AT therapy is recommended for those at intermediate- to high-risk.

EARLY INVASIVE STRATEGY

This approach is based on the theory that knowledge of a patient's coronary anatomy followed by revascularization performed in an expeditious manner will facilitate care of these often unstable patients. If an early invasive approach is pursued, any AT therapy (LMWH or UH) initiated prior to PCI could be continued through the intervention with a similar outcome [20]. In addition, it would be prudent to initiate GP IIb/IIIa inhibition (in addition to aspirin and clopidogrel) either prior to or during percutaneous revascularization with the 'up-front' use of these agents reserved for those at highest risk. This strategy is particularly important for these patients if there is a perceived substantial delay in getting these patients to the catheterization laboratory [23, 34, 58]. Alternatively, the 'up-front' use of bivalirudin in these patients may provide a seamless transition from the early medical to the early invasive approach in these patients.

EARLY CONSERVATIVE STRATEGY

This approach has been based on the theory that plaque stabilization is not only possible in this clinical setting but also allows for more scrutinized selection of 'appropriate' patients for invasive therapy. Unfortunately, the medical literature has been peppered with studies both for and against this strategy. While one recent clinical trial could not demonstrate a clinical benefit with an early invasive vs a selectively invasive strategy [53], several other contemporary trials of invasive vs conservative strategies have revealed a favorable outcome for patients assigned to an early invasive approach [43, 44, 54–56]. Furthermore, the theoretically beneficial approach of plaque stabilization or 'cooling off,' of patients has not been shown to provide benefit when compared with early invasive therapy [57].

If an early conservative approach was pursued, then a LMWH (in addition to aspirin and a thienopyridine) would be preferable over UH as the AT backbone of therapy [40, 42]. Furthermore, GP IIb/IIIa inhibition would be reasonable in patients at intermediate and high risk.

10.4 RECOMMENDATIONS

Risk stratification remains central to choosing the most appropriate antithrombotic regimen for patients presenting with NSTE ACS (Figure 10.2 and Table 10.7). Based on the currently

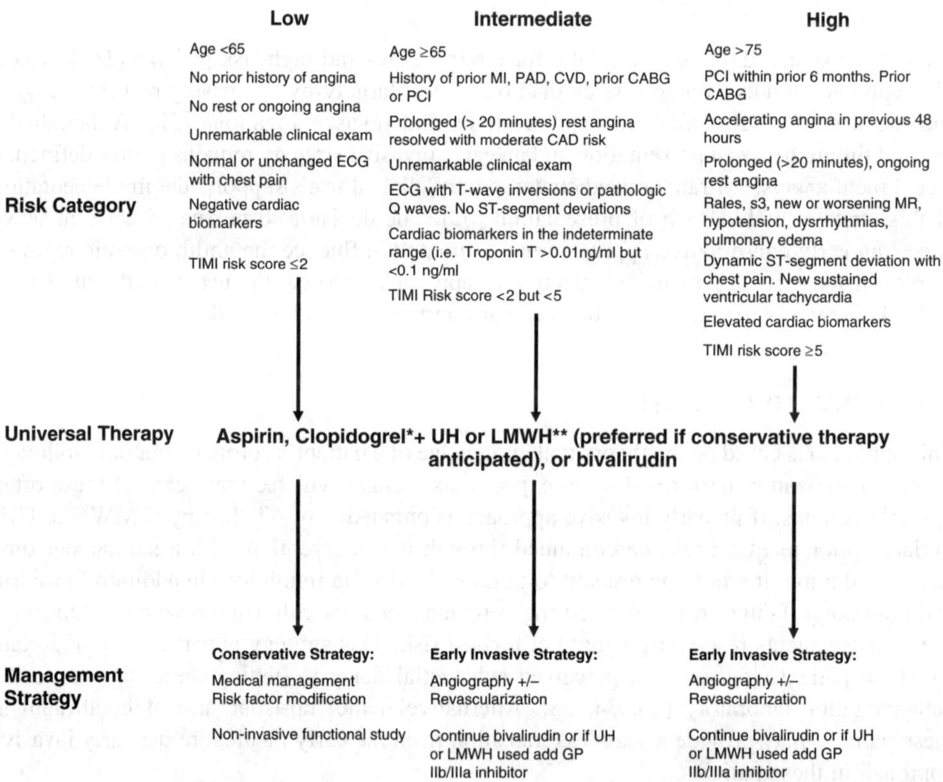

Figure 10.2 A proposed algorithm for the approach to patients with non-ST-segment elevation ACS. Universal therapy for patients with a definite non-ST-segment elevation ACS should include aspirin, clopidogrel, and an antithrombin agent. Additional therapies for selected intermediate- and high-risk patients include an early invasive strategy and for those initially treated with UH or LMWH, the use of GP IIb/IIIa inhibitors. *Reserve for peri-procedural administration in patients at high risk for surgical CAD; ** Both enoxaparin and dalteparin FDA approved for this indication; ECG = electrocardiogram; EF = ejection fraction; PAD = peripheral artery disease

Table 10.7 Recommended antithrombotic therapy for non-ST-segment elevation ACS

Agent	Comments
Antiplatelet Agents	
Aspirin	• All patients indefinitely – 162–325 mg initial dose – 75–160 mg daily thereafter
ADP receptor antagonists (i.e. clopidogrel)	• 600 mg load then 75 mg daily • All patients except: – Anticipated urgent CABG – Elective CABG within 5 days • Duration – 1 year*
GP IIb/IIIa antagonists	• All high-risk patients (see Table 10.6) • Abciximab: 0.25 mg/kg bolus then 0.125 μg/kg per min for 12 h • **Medical management****: Eptifibatide: 180 μg/kg bolus then 2 μg/kg per min × 72–96 h • **PCI****: Eptifibatide: 180 μg/kg bolus followed by repeat 180 μg/kg bolus in 10 minutes. Infusion 2 μg/kg per min • Tirofiban***: 0.4 μg/kg per min × 30 min then 0.1 μg/kg per min × 48–96 h • Avoid abciximab if PCI not planned
Antithrombin agents	
UH	• Agent of choice for patients managed with an early invasive strategy • 60 IU/kg (max 5000 IU) bolus then 12 (max 1000 IU) IU/kg per h • Goal aPTT 50–70 sec
LMWH	• Alternative to UH for patients managed with an early invasive strategy • Agent of choice for conservative strategy – Enoxaparin: 1 mg/kg SC twice a day – Dalteparin: 120 IU/kg SC twice a day • Avoid in CKD (i.e. CrCl <30 mL/min for enoxaparin) • Avoid in anticipated urgent CABG
DTIs	• Alternative to UH and LMWH in patients with HIT

*At least one year, although optimal duration for patients receiving drug-eluting stents unknown
**For CrCl <50mL/min: 180 μg/kg bolus × 1 then 1 μg/kg per min. 22.6 mg max bolus and 15 mg/h max infusion
***Continue 12–24 h after PCI. Decrease dose by 50% for CrCl <30 mL/min
CrCl = creatinine clearance

available data, the management of definite NSTE ACS can be divided into therapies beneficial to all patients and to therapies most useful for those at intermediate and high risk. The approach to patients at the extremes of risk, low- and high-risk, remains the most straight forward: background aspirin, clopidogrel and an antithrombin agent for both, with the difference being that the high-risk patients should also have concomitant GP IIb/IIIa inhibition and an early invasive strategy. For the low-risk patients, medical optimization and further risk stratification may be the best strategy.

Whereas patients at intermediate risk were previously stabilized, with aspirin, clopidogrel and an AT agent affording the opportunity for further risk stratification, the current guidelines favor a more aggressive approach for these patients which includes the use of an early invasive strategy and a low threshold to add a GP IIb/IIIa inhibitor. It should be noted that irrespective of the patient's risk, if there is significant preprocedural suspicion that surgical atherosclerotic disease may be present, it would be prudent to reserve clopidogrel dosing for the possible peri-intervention period and to use UH as the antithrombin agent.

10.5 CONCLUSIONS

Unlike patients with an STEMI, where the treatment paradigm is clear – complete and rapid restoration of antegrade coronary perfusion – the treatment paradigm for NSTE ACS remains one in evolution. This can be attributed to the heterogeneous nature of this patient population, an incomplete and at times contradictory body of literature, personal preferences or a combination of these factors. Nevertheless, what remains integral to the management of these patients is the utility of potent antiplatelet and AT therapy in addition to aggressive risk factor modification. Although the likelihood of a universally beneficial cocktail may not be possible for these patients, ongoing studies assessing the likelihood of seamless antithrombotic therapy that can bridge the medical and interventional worlds and different regimen permutations will hopefully come close. Ultimately, individualized care will be the answer.

REFERENCES

[1] Antman, E.M., *et al.*, (2000) The TIMI risk score for unstable angina/non-ST elevation MI: A method for prognostication and therapeutic decision making. *JAMA*, 284(7):835–42.
[2] Boersma, E., *et al.*, (2000) Predictors of outcome in patients with acute coronary syndromes without persistent ST-segment elevation. Results from an international trial of 9461 patients. The PURSUIT Investigators. *Circulation*, 101(22):2557–67.
[3] Sabatine, M.S., *et al.*, (2002) Identification of patients at high risk for death and cardiac ischemic events after hospital discharge. *Am Heart J*, 143(6):966–70.
[4] Budaj, A., *et al.*, (2002) Benefit of clopidogrel in patients with acute coronary syndromes without ST-segment elevation in various risk groups. *Circulation*, 106(13):1622–6.
[5] Scirica, B.M., *et al.*, (2002) Validation of the thrombolysis in myocardial infarction (TIMI) risk score for unstable angina pectoris and non-ST-elevation myocardial infarction in the TIMI III registry. *Am J Cardiol*, 90(3):303–5.
[6] Samaha, F.F., *et al.*, (2002) Usefulness of the TIMI risk score in predicting both short- and long-term outcomes in the Veterans Affairs Non-Q-Wave Myocardial Infarction Strategies In-Hospital (VANQWISH) Trial. *Am J Cardiol*, 90(9):922–6.
[7] Mega, J.L., *et al.*, (2005) Correlation between the TIMI risk score and high-risk angiographic findings in non-ST-elevation acute coronary syndromes: observations from the Platelet Receptor Inhibition in Ischemic Syndrome Management in Patients Limited by Unstable Signs and Symptoms (PRISM-PLUS) trial. *Am Heart J*, 149(5):846–50.
[8] Soiza, R.L., *et al.*, (2006) Risk stratification in acute coronary syndromes–does the TIMI risk score work in unselected cases? *QJM*, 99(2):81–7
[9] Antman, E.M., *et al.*, (1996) Cardiac-specific troponin I levels to predict the risk of mortality in patients with acute coronary syndromes. *N Eng J Med*, 335(18):1342–9.
[10] Lewis, H.D., Jr., *et al.*, (1983) Protective effects of aspirin against acute myocardial infarction and death in men with unstable angina. Results of a Veterans Administration Cooperative Study. *N Eng J Med*, 309(7):396–403.
[11] Cairns, J.A., *et al.*, (1985) Aspirin, sulfinpyrazone, or both in unstable angina. Results of a Canadian multicenter trial. *N Eng J Med*, 313(22):1369–75.

[12] The RISC group, (1990) Risk of myocardial infarction and death during treatment with low dose aspirin and intravenous heparin in men with unstable coronary artery disease. The RISC Group. *Lancet*, 336(8719):827–30.

[13] Theroux, P., *et al.*, (1988) Aspirin, heparin, or both to treat acute unstable angina. *N Eng J Med*, 319(17):1105–11.

[14] Braunwald, E., *et al.*, (2002) ACC/AHA 2002 guideline update for the management of patients with unstable angina and non-ST-segment elevation myocardial infarction—summary article: a report of the American College of Cardiology/American Heart Association task force on practice guidelines (Committee on the Management of Patients With Unstable Angina). *J Am Coll Cardiol*, 40(7):1366–74.

[15] Antithrombotic trialists' collaboration, (2002) Collaborative meta-analysis of randomised trials of antiplatelet therapy for prevention of death, myocardial infarction, and stroke in high risk patients. *Br Med J*, 324(7329):71–86.

[16] The CAPRIE Steering Committee. (1996) A randomised, blinded, trial of clopidogrel versus aspirin in patients at risk of ischaemic events (CAPRIE). *Lancet*, 348(9038):1329–39.

[17] Yusuf, S., *et al.*, (2001) Effects of clopidogrel in addition to aspirin in patients with acute coronary syndromes without ST-segment elevation. *N Eng J Med*, 345(7):494–502.

[18] Steinhubl, S.R., *et al.*, (2002) Early and sustained dual oral antiplatelet therapy following percutaneous coronary intervention: a randomized controlled trial. *JAMA*, 288(19):2411–20.

[19] Mehta, S.R., Yusuf, S., (2003) Short- and long-term oral antiplatelet therapy in acute coronary syndromes and percutaneous coronary intervention. *J Am Coll Cardiol*, 41(4 Suppl S):79S–88S.

[20] Ferguson, J.J., *et al.*, (2004) Enoxaparin vs unfractionated heparin in high-risk patients with non-ST-segment elevation acute coronary syndromes managed with an intended early invasive strategy: primary results of the SYNERGY randomized trial. *JAMA*, 292(1):45–54.

[21] The EPIC investigators, (1994) Use of a monoclonal antibody directed against the platelet glycoprotein IIb/IIIa receptor in high-risk coronary angioplasty. The EPIC Investigation. *N Eng J Med*, 330(14):956–61.

[22] The EPILOG Investigators, (1997) Platelet glycoprotein IIb/IIIa receptor blockade and low-dose heparin during percutaneous coronary revascularization. *N Eng J Med*, 336(24):1689–96.

[23] The CAPTURE investigators, (1997) Randomised placebo-controlled trial of abciximab before and during coronary intervention in refractory unstable angina: the CAPTURE Study. *Lancet*, 349(9063):1429–35.

[24] Randomised placebo-controlled trial of effect of eptifibatide on complications of percutaneous coronary intervention: IMPACT-II. Integrilin to Minimise Platelet Aggregation and Coronary Thrombosis-II, (1997) *Lancet*, 349(9063):1422–8.

[25] The RESTORE investigators, (1997) Effects of platelet glycoprotein IIb/IIIa blockade with tirofiban on adverse cardiac events in patients with unstable angina or acute myocardial infarction undergoing coronary angioplasty. Randomized Efficacy Study of Tirofiban for Outcomes and REstenosis. *Circulation*, 96(5):1445–53.

[26] The PRISM study investigators, (1998) A comparison of aspirin plus tirofiban with aspirin plus heparin for unstable angina. Platelet Receptor Inhibition in Ischemic Syndrome Management (PRISM). *N Eng J Med*, 338(21):1498–505.

[27] The PARAGON investigators, (1998) International, randomized, controlled trial of lamifiban (a platelet glycoprotein IIb/IIIa inhibitor), heparin, or both in unstable angina. Platelet IIb/IIIa Antagonism for the Reduction of Acute coronary syndrome events in a Global Organization Network. *Circulation*, 97(24):2386–95.

[28] The PRISM-PLUS investigators, (1998) Inhibition of the platelet glycoprotein IIb/IIIa receptor with tirofiban in unstable angina and non-Q-wave myocardial infarction. Platelet Receptor Inhibition in Ischemic Syndrome Management in Patients Limited by Unstable Signs and Symptoms (PRISM-PLUS). *N Eng J Med*, 338(21):1488–97.

[29] The PURSUIT trial investigators, (1998) Inhibition of platelet glycoprotein IIb/IIIa with eptifibatide in patients with acute coronary syndromes. Platelet Glycoprotein IIb/IIIa in Unstable Angina: Receptor Suppression Using Integrilin Therapy. *N Eng J Med*, 339(7):436–43.

[30] Simoons, M.L., (2001) Effect of glycoprotein IIb/IIIa receptor blocker abciximab on outcome in patients with acute coronary syndromes without early coronary revascularisation: the GUSTO IV-ACS randomised trial. *Lancet*, 357(9272):1915–24.

[31] Januzzi, J.L., *et al.*, (2001) Elevation in serum troponin I predicts the benefit of tirofiban. *J Thromb Thrombolysis*, 11(3):211–15.
[32] Januzzi, J.L., *et al.*, (2001) Optimizing glycoprotein IIb/IIIa receptor antagonist use for the non-ST-segment elevation acute coronary syndromes: risk stratification and therapeutic intervention. *Am Heart J*, 146(5):764–74.
[33] O'Rourke, R.A., *et al.*, (2001) New approaches to diagnosis and management of unstable angina and non-ST-segment elevation myocardial infarction. *Arch Intern Med*, 161(5):674–82.
[34] Roffi, M., *et al.*, (2001) Platelet glycoprotein IIb/IIIa inhibitors reduce mortality in diabetic patients with non-ST-segment-elevation acute coronary syndromes. *Circulation*, 104(23): 2767–71.
[35] Boersma, E., *et al.*, (2002) Platelet glycoprotein IIb/IIIa inhibitors in acute coronary syndromes: a meta-analysis of all major randomised clinical trials. *Lancet*, 359(9302):189–98.
[36] Lim, M.J., *et al.*, (2005) Treating patients with acute coronary syndromes with aggressive antiplatelet therapy (from the Global Registry of Acute Coronary Events). *Am J Cardiol*, 96(7):917–21.
[37] Neri Serneri, G.G., *et al.*, (1990) Effect of heparin, aspirin, or alteplase in reduction of myocardial ischaemia in refractory unstable angina. *Lancet*, 335(8690):615–18.
[38] Telford, A.M., Wilson, C., (1981) Trial of heparin versus atenolol in prevention of myocardial infarction in intermediate coronary syndrome. *Lancet*, 1(8232):1225–8.
[39] Tolleson, T.R., *et al.*, (2003) Relationship between heparin anticoagulation and clinical outcomes in coronary stent intervention: observations from the ESPRIT trial. *J Am Coll Cardiol*, 41(3): 386–93.
[40] Antman, E.M., *et al.*, (1999) Enoxaparin prevents death and cardiac ischemic events in unstable angina/non-Q-wave myocardial infarction. Results of the thrombolysis in myocardial infarction (TIMI) 11B trial. *Circulation*, 100(15):1593–601.
[41] Antman, E.M., *et al.*, (1999) Assessment of the treatment effect of enoxaparin for unstable angina/non-Q-wave myocardial infarction. TIMI 11B-ESSENCE meta-analysis. *Circulation*, 100(15):1602–8.
[42] Cohen, M., *et al.*, (1997) A comparison of low-molecular-weight heparin with unfractionated heparin for unstable coronary artery disease. Efficacy and Safety of Subcutaneous Enoxaparin in Non-Q-Wave Coronary Events Study Group. *N Eng J Med*, 337(7):447–52.
[43] Invasive compared with non-invasive treatment in unstable coronary-artery disease: FRISC II prospective randomised multicentre study. FRagmin and Fast Revascularisation during InStability in Coronary artery disease Investigators, (1999) *Lancet*, 354(9180): 708–15.
[44] Cannon, C.P., *et al.*, (2001) Comparison of early invasive and conservative strategies in patients with unstable coronary syndromes treated with the glycoprotein IIb/IIIa inhibitor tirofiban. *N Eng J Med*, 344(25):1879–87.
[45] Blazing, M.A., *et al.*, (2004) Safety and efficacy of enoxaparin vs unfractionated heparin in patients with non-ST-segment elevation acute coronary syndromes who receive tirofiban and aspirin: a randomized controlled trial. *JAMA*, 292(1):55–64.
[46] Direct Thrombin Inhibitor trialists' collaborative group. (2002) Direct thrombin inhibitors in acute coronary syndromes: principal results of a meta-analysis based on individual patients' data. *Lancet*, 359(9303):294–302.
[47] Lincoff, A.M., *et al.*, (2003) Bivalirudin and provisional glycoprotein IIb/IIIa blockade compared with heparin and planned glycoprotein IIb/IIIa blockade during percutaneous coronary intervention: REPLACE-2 randomized trial. *JAMA*, 289(7):853–63.
[48] Gibson, C.M., *et al.*, (2006) A randomized trial to evaluate the relative protection against post-percutaneous coronary intervention microvascular dysfunction, ischemia, and inflammation among antiplatelet and antithrombotic agents: the PROTECT-TIMI-30 trial. *J Am Coll Cardiol*, 47(12):2364–73.
[49] Simoons, M.L., *et al.*, (2004) A dose-finding study of fondaparinux in patients with non-ST-segment elevation acute coronary syndromes: the Pentasaccharide in Unstable Angina (PENTUA) Study. *J Am Coll Cardiol*, 43(12):2183–90.
[50] Yusuf, S., *et al.*, (2006) Comparison of fondaparinux and enoxaparin in acute coronary syndromes. *N Eng J Med*, 354(14):1464–76.

[51] Mehta, S.R., *et al.*, (2005) Routine vs selective invasive strategies in patients with acute coronary syndromes: a collaborative meta-analysis of randomized trials. *JAMA*, 293(23): 2908–17.

[52] Bavry, A.A., *et al.*, (2006) Benefit of early invasive therapy in acute coronary syndromes: a meta-analysis of contemporary randomized clinical trials. *J Am Coll Cardiol*, 48(7): 1319–25.

[53] de Winter, R.J., *et al.*, (2005) Early invasive versus selectively invasive management for acute coronary syndromes. *N Eng J Med*, 353(11):1095–104.

[54] Fox, K.A., *et al.*, (2002) Interventional versus conservative treatment for patients with unstable angina or non-ST-elevation myocardial infarction: the British Heart Foundation RITA 3 randomised trial. Randomized Intervention Trial of unstable Angina. *Lancet*, 360(9335): 743–51.

[55] Boden, W.E., (2003) 'Routine invasive' versus 'selective invasive' approaches to non-ST-segment elevation acute coronary syndromes management in the post-stent/platelet inhibition era. *J Am Coll Cardiol*, 41(4 Suppl S):113S–22S.

[56] Fox, K.A., *et al.*, (2005) 5-year outcome of an interventional strategy in non-ST-elevation acute coronary syndrome: the British Heart Foundation RITA 3 randomised trial. *Lancet*, 366(9489):914–20.

[57] Neumann, F.J., *et al.*, (2003) Evaluation of prolonged antithrombotic pretreatment ('cooling-off' strategy) before intervention in patients with unstable coronary syndromes: a randomized controlled trial. *JAMA*, 290(12):1593–9.

[58] Topol, E.J., (2003) A guide to therapeutic decision-making in patients with non-ST-segment elevation acute coronary syndromes. *J Am Coll Cardiol*, 41(4 Suppl S):S123–9.

[59] Cohen, M., *et al.*, (1990) Usefulness of antithrombotic therapy in resting angina pectoris or non-Q-wave myocardial infarction in preventing death and myocardial infarction (a pilot study from the Antithrombotic Therapy in Acute Coronary Syndromes Study Group). *Am J Cardiol*, 66(19):1287–92.

[60] Theroux, P., *et al.*, (1993) Aspirin versus heparin to prevent myocardial infarction during the acute phase of unstable angina. *Circulation*, 88(5 Pt 1):2045–8.

[61] Cohen, M., *et al.*, (1994) Combination antithrombotic therapy in unstable rest angina and non-Q-wave infarction in nonprior aspirin users. Primary end points analysis from the ATACS trial. Antithrombotic Therapy in Acute Coronary Syndromes Research Group. *Circulation*, 89(1):81–8.

[62] Holdright, D., *et al.*, (1994) Comparison of the effect of heparin and aspirin versus aspirin alone on transient myocardial ischemia and in-hospital prognosis in patients with unstable angina. *J Am Coll Cardiol*, 24(1):39–45.

[63] Gurfinkel, E.P., *et al.*, (1995) Low molecular weight heparin versus regular heparin or aspirin in the treatment of unstable angina and silent ischemia. *J Am Coll Cardiol*, 26(2):313–18.

[64] Neri Serneri, G.G., *et al.*, (1995) Randomised comparison of subcutaneous heparin, intravenous heparin, and aspirin in unstable angina. Studio Epoorine Sottocutanea nell'Angina Instobile (SESAIR) Refrattorie Group. *Lancet*, 345(8959):1201–4.

[65] Becker, R.C., *et al.*, (1999) A randomized, multicenter trial of weight-adjusted intravenous heparin dose titration and point-of-care coagulation monitoring in hospitalized patients with active thromboembolic disease. Antithrombotic Therapy Consortium Investigators. *Am Heart J*, 137(1):59–71.

[66] Rabah, M.M., *et al.*, (1999) Usefulness of intravenous enoxaparin for percutaneous coronary intervention in stable angina pectoris. *Am J Cardiol*, 84(12):1391–5.

[67] Karsch, K.R., *et al.*, (1996) Low molecular weight heparin (reviparin) in percutaneous transluminal coronary angioplasty. Results of a randomized, double-blind, unfractionated heparin and placebo-controlled, multicenter trial (REDUCE trial). Reduction of Restenosis After PTCA, Early Administration of Reviparin in a Double-Blind Unfractionated Heparin and Placebo-Controlled Evaluation. *J Am Coll Cardiol*, 28(6):1437–43.

[68] Martin, J.L., *et al.*, (2004) Reliable anticoagulation with enoxaparin in patients undergoing percutaneous coronary intervention: The pharmacokinetics of enoxaparin in PCI (PEPCI) study. *Catheter Cardiovasc Interv*, 61(2):163–70.

[69] Kereiakes, D.J., *et al.*, (2001) Enoxaparin and abciximab adjunctive pharmacotherapy during percutaneous coronary intervention. *J Invasive Cardiol*, 13(4):272–8.

[70] Choussat, R., *et al.*, (2002) A unique, low dose of intravenous enoxaparin in elective percutaneous coronary intervention. *J Am Coll Cardiol*, 40(11):1943–50.

[71] Fox, K.A., *et al.*, (2002) Comparison of enoxaparin versus unfractionated heparin in patients with unstable angina pectoris/non-ST-segment elevation acute myocardial infarction having subsequent percutaneous coronary intervention. *Am J Cardiol*, 90(5):477–82.

[72] Collet, J.P., *et al.*, (2001) Percutaneous coronary intervention after subcutaneous enoxaparin pretreatment in patients with unstable angina pectoris. *Circulation*, 103(5):658–63.

[73] The FRISC II investigators, (1999) Long-term low-molecular-mass heparin in unstable coronary-artery disease: FRISC II prospective randomised multicentre study. FRagmin and Fast Revascularisation during InStability in Coronary artery disease. *Lancet*, 354(9180):701–7.

[74] Young, J.J., Kereiakes, D.J., Grines, C.L., (2000) Low-molecular-weight heparin therapy in percutaneous coronary intervention: the NICE 1 and NICE 4 trials. National Investigators Collaborating on Enoxaparin Investigators. *J Invasive Cardiol*, 12 Suppl E:E14–E18;discussion E18–E25.

[75] Kereiakes, D.J., *et al.*, (2001) Dalteparin in combination with abciximab during percutaneous coronary intervention. *Am Heart J*, 141(3):348–52.

[76] Bhatt, D.L., *et al.*, (2003) Safety of concomitant therapy with eptifibatide and enoxaparin in patients undergoing percutaneous coronary intervention: results of the Coronary Revascularization Using Integrilin and Single bolus Enoxaparin Study. *J Am Coll Cardiol*, 41(1):20–5.

[77] Ferguson, J.J., *et al.*, (2003) Combining enoxaparin and glycoprotein IIb/IIIa antagonists for the treatment of acute coronary syndromes: final results of the National Investigators Collaborating on Enoxaparin-3 (NICE-3) study. *Am Heart J*, 146(4):628–34.

[78] Klein, W., *et al.*, (1997) Fragmin in unstable angina pectoris or in non-Q-wave acute myocardial infarction (the FRIC Study). *Am J Cardiol*, 80(5A):30E–34E.

[79] The FRISC study group, (1996) Low-molecular-weight heparin during instability in coronary artery disease, Fragmin during Instability in Coronary Artery Disease (FRISC). *Lancet*, 347(9001):561–8.

[80] Comparison of two treatment durations (6 days and 14 days) of a low molecular weight heparin with a 6-day treatment of unfractionated heparin in the initial management of unstable angina or non-Q wave myocardial infarction: FRAX.I.S. (FRAxiparine in Ischaemic Syndrome), (1999) *Eur Heart J*, 20(21):1553–62.

11 Anticoagulation Strategies for Patients Undergoing Percutaneous Coronary Intervention

11.1 INTRODUCTION

The use of optimal antiplatelet and antithrombotic strategies is pivotal in reducing adverse events among patients undergoing PCI. Indeed, a number of novel pharmaceuticals have been introduced since the mid-1990s which has led to improved angiographic and, more importantly, clinical outcomes. Within this chapter we attempt to review the current evidence regarding the efficacy of available adjunctive agents for anticoagulating patients undergoing percutaneous coronary revascularization, and to delineate a treatment algorithm for both elective and acute cases.

Certainly, each of the following recommendations can be debated; we recognize that there exist no universally accepted guidelines for anticoagulation. Indeed, a number of variables must always be taken into account prior to prescribing an antithrombotic regimen for any individual patient. Patients undergoing PCI in the midst of an acute coronary event frequently require more aggressive anticoagulation and platelet aggregation inhibition than lower-risk patients undergoing elective PCI for stable angina pectoris. Risk, of course, is a relatively subjective metric; different interventional cardiologists will have different definitions of high-risk lesions and high-risk patients. Similarly, generalizing antithrombotic regimen safety data to a wide spectrum of catheter-based therapeutic devices should be avoided. A level of anticoagulation that is safe and effective for angioplasty and stent placement may not be sufficient for devices with longer intracoronary dwell times, such as wire-control or thrombus extraction catheters. Nonetheless, the compilation of recently released randomized clinical trial data does provide for several broader recommendations.

11.2 ANTIPLATELET THERAPY

ASPIRIN

The cornerstone of antiplatelet therapy is aspirin, or ASA. It remains the most widely studied antiplatelet drug, with >100,000 patients included in randomized trials against placebo [1]. Although no trials have been completed that specifically compare different doses of ASA in the setting of PCI, the ability of ASA to inhibit platelet aggregation and prevent thrombotic cardiovascular events makes its administration essential from both risk-benefit and cost-benefit standpoints.

Two placebo-controlled randomized trials have demonstrated the ability of ASA to reduce ischemic complications among patients undergoing elective PCI [2,3]. Both studies noted a reduction in their respective primary endpoints (STEMI or acute vessel closure) for patients routinely administered ASA. As such, all patients undergoing percutaneous intervention of any kind, whether coronary or peripheral, should receive an empiric ASA at least 2 h before the procedure; thereafter it should be continued indefinitely. If a stent is deployed in the course of the procedure, a minimum dose of 325 mg daily is advised for at least one month prior to reducing to 81 mg daily. Although no randomized data comparing low and higher doses of ASA in PCI exists, a *post hoc* analysis of the CURE trial demonstrated a comparable reduction in the primary endpoint (death/MI/stroke) in over 5300 patients receiving low dose (<100 mg), intermediate dose (101–199 mg), or high dose (>200 mg) ASA [4]. However, the higher doses of ASA were associated with a statistically significant increase in major bleeding.

Numerous randomized controlled trials showed decreased mortality rates when ASA (75–325 mg) was given to hospitalized patients with an ACS [5]. In the setting of an ACS, a dose of 162 mg or more produces a rapid clinical antithrombotic effect caused by immediate and near-total inhibition of thromboxane A2 production. Chewed non-enteric-coated ASA provides more rapid bioavailability than swallowed tablets [6]. The earlier ASA is given, the greater the reduction in risk of mortality [7]. Therefore, it is reasonable for dispatchers to routinely administer a single dose (160–325 mg) of ASA to all out-of-hospital patients with suspected ACS and without a true aspirin allergy, regardless of planned transfer direct to the catheterization laboratory.

The issue of ASA resistance has confounded many physicians, specifically regarding appropriate dosing and loading time [8]. The majority of studies assessing ASA efficacy have relied on relatively non-specific assays, including the effect on bleeding times, or the ability to inhibit platelet aggregation, as measured by whole blood aggregometry, or a rapid platelet function assay. Using these techniques, it is estimated that between 10 and 40% of patients demonstrate some ASA antiplatelet resistance. However, the use of qualified and direct measurements of ASA efficacy such as AA-induced light transmittance platelet aggregation (LTA) and thrombelastography (TEG), has suggested that the true incidence of ASA resistance may be quite low [9]. As such, until the definition and treatment of aspirin 'resistance' is more clearly delineated, routine testing of bleeding times or other parameters is not advocated. Similarly, the recommended dosing should remain static.

THIENOPYRIDINES

The thienopyridines permanently inhibit the platelet 2-methythio-ADP-binding receptor, thereby irreversibly inactivating exposed mature platelets for the duration of their lifespan (7–10 days) [[10]. The only two thienopyridines available for use are ticlopidine, approved in the United States in 1991, and clopidogrel, approved in 1998. The combination of ticlopidine and aspirin is a safe and effective means of preventing stent thrombosis in patients [[11]. However, because of its prominent and feared side effects, namely reversible neutropenia (0.8%) and thrombotic thrombocytopenic purpura (approximately 1 in 1600 patients) [12], ticlopidine has almost completely been replaced by clopidogrel both within and outside the catheterization laboratory. Although the FDA still has not officially approved routine clopidogrel administration for adjunctive antiplatelet therapy, it has nonetheless become the standard of care in patients undergoing PCI. Clopidogrel is biotransformed and activated in the liver via the CP450 system [10]. The parent compound is rapidly absorbed, with peak serum concentrations achieved within 1 h after oral ingestion. Steady-state concentrations are achieved after approximately 4–7 days of consecutive dosing (50–100 mg). Recent data suggests that a high loading dose of clopidogrel (300–600 mg) given two or more hours prior to an interventional procedure may reduce acute ischemic events at the time of PCI.

The definitive trial in elective coronary stenting, CREDO [13], examined the benefit of clopidogrel pretreatment and the efficacy of long-term treatment (12 months). In this trial of 2116 patients, 90% of whom received stents, a 26.9% RR reduction (8.5% vs 11.5%; p-value = 0.02) in the primary endpoint (composite death, MI, stroke) was observed among patients randomized to receive clopidogrel for one year following PCI compared with those randomized to placebo.

Although questions remained regarding the utility of clopidogrel pretreatment, the subgroup analysis of the CREDO trial suggested that pretreatment given more than 6 h before elective stent deployment may be necessary to improve short-term outcomes [14]. This idea was recently addressed in a randomized controlled trial comparing high (600 mg) vs standard (300 mg) loading doses of clopidogrel given 4–8 h before elective PCI [15]. Not only was pretreatment with a high loading dose associated with improved 30-day clinical outcomes, it was as safe as the standard dose loading regimen. Combined with recent trials suggesting a 600 mg loading dose of clopidogrel given at least 2 h prior to PCI may obviate the need for adjunctive GP IIb/IIIa inhibition with abciximab in low- to intermediate-risk non-diabetic (ISAR-REACT) [16] and diabetic (ISAR-SWEET) [17] patients, these data support the high loading dose of clopidogrel and should influence contemporary practice.

Given the benefit of a 600 mg loading dose over a 300 mg loading dose, the logical next step was to ascertain whether or not even higher loading doses would exert additional suppression of platelet function. The recently released ISAR-CHOICE [18] trial assessed the effects of increasing loading doses of clopidogrel (300, 600 or 900 mg) on the plasma concentrations of the active thiol metabolite, unchanged clopidogrel and the inactive carboxyl metabolite of clopidogrel as well as on parameters of platelet aggregation. Loading with 600 mg resulted in higher plasma concentrations of the active metabolite, clopidogrel and the carboxyl metabolite, and improved inhibition of platelet aggregation compared with loading with 300 mg. In addition, no incremental difference was noted with the 900 mg loading dose.

The beneficial effects of clopidogrel have also been observed in patients with ACS undergoing PCI. The PCI-CURE substudy [19], derived from the larger CURE cohort, randomized 2658 ACS patients undergoing PCI to either clopidogrel (300 mg loading bolus, followed by 75 mg daily) or placebo. The primary endpoint, a composite of death, MI and urgent revascularization, was significantly reduced in the clopidogrel group (4.5%) vs placebo (6.4%) at 12 months. The median duration between initiation of therapy and PCI was 10 days.

The question of optimal loading dose in the ACS population was recently addressed in the ALBION study [20], which was designed to determine the effectiveness of these three different loading doses of clopidogrel in 103 patients with UA/NSTEMI undergoing PCI (publication pending). Similar to the results seen in the elective setting, the onset of action and level of platelet inhibition was achieved faster with the 600 mg and 900 mg loading doses of clopidogrel compared to the 300 mg loading dose with no significant difference between the 600 mg and the 900 mg loading doses. Although the study was not powered to detect differences in clinical endpoints, the bleeding rates were similar among treatment groups.

Accordingly, current common clinical practice is pretreatment with a 300 mg or 600 mg loading dose of clopidogrel at least 4 h before the procedure in those undergoing elective intervention, and those presenting with ACS whenever possible. In low- to intermediate-risk patients, clopidogrel pretreatment and a maintenance dose of aspirin and clopidogrel for at least one year after PCI are supported by the data, although the optimal duration of clopidogrel treatment beyond one year remains contested. It is reasonable to preload appropriately selected patients with clopidogrel prior to transfer for PCI at another facility, or if PCI is planned at a future time. If staged PCI is scheduled for a later date, clopidogrel 75 mg daily should be initiated least 3–5 days prior to the procedure, in order to achieve maximal inhibition of platelet aggregation. In addition, all patients undergoing *ad hoc* PCI and not at high risk for bleeding should receive at least a 300 mg loading dose just prior to stent deployment.

Pretreatment is not without risk, of course. For patients who undergo CABG surgery within 5 days after being treated with clopidogrel, there is an increased risk of bleeding, a greater need for transfusions, and an increased length of hospital stay [21]. Therefore, open-heart surgery should be delayed while clopidogrel is held for at least 5–7 days whenever possible in this circumstance. Only a fraction of patients who present with ACS will need urgent or emergent CABG; consequently clopidogrel bolus should rarely be withheld. The potential 'upstream' cardiac benefit outweighs the increased risk of bleeding should CABG become necessary.

In patients who have undergone PCI, clopidogrel 75 mg daily should be given for at least 1 month after bare-metal stent implantation, 3 months after sirolimus-eluting stent implantation, and 6 months after paclitaxel-eluting stent implantation, and ideally up to 12 months in patients not at high risk of bleeding [22]. In contrast to the number of investigations with different loading doses, no trials have been performed comparing different clopidogrel maintenance doses (>75 mg daily), although such trials are expected.

Given the cost of clopidogrel, patients frequently stop taking the pill regularly before the planned 12 months. Physicians must be mindful of this potential pitfall, as the risk of sub-acute stent thrombosis remains elevated through the first year. In addition, a cost analysis of the CREDO trial [23] suggested that clopidogrel loading before PCI followed by therapy for one year is cost-effective. Assuming that clopidogrel 75 mg costs $3.22, the incremental cost-effectiveness ratios based on Framingham data ranged from $3685 to $4353/ life year gained.

GLYCOPROTEIN IIB/IIIA INHIBITORS

Given the central role of platelets in atherothrombosis and the relatively incomplete platelet inhibition with aspirin and the thienopyridines, the development of drugs targeting the final pathway for platelet aggregation, the GP IIb/IIIa receptor, ensued. In primate animal studies [24], these agents markedly diminished thrombus formation and platelet aggregates in injured coronary arteries, paving the way for numerous, largely successful, clinical trials.

Abciximab (ReoPro™) is a chimeric mouse–human monoclonal antibody directed against the GP IIb/IIIa receptor; its mechanism of action is thought to be due to steric hindrance of the receptor [25]. It also inhibits the vitronectin ($\alpha_v\beta_3$) receptor, which mediates platelet coagulation as well as endothelial and vascular smooth muscle cell proliferation. While aciximab has a short plasma half-life, owing to its strong affinity to platelet receptors, it may occupy some receptors for weeks. In practice, platelet aggregation gradually returns to normal about 24 to 48 h after discontinuation of the drug, but low levels of GP IIb/IIIa receptor blockade are present for up to 15 days following completion of drug infusion.

Eptifibatide (Integrilin™) [25] is an intravenous cyclical heptapeptide that selectively blocks the platelet GP IIb/IIIa receptor. It reversibly binds to platelets, has a half-life of about 2.5 h and is renally cleared. Tirofiban [25] is a non-peptide small molecule inhibitor of the platelet GP IIb/IIIa receptor. In patients with severe renal impairment or on hemodialysis, the dosing should be cut in half. It has a serum half-life of about two hours.

GP IIb/IIIa antagonists are undeniably cardioprotective, both in the use of elective PCI and in patients presenting with ACS undergoing PCI [26]. In fact, starting with the first large clinical trial substantiating the efficacy of GP IIb/IIIa antagonists, the EPIC trial [27], which included 2099 patients undergoing high-risk angioplasty (acute MI within 12 h, UA and high-risk morphology), the benefit of these agents in subsequent trials has consistently been robust and durable.

Hemorrhagic complications were significantly increased by abciximab in the EPIC trial [28], however, raising concerns regarding the safety of these agents. Compared with placebo, the bolus and infusion of abciximab resulted in a doubling in the rates of major bleeding (7 vs 14%, p-value = 0.001) and red blood cell transfusions (7% vs 15%, p-value <0.001). Conjunctive heparin therapy appeared to have played a key role in the pathogenesis of bleeding among these patients. Heparin dosages in EPIC were not weight-adjusted [29], and a relationship was observed between the risk of bleeding and lighter body weight, total heparin dose and the intensity of anticoagulation as measured by peak ACT. Moreover, femoral artery vascular access sheaths had been left in place for the 12-h abciximab infusion, requiring ongoing heparin during that period.

The increased rates of bleeding complications were addressed in the subsequent EPILOG trial [30] in which weight adjustment of heparin dosage and a policy of early sheath removal eliminated the excess of bleeding complications with abciximab. In 2792 patients undergoing urgent or elective angioplasty, the 30-day rate of death, myocardial infarction or urgent revascularization was 5.2% with abciximab and low-dose heparin compared with 11.7% with placebo and standard-dose heparin. More recently, the EPISTENT [31] investigators demonstrated that the same primary endpoint was less common in patients undergoing stenting with abciximab–heparin (5.3%) than with balloon angioplasty plus abciximab–heparin (6.9%) or stenting plus placebo–heparin (10.8%).

In PURSUIT [32] and PRISM-PLUS [33], testing eptifibatide and tirofiban respectively, the majority of patients did not undergo percutaneous revascularization during their initial hospitalization. However, these patients still derived clinical benefit from receiving GP IIb/IIIa antagonists. In a meta-analysis [34] of PRISM-PLUS, PURSUIT and CAPTURE, a statistically significant absolute RR in death/MI of 1.4% was observed with GP IIb/IIIa inhibition during the period of pharmacologic therapy initiated 'upstream' before PCI. The absolute RR observed during the first 48 h after intervention was 3.1%, suggesting that a large portion of benefit attributed to GP IIb/IIIa inhibition was noted during PCI. As a result of these trials, eptifibatide or tirofiban may be used for the medical management of high-risk patients regardless of whether mechanical intervention is planned.

Abciximab has been shown to improve the results of the primary PCI in acute STEMI. Montalescot and colleagues [35], in the ADMIRAL trial, found that the use of abciximab given before stenting in patients with acute MI improved outcomes, resulting in better TIMI flow immediately following stenting and at 6 months, better recovery of left ventricular function at 6 months, and lower MACE at 30 days and 6 months. The benefit of peri-procedural abciximab was also observed in the recently completed CADILLAC trial, which evaluated the combined role of routine stent deployment and abciximab administration in the management of acute MI, achieving the lowest adverse event rates of any acute MI trial to date (30-day mortality 2.0%, MI 0.7%, TVR 3.3%, stroke 0.2%) [36]. CADILLAC, like ADMIRAL, found that abciximab was associated with fewer peri-procedural ischemic events, and reduced 30-day adverse events. This benefit was seen mostly in non-stented patients and the benefit was not as pronounced as in the ADMIRAL trial, which consisted of a higher risk patient cohort and gave abciximab 'upstream' from PCI.

Despite the evidence supporting 'upstream' GP IIb/IIIa inhibitor administration, in actual practice these agents are most commonly administered in the catheterization laboratory, immediately prior to proposed PCI. One deterrent may be the referring physician's reluctance to administer the drug owing to lack of familiarity. Another concern is that higher-risk patients might ultimately need emergent open-heart surgery. Early surgical experience with abciximab and other GP IIb/IIIa receptor antagonists suggested a tendency toward excessive bleeding in patients treated with these agents [37]. Fortunately, the percentage of patients who need CABG in the acute phase of MI is actually relatively modest. Nonetheless, in certain circumstances, such as failed PCI, sudden reocclusion, or cardiogenic shock, surgical revascularization may become necessary. Patients may safely undergo CABG within 2 h of discontinuation of eptifibatide. The PURSUIT investigators did not observe an increase in adverse clinical effects (including transfusions) with eptifibatide infusion in the immediate preoperative period; in fact a significant decrease in the incidence of peri-operative MI was noted [38]. Transfusion requirements are clearly higher for patients who undergo emergent CABG after having received abciximab [37]. However, the occurrence of in-hospital adverse cardiac events is comparable to patients who do not receive abciximab. Contemporary reports have not noted increased bleeding when incorporating exacting heparin management during cardiopulmonary bypass plus early platelet transfusion, if required [39]. Although the majority of GP IIb/IIIa trials largely incorporated higher-risk patients, the ESPRIT [40] trial collaborators sought to examine the benefit of eptifibatide in elective coronary stent placement. They randomized just over 2000 patients to a double-bolus eptifibatide regimen (two 180 mg/kg boluses 2 min apart, followed by a 2 mg/kg per min infusion for 18–24 h) vs placebo, and found that the patients receiving eptifibatide had a significant 37% reduction in the combined endpoint of death, MI or target vessel revascularization at 30 days. A recent systematic overview [41] of 19 randomized, placebo-controlled trials, including more than 20,000 patients, noted a significant reduction in all-cause mortality at 30 days and 6 months for those patients receiving GP IIb/IIIa antagonists. The relative RR was similar in patients with or without ACS.

Importantly, the only subset of patients who appear to derive no benefit from GP IIb/IIIa inhibition are those who need aortocoronary saphenous vein graft intervention. A pooled analysis [42] of five trials including 627 patients undergoing graft intervention did not observe a benefit in terms of adverse event reduction with routine administration of GP IIb/IIIa antagonist either at 30 days or at 6 months. Vein graft disease is mostly composed of friable plaque at specifically high risk for embolization [43], and platelet inhibition may be of secondary importance compared to routine application of distal protection. Instead, these interventions should be performed under cover of aggressive boluses of antithrombotic agents (i.e. UH for a target ACT >300 sec).

Is a GP IIb/IIIa antagonist otherwise necessary for all patients? The results of ISAR-SWEET17 challenge a strategy of routine administration of GP IIb/IIIa inhibitors, even in diabetic patients. Patients undergoing elective PCI who have been appropriately pretreated with aspirin and clopidogrel can probably be safely anticoagulated at time of procedure with just heparin or bivalirudin, utilizing provisional GP IIb/IIIa blockers as needed. Similarly, they should be considered in patients with higher-risk lesions (Type B or C), or if multiple PCIs in the same patient are anticipated. GP IIb/IIIa inhibitor administration is still recommended routinely for patients with UA/NSTEMI in whom a catheterization and PCI are planned and may be administered just before PCI, or 'upstream' in the emergency room or at the referring hospital. For patients presenting with acute MI, the largest experience lies with abciximab [44]; it should be used preferentially in this setting.

Few prospective randomized data are available testing the combined administration of LMWH and GP IIb/IIIa blockers. That LMWH does not activate platelets like UH may be a theoretical advantage and, as such, GP IIb/IIIa inhibition may be synergistically enhanced when combined with these agents. A Canadian study [45] randomized 200 patients to receive open-label enoxaparin (0.75 mg/kg intravenous bolus) or UH (60 U/kg intravenous bolus) and eptifibatide or tirofiban before elective PCI. The investigators noted similar levels of anticoagulation and platelet inhibition with enoxaparin and UH when concomitant therapy with eptifibatide or tirofiban was used with PCI, without an observed increase in early bleeding events or peri-procedural ischemic complications.

The GUSTO-IV [46] ACS trial provided preliminary evidence for the safety of combining LMWH with GP IIb/IIIa antagonists in UA/NSTEMI. In a prospectively defined substudy [47], 974 patients who received dalteparin were randomized to treatment either with 24 h of abciximab, 48 h of abciximab or placebo. In the trial as a whole, the incidence of bleeding complications was increased in patients receiving abciximab compared with those receiving placebo; however, the magnitude of this increase was similar in the subgroups receiving either dalteparin or UH, providing indirect evidence that the combination of abciximab and dalteparin does not increase risk for major bleeding compared with the combination of abciximab and UH. Although these data suggest relative safety for concomitant use of LMWH with GP IIb/IIIa inhibitors, one should not lose sight of the need for prospective randomized clinical trials that compare LMWH with UH in combination with these agents. Data on this question will be provided when the results of the NICE-5 Trial, a prospective randomized multicenter study of approximately 8000 patients presenting with ACS undergoing a planned invasive treatment strategy, become available. In this trial patients will be randomized to either UH or enoxaparin and will receive concomitant anti-platelet therapy with a GP IIb/IIIa inhibitor.

Similarly, few data exist on the use of combination therapy with thienopyridines and GP IIb/IIIa inhibitors in higher-risk patients with an ACS. However, a retrospective analysis of the multinational GRACE trial [48], which included 8081 patients with UA/NSTEMI, noted a significantly increased risk of major bleeding during hospitalization for patients receiving 'triple' antiplatelet therapy (aspirin + thienopyridine + GP IIb/IIIa) vs those receiving just aspirin and a thienopyridine. No difference was noted for in-hospital mortality. A trial designed to assess the value of abciximab in acute MI patients undergoing PCI after clopidogrel pretreatment (600 mg bolus >2 h before PCI) is currently underway, but completion of enrollment is not expected until August 2007.

11.3 ANTITHROMBOTIC THERAPY

UH

UH is the most widely used anticoagulant during PCI, and has served as the backbone anticoagulant for nearly 50 years. UH is a heterogeneous mixture of polysaccharide chains, ranging in size from 5000 to 40,000 Da that potentiate the ability of AT to inactivate thrombin (Factor IIa) and Factor Xa. Although UH is nearly universally utilized, it has several important pharmacokinetic and clinical limitations (Chapter 5). Particularly important limitations for an interventional cardiologist include UH's ability to paradoxically stimulate platelet aggregation, and inability to neutralize fibrin-bound thrombus. Also, platelet factor 4 binding may blunt its efficacy, and it confers a significant risk of HIT and/or HITTS [49].

UH administration should be carefully monitored, although the ideal level of anticoagulation, as determined by ACT, has yet to be consensually defined. According to the guidelines [22] for antithrombotic therapy in patients undergoing PCI recently published by ACC and AHA, target ACT values are 250–300 sec with the HemoTec (Medtronics, Minneapolis, Minn) device and 300–350 sec with the Hemachron (International Technidyne, Edison, NJ) device. A weight-adjusted initial bolus of 60–100 U/kg UH is recommended. When GP IIb/IIIa receptor antagonists are added, the target ACT is reduced to 200–250 sec with either device; the recommended initial bolus is 50–70 U/kg UH.

Weight-adjusted UH dosing became the standard after trials utilizing fixed-dose boluses of UH had inconsistent results. Most notably, the landmark EPIC trial observed that routine administration of higher-dose boluses (10,000 IU) of UH was associated with higher rates of hemorrhagic complications [28]. In contrast, several observational series using fixed low-dose UH have demonstrated relatively consistent efficacy and safety. Excellent angiographic success rates have been documented with fixed UH doses ranging from 1000 to 5000 IU with significantly reduced bleeding complication rates across broad patient populations including those with ACS [50–52]. Importantly, none of these series were randomized or controlled, but the results challenge the concept that high doses of UH are routinely necessary to achieve therapeutic benefit.

A meta-analysis [53] composed of pooled data from six randomized trials of varying anticoagulants suggested that an ACT of 300–375 sec was associated with the lowest risk of adverse ischemic events. However, the majority of these patients underwent balloon angioplasty only. A more recent analysis [54] of 2064 patients in the ESPRIT trial, all of whom received a stent, noted that an ACT target of 200–250 sec was safe and effective, regardless of whether or not an adjunctive IIb/IIIa was administered. Approximately 97% of ESPRIT patients received a thienopyridine, and the vast majority had a stent deployed, making these results particularly applicable to contemporary PCI. Thus, in contemporary practice, a target ACT of 200–250 sec may be sufficient, especially if the patient has been appropriately preloaded with clopidogrel. A more conservative UH bolus of 50–70 IU/kg is still advised whenever a GP IIb/IIIa inhibitor is concurrently administered.

LOW-MOLECULAR-WEIGHT HEPARIN

LMWHs are derived from UH through either chemical or enzymatic depolymerization, resulting in shorter molecules of about 4000–5000 Da. The LMWHs also bind AT via the same pentasaccharide sequence as UH, but only about 25–50% of the chains are long enough to do so. As such, the anticoagulant effect of LMWH is largely due to Factor Xa inhibition; the LMWHs have anti-Xa to anti-IIa ratios between 2:1 and 4:1 [55]. LMWH binds less strongly to protein, has enhanced and relatively predictable bioavailability, stimulates platelets to a lesser extent, and is more resistant to platelet factor 4 inhibition than UH. Furthermore, immune-mediated thrombocytopenia is rarely associated with short-term use of LMWH. The relative disadvantages of LMWH compared to UH include cost, lack of an easily interpretable and standardized point-of care-test and inability to rapidly reverse its anticoagulant effect. Protamine sulfate reverses only about 60% of LMWH's anti-Xa activity. An ever-growing body of evidence supports the use of LMWH during PCI, although concerns remain regarding bleeding complications.

Extensive data demonstrate that PCI can be performed safely and effectively under LMWH cover in ACS patients with and without GP IIb/IIIa inhibitors. In fact, the current ACC/AHA guidelines suggest that enoxaparin may be preferable (Class IIa) to UH [22]. However, many proceduralists continue to use LMWH reluctantly, in part because, until recently, the majority of trial evidence, including the results of ESSENCE [56] and TIMI-11B [57], had for the most part included patients who were managed conservatively. In contrast, the official guidelines had increasingly advocated an early invasive therapy, followed by rapid revascularization whenever applicable. Two large randomized trials were recently completed addressing the role of LMWH in ACS patients destined for an early invasive strategy; SYNERGY [58], comparing UH with enoxaparin for high-risk ACS patients undergoing an early invasive strategy, and the A branch of the A-to-Z [59], comparing UH and enoxaparin in the context of NSTEMI patients also treated with tirofiban. Whereas SYNERGY noted essentially no differences in outcomes with a statistically significant increase in TIMI major bleeding (9.1% vs 7.6%), the A to Z trial investigators reported a 1% absolute RR in the risk of death/MI/recurrent ischemia at 7 days with a statistically insignificant difference in bleeding with enoxaparin.

An accompanying large meta-analysis [60], incorporating the results of SYNERGY and A-to-Z along with four older trials, noted a 0.9% absolute reduction in the combined risk of death/MI at 30 days. This benefit was completely driven by a reduction in MI; the rate of death after 30 days was 3% for both enoxaparin and UH. While no significant difference in major bleeding was observed, minor bleeding was increased in the LMWH group.

There remains uncertainty regarding the choice of antithrombotic in the catheterization laboratory for patients who require PCI while on enoxaparin. In the ESSENCE [56] and TIMI-11B [57] trials, LMWH therapy was discontinued before catheterization, and interventional procedures were performed using UH. In both trials, patients receiving enoxaparin had rates of major hemorrhage similar to those seen in patients receiving UH. Perhaps as a result, many interventionalists became comfortable with a 'cross-over' strategy when anticoagulating their own patients. This may explain why, in the SYNERGY [58] trial, nearly 800 patients received postrandomization 'cross-over' therapy before PCI. Importantly, this group experienced a markedly elevated risk of adverse events; the risk of receiving a blood transfusion more than doubled (15.2% vs 31.5%) while the 30-day incidence of death/ MI increased from 13.9% to 18.5%. Thus, every attempt should be made to maintain ACS patients on the antithrombin agent initiated upstream when they undergo percutaneous revascularization.

GP IIb/IIIa inhibitors may be used as clinically indicated without concern for increased bleeding in patients receiving LMWH. The NICE-3 registry [61] specifically examined the safety of enoxaparin in conjunction with GP IIb/IIIa administration in 661 patients presenting with ACS with the specific GP IIb/IIIa used left to the discretion of the operator. If enoxaparin had been given within the prior 8 h, no additional LMWH was administered. If a dose had been given more than 8 h earlier, an additional 0.3 mg/kg intravenously was prescribed. For those patients undergoing PCI, the researchers reported an observed primary endpoint (major bleeding) of 1%, which compared favorably to historical controls. Event rates for transfusion, minor bleeding or death/MI in PCI patients were not reported.

Collet *et al.* [62] evaluated the strategy for transition to PCI in 451 'real-world' patients with UA/NSTEMI receiving enoxaparin (1 mg/kg SC twice daily). Coronary angiography and *ad hoc* PCI were performed after 48 h of LMWH therapy and were performed within 8 h of the morning dose. No additional LMWH or UFH was administered at the time of PCI, and vascular access sheaths were routinely removed 10 h after the last LMWH injection. Ultimately only 132 patients underwent PCI. However, in this subset, there were no in-hospital adverse peri-procedural events. At 30 days, the incidence of death/MI and major bleeding in those patients who underwent PCI was 3% and 0.8% respectively, compared to 6.2% and 1.3% in those patients treated medically. These data compare favorably with the results of other landmark randomized trials, thereby validating a strategy of taking patients with UA/NSTEMI who have received enoxaparin within the past 8 h to the catheterization laboratory and performing PCI if needed without additional anticoagulation.

The role of LMWH in elective PCI is still evolving, although support for its utilization is growing. In a large, randomized trial that compared LMWH and UH specifically during elective cardiac catheterization, 612 patients undergoing single-vessel PCI were randomly assigned to receive either reviparin (7000 IU intravenously followed by an 18- to 24-hour infusion) or UH (10,000 IU followed by an IV infusion) [63]. Reviparin was subsequently continued as a twice-daily SC injection for 28 days, with the UH-treated group receiving matching placebo injections. In reviparin-treated patients, the requirement for bailout intervention was significantly reduced (2.0% vs 6.9% with UFH treatment, p-value $= 0.003$), as was the occurrence of major ischemic complications during the first few days of the trial. At 30 weeks, the composite endpoint of death, MI or need for repeat intervention was similar in both groups (33% for reviparin vs 32% for UH), as was the incidence of major hemorrhage (2.5% for reviparin vs 2.6% for UH).

One study examined the efficacy and safety of a prespecified low dose of intravenous enoxaparin (0.5 mg/kg) in 242 patients undergoing elective PCI [64]. These patients were enrolled consecutively, regardless of age, weight, renal function or use of GP IIb/IIIa inhibitors (26%). Sheaths were pulled immediately after the procedure in those patients receiving only enoxaparin, and 4 h after the procedure in those also treated with eptifibatide. A consistent prespecified anticoagulation level was achieved, regardless of advanced age, renal failure, obesity and eptifibatide use. In addition, the incidence of bleeding complications was relatively low, as was the incidence of ischemic complications. While these results are reassuring, they probably need to be duplicated in a larger trial before widespread utilization can be recommended.

A recent meta-analysis [65] assessed efficacy and safety endpoints with intravenous LMWH compared with UH in patients undergoing PCI. The study included data from eight randomized trials in which patients received LMWH ($n = 1037$) or UH ($n = 978$) and data on LMWH from seven additional non-randomized studies/registries. The analysis of pooled data noted a trend towards improved efficacy (5.8% vs 7.6%) and reduced major bleeding (0.6% vs 1.8%) with LMWH compared with UH. Combined with the results presented from the STEEPLE [66] trial, which demonstrated significantly fewer bleeding complications with enoxaparin compared with UH in 3528 patients undergoing non-urgent PCI, it appears that LMWH is at least as safe and efficacious as UH for patients undergoing elective PCI.

In short, LMWHs have a more predictable anticoagulant effect than UH, and may be preferred in NSTEMI/UA patients. Factor Xa levels are effectively inhibited within 30 min and remain so for at least eight hours after injection of a single 1 mg/kg SC dose of enoxaparin. Therefore, in ACS patients who have received enoxaparin, PCI may be safely performed within this 8-hour window without additional dosing. If the procedure takes place within 8–12 h, an additional 0.3 mg/kg intravenous injection is advised. 'Cross-over' anticoagulation from UH to LMWH or vice versa should be avoided; the anticoagulant that the patient received prior to arriving in the catheterization laboratory should be continued. Elderly patients, or patients with impaired renal function, should preferably receive UH or bivalirudin.

BIVALIRUDIN

DTIs, namely hirudin and its analogues, have several theoretical advantages over heparin. These agents bind specifically and reversibly to both fibrin-bound and unbound thrombin, do not require a cofactor such as antithrombin III and have no known natural inhibitors, such as platelet factor 4 [67,68]. Bivalirudin (Angiox™, Angiomax™), a synthetic 20-amino acid peptide analogue of hirudin, has been approved in Europe for use as an anticoagulant in patients undergoing PCI. In the United States, bivalirudin is approved in patients undergoing PCI in conjunction with ASA administration, and has recently been approved for use with provisional GP IIb/IIIa inhibition.

Bivalirudin appears to be an attractive and, in certain populations, superior option to UH in PCI. The BAT trial [69] enrolled 4312 patients with UA/NSTEMI undergoing PCI to either bivalirudin or conventional dosing of UH. For the group receiving bivalirudin, a 22% relative RR in the primary composite endpoint, death, MI and repeat revascularization at 7 days, was noted in addition to a significant decrease in bleeding complications (3.5% vs 9.3%) compared to UH. The BAT trial, however, was completed before the widespread use of stents and GP IIb/IIIa antagonists.

The contemporary REPLACE-2 [70] study showed that bivalirudin plus provisional GP IIb/IIIa inhibition was non-inferior to heparin plus planned GP IIb/IIIa inhibition, and confirmed that bivalirudin was associated with a reduced risk of bleeding complications. Briefly, this large ($n = 6010$) randomized and well-controlled study noted that an anticoagulation strategy of bivalirudin (0.75 mg/kg bolus before PCI, then a 1.75 mg/kg per h infusion for the duration of PCI) and provisional GP IIb/IIIa inhibitor resulted in a numerically reduced incidence of the composite endpoint (death, MI, revascularization, major bleeding) when compared to UH (pre-PCI bolus 65 U/kg) and routine GP IIb/IIIa inhibition. The incidence of major bleeding, need for transfusion and thrombocytopenia was significantly lower in the bivalirudin cohort. All patients were treated with aspirin therapy, and more than 85% received pretreatment with a thienopyridine. A trend towards decreased death rates was observed in patients who received bivalirudin at 1 year follow-up.

Expanding the use of bivalirudin for patients with ACS as a feasible, seamless transition from medical to percutaneous management was recently demonstrated. The ACUITY trial [71] randomized 13,819 patients with moderate- to high-risk ACS to one of three arms: UFH or enoxaparin plus routine GP IIb/IIIa inhibition; bivalirudin plus routine GP IIb/IIIa inhibition; or bivalirudin alone, with GP IIb/IIIa inhibition only given as bailout (in this arm, around 7% of patients actually received a bailout GP IIb/IIIa inhibitor). Bivalirudin was associated with significantly less bleeding (3.0% vs 5.7%, p-value <0.001) and a similar rate of ischemic events (7.8% vs 7.3%, p-value $= 0.32$) as a combination of heparin or enoxaparin plus a GP IIb/IIIa inhibitor. However, bivalirudin plus a GP IIb/IIIa inhibitor failed to show superiority over heparin/enoxaparin plus a GP IIb/IIIa inhibitor, primarily resulting from attenuation of the benefit in bleeding complications seen with bivalirudin alone [72].

Bivalirudin may be particularly beneficial in higher-risk populations, specifically women, elderly patients (>65 years) and patients with renal impairment (serum creatinine >1.2 mg/dL) [73]. It should therefore be considered preferentially as an alternative to heparin plus planned GP IIb/IIIa inhibition in any patient undergoing urgent or elective PCI, especially in any patient with a high risk of bleeding complications. In addition, bivalirudin may be the anticoagulant of choice in patients with a history of HIT/HITTS [74]. Up to 5% of patients given heparin experience HIT/HITTS, the development of which is associated with a dramatic increase in morbidity and mortality. The ATBAT trial [75] evaluated the safety and efficacy of direct thrombin inhibition with bivalirudin during PCI in patients with HIT or HITTS. Over four years, this multicenter trial recruited 52 patients; the investigators reported a low incidence of major (one patient) and minor (seven patients) bleeding complications. None of the patients developed thrombocytopenia. In December 2005 the FDA approved the use of bivalirudin in patients with or at risk of HIT/HITTS undergoing PCI.

Bivalirudin demonstrates linear pharmacokinetics, allowing for a direct correlation between dose and anticoagulation activity. The drug is cleared through a combination of proteolytic cleavage and renal elimination. Bivalirudin is dialyzable; approximately 25% is cleared by hemodialysis. Accordingly, dosage adjustments are recommended in patients with moderate to severe renal impairment and in dialysis-dependent patients [73].

11.4 SPECIAL POPULATIONS

WOMEN

Even though more women than men die every year from coronary heart disease, women tend to be referred less frequently for diagnostic cardiac catheterization [76,77]. As a result, only about one-third of the 1.2 million PCIs completed annually in the United States are done in women [76]. Even more disturbingly, women tend to have higher rates of complications and in-hospital mortality after both elective and emergent PCI, although much of this difference is attributable to higher risk clinical characteristics [78–80]. Beyond the acute hospitalization, adjusted long-term mortality rates after PCI are similar for women and men [81,82].

Compared to men, women have a two- to four-fold increased risk of vascular complications such as arteriotomy associated hematomas, blood transfusion and retroperitoneal bleeds [83]. Many proceduralists are acutely aware of this discrepancy, and attempt to reduce this risk by whatever means possible. In an effort to balance risk, female patients will frequently receive relatively modest doses of peri-procedural anticoagulation.

The ACC/AHA guidelines [22] advise that lower doses of UH should be used in patients undergoing PCI at high risk of bleeding, including women and older adults. More conservative dosing is particularly recommended when combined with GP IIb/IIIa inhibitors.

Although LMWH and UH have not been formally compared in an exclusively female population, about 30% of the patients enrolled in the SYNERGY [58] and A-to-Z [59] acute coronary syndrome trials were female. Again, neither study noted a significant benefit for either therapy in either men or women, but LMWH was associated with a small increase in risk of bleeding.

Similarly, the safety and efficacy of bivalirudin have not been evaluated in an exclusively female cohort, but about 26% of the patients in the REPLACE-2 [70] trial were women. The incidence of peri-procedural ischemic complications was similar in both arms, but bivalirudin was associated with a significant reduction in major bleeding complications. These findings were substantiated in women, in whom major and minor bleeding was significantly reduced (p-value <0.0001) from 34.1% with UFH plus GP IIb/IIIa inhibitor to 19.7% with bivalirudin.

There exist no data that suggest antiplatelet therapy should be specifically modified for women undergoing PCI. The CREDO trial [13] ($n = 2116$, 29% women), which treated patients undergoing PCI with clopidogrel for up to one year noted a non-significant 32% relative RR in the combined endpoint of stroke, MI or death in women. In the ISAR-REACT trial [16] ($n = 2159$, 24% women), no additional benefit for the GP IIb/IIIa inhibitor abciximab was found for low-risk PCI patients pretreated with a 600 mg loading dose of clopidogrel. The combined endpoint, death, MI and target vessel revascularization at 30 days, did not differ between the two groups in either the entire cohort or specifically in the female subset.

GP IIb/IIIa inhibitor administration is clearly beneficial in women undergoing PCI. A meta-analysis of ten randomized placebo-controlled trials of GP IIb/IIIa inhibitors as peri-procedural antiplatelet therapy ($n = 13{,}166$, 26% women) noted a significant reduction in the combined endpoint of death or non-fatal MI six months after PCI [84]. Importantly higher risk patients, including elderly women, appeared to derive the greatest benefit [85,86]. Contrary to popular belief, GP IIb/IIIa inhibitors are not associated with an increase in major bleeding complications or vascular complications in women. They are associated with an increase in minor bleeding, however [85].

ELDERLY PATIENTS

Elderly patients require special consideration when administered anticoagulants because of age-related alterations in renal function, protein binding and increased bleeding and vascular complication risk [87]. Regrettably, elderly patients (age >75 years) are frequently excluded from enrollment in clinical trials so clinical data on this population is sparse. Procedure-related bleeding is common in these patients, which is at least partially due to the elevated prevalence of comorbidities such as uncontrolled hypertension, peripheral vascular disease and cerebrovascular disease. In addition, elderly patients are more likely to have significant left ventricular dysfunction, impaired renal function, increased lesion complexity and multivessel disease. Paradoxically, in an effort to prevent major bleeding, especially ICH, such patients frequently receive inadequate antiplatelet and antithrombotic dosing.

The most important limitation of anticoagulant dosing in elderly patients relates to renal impairment. UH can be used for such patients, although difficulties with dosing and monitoring often lead to supra-therapeutic levels of anticoagulation. LMWH has more predictable pharmacokinetics than conventional UH, but requires careful weight adjustments, especially with renal impairment. The small-molecule GP IIb/IIIa inhibitors (eptifibatide and tirofiban), together with bivalirudin, must also be adjusted for renal dysfunction.

The use of appropriate anticoagulant therapies should not be withheld in elderly patients at risk for ACS. Elderly patients with a moderate risk for ACS, defined as prior coronary disease or recurrent pain despite the use of anti-ischemic therapies, UH or enoxaparin should be treated with aspirin. In elderly patients with high-risk clinical features, such as dynamic electrocardiographic changes or positive cardiac biomarkers, GP IIb/IIIa inhibitors therapy should be added to aspirin and heparin [88].

PATIENTS WITH CHRONIC KIDNEY DISEASE

Patients with CKD are at increased risk of both thrombotic and bleeding complications [89,90]. Patients with CKD who undergo primary PCI in the setting of an acute MI are especially vulnerable; they incur a markedly increased risk of mortality, as well as acute reocclusion and major hemorrhage [91, 92]. Estimation of renal function is advised whenever prescribing antithrombotic or antiplatelet drugs to patients with renal dysfunction. Specifically, dose adjustment of many anticoagulants is indicated when the creatinine clearance falls below 30 mL/min. While dosing is usually appropriately made in patients with elevated serum creatinine, elderly patients, who, because of age-related renal dysfunction and smaller body mass index, often have reduced creatinine clearance may be inadvertently overlooked. Consequently, a creatinine clearance (or glomerular filtration rate) should be calculated routinely for every patient who presents for a catheterization laboratory procedure.

Generally, UH generally does not require dose adjustment in patients with CKD. Close monitoring of anticoagulation is recommended, however, because these patients are vulnerable to bleeding complications with higher levels of UH. LMWH, danaparoid sodium, hirudins and bivalirudin all undergo renal clearance. Lower doses and closer anticoagulation monitoring is advisable when these agents are used in patients with CKD. LMWHs are cleared almost exclusively via the kidneys [93]. The serum half-life of LMWH averages about 2–4 h after IV injection, and 3–6 h following SC injection [55]. The dosage of the subcutaneous LMWH enoxaparin in UA patients undergoing coronary angiogram and coronary angioplasty should be reduced by at least 50% of the standard dose (1 mg/kg per 12 h) in patients with severe CKD. A modestly sized ($n = 170$) single hospital pharmacokinetic study [94] attempted to adjust enoxaparin dosing in response to serum anti-Xa levels. After a bolus of enoxaparin 1 mg/kg subcutaneously, patients with a creatinine clearance of 30 to 60 mL received subsequent boluses of 0.75 mg/kg subcutaneously every 12 h, while those with a creatinine clearance of 30 mL/min or less received a 0.50 mg/kg per dose subcutaneously every 12 h. The investigators noted that about 80% of patients with moderate CKD and 60% of the patients with severe CKD were in the therapeutic anti-Xa range after the third dose. A dose-adjustment ratio {New dose = [(Current dose) × (Goal anti-Xa level)]/(Current anti-Xa level)} was used to adjust doses in patients whose levels were outside the therapeutic range. This formulation reliably placed patients in the therapeutic range established by consensus guidelines; the incidence of bleeding was noted to be equivalent to age-adjusted patients with normal renal function. Obviously, this cleverly designed protocol will need to be validated in larger studies, but the concept of pharmacokinetic-based adjustments in CKD seems reasonable.

Clinical trials that specifically address the efficacy of aspirin among patients with CKD undergoing PCI have not been performed. Aspirin is both hepatically metabolized and, to a lesser extent, renally excreted. Given aspirin's proven track record, however, it is difficult to advise adjusting the dose in patients with CKD. Importantly, ASA is significantly dialyzed. Post-dialysis dosing is recommended in patients acutely requiring consistent aspirin therapy (e.g. recent stent placement). Clopidogrel and ticlopidine are hepatically metabolized; dose adjustment is not required in patients with renal impairment

There exist few data supporting the efficacy and safety of GP IIb/IIIa inhibitors use in patients with significant renal failure [93]. The small-molecule agents (i.e. tirofiban and eptifibatide) are excreted predominantly via the kidneys, and randomized trials have largely excluded patients with CKD [25]. In contrast, abciximab, a monoclonal antibody fragment, undergoes almost no renal excretion and is eliminated through platelet degradation by the reticuloendothelial system [25]. In the EPIC [27] and EPISTENT [31] trials, abciximab therapy did not confer a significant bleeding risk on patients with mild renal dysfunction; however, safety data among patients with marked reductions in creatinine clearance are not available from these trials. A retrospective analysis of 4158 patients undergoing PCI at the Mayo Clinic did not note an association between abciximab administration, major bleeding and creatinine clearance on a multiplicative scale [95]. The researchers concluded that abciximab might be given safely in patients with CKD who are undergoing PCI.

Bivalirudin undergoes important renal excretion; dose adjustment is required in patients with moderate to severe CKD (creatinine clearance <30 mL/min) [73]. The half-life of bivalirudin is about 25 min in patients with normal renal function, about 34 min in those with moderate CKD and 57 min in those with severe CKD. Clinical support for the use of bivalirudin in patients with CKD may be derived from a retrospective analysis of the BAT trial [69] in which bivalirudin was compared with UH therapy among 4312 patients undergoing angioplasty. Nearly 75% of the enrolled patients had some degree of CKD. No matter the degree, bivalirudin-treated patients experienced both fewer bleeding complications and fewer ischemic complications than patients treated with UH. Considering the pathological derangements associated with renal impairment, including evidence of ongoing thrombin generation, a particular emphasis on direct thrombin inhibition seems justified in patients with CKD.

11.5 RECOMMENDATIONS

The choice of peri-procedural anticoagulation is, in part, dictated by the clinical scenario; elective PCI, UA/NSTEMI or STEMI. Irrespective of the clinical situation, the use of both antiplatelet and AT therapies remains central to management of these patients (Figure 11.1). Antiplatelet agents that are universally employed across the spectrum of CVDs include aspirin and clopidogrel. The GP IIb/IIIa inhibitors are reserved for those patients at intermediate and high risk undergoing PCI in addition to either UH or LMWH. The incremental benefit of concomitant GP IIb/IIIa inhibitors in patients already receiving bivalirudin is questionable with an attenuation of the beneficial effects with respect to hemorrhagic complications. Although theoretically beneficial, the use of 'triple' antiplatelet therapy may be minimally more beneficial than dual therapy albeit at an increased bleeding risk.

The AT agents currently utilized in the peri-procedural setting include UH, LMWH and bivalirudin. Important points to consider when selecting one of these agents include which agent was initiated prior to PCI (crossing over from UH to LMWH is not recommended), the use of concomitant GP IIb/IIIa inhibitors, the clinical condition for which the use of

Before procedure:

- Aspirin 81–325 mg once daily; first dose at least 2 hours before procedure*.
- Clopidogrel 75 mg once daily at least 3–5 days before the procedure**. A 600 mg oral bolus at least 2 hour before the procedure may be administered if PCI is planned on the same day.

During procedure:

- Heparin bolus to achieve activated clotting time (ACT) 250–300 seconds. Give 70–100 U/kg or 7000 U for women and 8000 U for men. If ACT target is not achieved give extra bolus of 2500–5000 U. When GP IIb/IIIa receptor antagonists are added, the target ACT is reduced to 200–250 seconds; the recommended initial bolus is 50–70 U/kg.***
- Bivalirudin may be substituted for UH or LMWH for low-risk patients and those with a history of HIT/HITTS. In addition, it should be considered preferentially in elderly patients (especially women), in patients with a history of renal failure, and in patients not adequately pretreated with clopidogrel.
- For intermediate and high-risk patients, high-risk stenosis, or multivessel PCI consider adding a GP IIb/IIIa receptor blocker·. If indicated, the bolus should be initiated at least 10 minutes before balloon inflation/stent deployment.

After procedure:

- Remove femoral sheath as soon as ACT falls below 150–180 seconds. Heparin infusions postprocedure should not be necessary for uncomplicated PCI.
- Bivalirudin may be discontinued at time of procedure completion.
- GP IIb/IIa inhibitor infusions conclude within 12–24 hours.
- ASA 325 mg daily for 1 month followed by 81 mg daily indefinitely.
- Clopidogrel 75 mg daily should be given for at least one month after bare-metal stent implantation, three months after sirolimus-eluting stent implantation, and six months after paclitaxel-eluting stent implantation. For patients not at high risk for bleeding, clopidogrel should ideally be continued for at least 12 months.§

*In the ACS setting the administration of 325 mg ASA is recommended
**Patients who are clopidogrel intolerant may be preloaded with ticlopidine 500 mg orally bid X 48 hours. For patients with ACS at high-risk of having surgical CAD, may reserve the administration of clopidogrel until anatomy is defined.
***Enoxaparin anticoagulation for elective PCI is not supported by evidence to date. However, this strategy preliminarily appears to be safe and effective; ongoing trials are pending.
·No significant benefit to "upstream" administration in patients with NSTE ACS
§Optimal duration of therapy unknown

Figure 11.1 Proposed Algorithm: Periprocedural Anticoagulation

anticoagulation is indicated and clinical characteristics, e.g. presence of CKD. Emerging data regarding the use of bivalirudin in ACS patients has brought this agent to the forefront in the management of these patients, given its effective and seamless delivery with a significant reduction in hemorrhagic complications. Nevertheless, more data regarding the efficacy and safety of bivalirudin is required before this agent can develop into the agent of choice for peri-procedural anticoagulation.

When pursuing PCI in the setting of an STEMI it is important to identify the goals of antithrombotic therapy, primary reperfusion or adjunctive therapy for primary PCI. With respect to antiplatelet therapies, aspirin remains a cornerstone. Aspirin should be given at a dose of 162–325 mg at initial evaluation and 75 to 162 mg/day indefinitely thereafter unless contraindications exist. Clopidogrel should be added to patients less than 75 years of age at the load dose of 300 mg with 75 mg daily doses thereafter. This dosing regimen may also be used as an alternative to aspirin in allergic patients. In patients older than 75 years of age, clopidogrel at 75 mg daily without a loading bolus should be employed. The GP IIb/IIIa inhibitors have also proven efficacious in this setting. UH remains the most widely utilized AT therapy for these patients, with the DTI bivalirudin reserved for patients with an STEMI.

11.6 CONCLUSIONS

While ASA and UH remain the stalwart and most widely used antiplatelet and antithrombotic therapies respectively, the armamentarium of newer agents continues to expand. The breadth of clinical data accumulated to date can seem frustrating to interpret, but a careful review will allow implementation of effective anticoagulation regimens in a wide array of patient subsets. As always, the relative potency of certain of these agents must be weighed against the possibility of systemic harm, most specifically major bleeding.

Given the central role of thrombin in both the pathogenesis of peri-procedural ischemic complications and ACS, there is persistent interest in the development and application of new antithrombotics that inhibit upstream targets in the coagulation cascade. One such agent, fondaparinux has been reported to be effective and safe in the management of patients with ACS undergoing PCI, while apparently reducing the incidence of bleeding [96]. Fondaparinux binds specifically to AT, allowing inhibition of factor Xa without interfering with other clotting factors, and is already established as an effective therapy in the prevention of asymptomatic and symptomatic venous thromboembolic events. Also, a number of oral direct factor Xa inhibitors as well as other oral DTIs are in clinical development for the prevention and treatment of thrombosis [97]. Whether these will lend themselves to peri-procedural anticoagulation remains to be seen. One such agent, DX-9065a, was shown to be effective and safe in smaller phase II clinical tests enrolling both stable angina and higher-risk patients [98]. Another agent, recombinant nematode anticoagulant protein c2 (rNAPc2) [99], a novel and potent inhibitor of the enzymatic complex composed of serum tissue factor and the serine protease factor VIIa (fVIIa/TF), is anticipated to be tested in ACS patients shortly. Hopefully, these agents will ultimately expand and improve current therapeutic strategies in reducing thrombotic complications during PCI.

Since the mid-1990s, there has been a remarkable increase in the clinical evaluation and therapeutic application of varied platelet inhibitor pharmaceuticals. Even now, several more drugs are being developed, aimed at inhibiting alternate platelet integrins and controlling different phases of platelet function such as platelet adhesion. The recent results of the four large trials of oral GP IIb/IIIa inhibitors portend a poor prognosis for this class. In fact, when the treatment arms from the four trials was analyzed together [100], a statistically significant increase in mortality was noted, making further development of other oral GP IIb/IIIa inhibitors extremely unlikely. Important lessons were learned from this experience, however, and will surely be applied towards the development of other agents.

Further research on peri-procedural pharmacotherapy will surely also reveal more on anti-inflammatory and hypolipidemic agents, specifically as to how pre-treatment with these drugs might attenuate both localized injury and systemic response to PCI. Beyond these exciting prospects, however, we should improve familiarity with the currently available therapeutic options. Regrettably, our focus and interest is too often on the correct application of transcatheter devices, and too little on appropriate pharmacology.

REFERENCES

[1] Antiplatelet Trialists' Collaboration, (1994) Collaborative overview of randomised trials of antiplatelet therapy - I: Prevention of death, myocardial infarction, and stroke by prolonged antiplatelet therapy in various categories of patients. *Br Med J*, 308:81–106.

[2] Schwartz, L., Bourassa, M.G., Lesperance, J., *et al.*, (1988) Aspirin and dipyridamole in the prevention of restenosis after percutaneous transluminal coronary angioplasty. *N Eng J Med*, 318(26):1714–19.

[3] Savage, M.P., Goldberg, S., Bove, A.A., *et al.*, (1995) Effect of thromboxane A_2 blockade on clinical outcome and restenosis after successful coronary angioplasty: Multi-hospital eastern Atlantic restenosis trial (M-HEART II). *Circulation*, 92:3194–200.

[4] Peters, R.J., Mehta, S.R., Fox, K.A., *et al.*, (2003) Effects of aspirin dose when used alone or in combination with clopidogrel in patients with acute coronary syndromes: observations from the Clopidogrel in Unstable angina to prevent Recurrent Events (CURE) study. *Circulation*, 108(14): 1682–7.

[5] Antithrombotic trialists' collaboration, (2002) Collaborative meta-analysis of randomised trials of antiplatelet therapy for prevention of death, myocardial infarction, and stroke in high risk patients. *Br Med J*, 324:71–86.

[6] Sagar, K.A., Smyth, M.R., (1999) A comparative bioavailability study of different aspirin formulations using on-line multidimensional chromatography. *J Pharm Biomed Anal*, 21:383–92.

[7] Eisenberg, M.J., Topol, E.J., (1996) Prehospital administration of aspirin in patients with unstable angina and acute myocardial infarction. *Arch Intern Med*, 156:1506–10.

[8] Hankey, G.J., Eikelboom, J.W., (2006) Aspirin resistance. *Lancet*, 367:606–17.

[9] Tantry, U.S., Bliden, K.P., Gurbel, P.A., (2005) Overestimation of platelet aspirin resistance detection by thrombelastograph platelet mapping and validation by conventional aggregometry using arachidonic acid stimulation. *J Am Coll Cardiol*, 46(9):1705–9.

[10] Kam, P.C., Nethery, C.M., (2003) The thienopyridine derivatives (platelet adenosine diphosphate receptor antagonists), pharmacology and clinical developments. *Anaesthesia*, 58(1): 28–35.

[11] Bhatt, D.L., Bertrand, M.E., Berger, P.B., *et al.*, (2002) Meta-analysis of randomized and registry comparisons of ticlopidine with clopidogrel after stenting. *J Am Coll Cardiol*, 39(1):9–14

[12] Hass, W.K., Easton, J.D., Adams, H.P. Jr, *et al.*, (1989) A randomized trial comparing ticlopidine hydrochloride with aspirin for the prevention of stroke in high-risk patients. *N Eng J Med*, 321:501–7.

[13] Steinhubl, S.R., Berger, P.B., Mann, J.T. 3rd, *et al.*, CREDO Investigators, (2002) Clopidogrel for the Reduction of Events During Observation. Early and sustained dual oral antiplatelet therapy following percutaneous coronary intervention: a randomized controlled trial. *JAMA*, 288(19):2411–20.

[14] Steinhubl, S.R., Darrah, S., Brennan, D., *et al.*, (2003) Optimal duration of pretreatment with clopidogrel prior to PCI: data from the CREDO trial. *Circulation*, 108:IV–374. Abstract.

[15] Patti, G., Colonna, G., Pasceri, V., *et al.*, (2005) Randomized trial of high loading dose of clopidogrel for reduction of periprocedural myocardial infarction in patients undergoing coronary intervention:results from the ARMYDA-2 (Antiplatelet therapy for Reduction of MYocardial Damage during Angioplasty) study. *Circulation*, 111(16):2099–106.

[16] Kandzari, D.E., Berger, P.B., Kastrati, A., *et al.*, (2004) Influence of treatment duration with a 600-mg dose of clopidogrel before percutaneous coronary revascularization. *J Am Coll Cardiol*, 44(11):2133–6.

[17] Mehilli, J., Kastrati, A., Schuhlen, H., *et al.*, (2004) Randomized clinical trial of abciximab in diabetic patients undergoing elective percutaneous coronary interventions after treatment with a high loading dose of clopidogrel. *Circulation*, 110(24):3627–35.

[18] von Beckerath, N., Taubert, D., Pogatsa-Murray, G., *et al.*, (2005) Absorption, metabolization, and antiplatelet effects of 300-, 600-, and 900-mg loading doses of clopidogrel: results of the ISAR-CHOICE (Intracoronary Stenting and Antithrombotic Regimen: Choose Between 3 High Oral Doses for Immediate Clopidogrel Effect) Trial. *Circulation*, 112(19): 2946–50.

[19] Mehta, S.R., Yusuf, S., Peters, R.J., *et al.*, (2001) Effects of pretreatment with clopidogrel and aspirin followed by long-term therapy in patients undergoing percutaneous coronary intervention: the PCI-CURE study. *Lancet*, 358(9281):527–33.

[20] Montalescot, G., on behalf of the Albion investigators, (2005) Assessment of the best loading dose of clopidogrel to blunt platelet activation, inflammation, and ongoing necrosis. Oral presentation EuroPCR Congress. May 24, 2005.

[21] Chu, M.W., Wilson, S.R., Novick, R.J., Stitt LW, Quantz MA, (2004) Does clopidogrel increase blood loss following coronary artery bypass surgery? *Ann Thor Surg*, 78(5):1536–41.

[22] Smith, S.C. Jr, Feldman, T.E., Hirshfeld, J.W. Jr, Jacobs AK, Kern MJ, King BS 3rd, *et al.*, (2006) ACC/AHA/SCAI 2005 guideline update for percutaneous coronary intervention: a report of the American College of Cardiology/American Heart Association Task Force on Practice Guidelines (ACC/AHA/SCAI Writing Committee to Update 2001 Guidelines for Percutaneous Coronary Intervention). *Circulation*, 113(7):e166–286.

[23] Beinart, S.C., Kolm, P., Veledar, E., Zhang, Z., Mahoney EM., Bouin, O., *et al.*, (2005) Long-term cost effectiveness of early and sustained dual oral antiplatelet therapy with clopidogrel given for up to one year after percutaneous coronary intervention: Results from the clopidogrel for the reduction of events during observation (CREDO) trial. *J Am Coll Cardiol*, 46:761–9.

[24] Rote, W.E., Nedelman, M.A., Mu, D.X., *et al.*, (1994) Chimeric 7E3 prevents carotid artery thrombosis in cynomolgus monkeys. *Stroke*, 25(6):1223–32.

[25] Kleiman, N.S., (1999) Pharmokinetics and pharmacodynamics of glycoprotein IIb/IIIa inhibitors. *Am Heart J*, 138:S263–75.

[26] Topol, E.J., Byzova, T.V., Plow, E.F., (1999) Platelet GPIIb-IIIa blockers. *Lancet*, 353:227–31.

[27] The EPIC investigators, (1994) Use of a monoclonal antibody directed against the platelet glycoprotein IIb/IIIa receptor in high-risk coronary angioplasty. *N Eng J Med*, 330(14):956–61.

[28] Aguirre, F.V., Topol, E.J., Ferguson, J.J., *et al.*, (1995) Bleeding complications with the chimeric antibody to platelet glycoprotein IIb/IIIa integrin in patients undergoing percutaneous coronary intervention. *Circulation*, 91:2882–90.

[29] Moliterno, D.J., Califf, R.M., Aguirre, F.V., *et al.*, (1995) Effect of platelet glycoprotein IIb/IIIa integrin blockade on activated clotting time during percutaneous transluminal coronary angioplasty or directional atherectomy (the EPIC trial). Evaluation of c7E3 Fab in the Prevention of Ischemic Complications trial. *Am J Cardiol*, 75(8):559–62.

[30] The EPILOG investigators, (1997) Platelet glycoprotein IIb/IIIa blockade with abciximab with low-dose heparin during percutaneous coronary revascularization. *N Eng J Med*, 336:1689–96.

[31] The EPISTENT investigators, (1998) Randomised placebo-controlled and balloon-angioplasty-controlled trial to assess safety of coronary stenting with use of platelet glycoprotein IIb/IIIa blockade. *Lancet*, 352:87–92.

[32] The PURSUIT trial investigators, (1998) Inhibition of platelet glycoprotein IIb/IIIa with eptifibatide in patients with acute coronary syndromes. *N Eng J Med*, 339:436–43.

[33] The PRISM-PLUS study investigators, (1998) Inhibition of the platelet glycoprotein IIb/IIIa receptor with tirofiban in unstable angina and non-Q-wave myocardial infarction. *N Eng J Med*, 338:1488–97.

[34] Boersma, E., Akkerhuis, K.M., Theroux, P., *et al.*, (1999) Platelet glycoprotein IIb/IIIa receptor inhibition in non-ST-elevation acute coronary syndromes: early benefit during medical treatment only, with additional protection during percutaneous coronary intervention. *Circulation*, 100(20):2045–8.

[35] Montalescot, G., Barragan, P., Wittenberg, O., *et al.*, (2001) Platelet glycoprotein IIb/IIIa inhibition with coronary stenting for acute myocardial infarction. *N Eng J Med*, 344(25): 1895–903.

[36] Stone, G.W., Grines, C.L., Cox, D.A., *et al.*, (2002) Comparison of angioplasty with stenting, with or without abciximab, in acute myocardial infarction. *N Eng J Med*, 346(13): 957–66.

[37] Silvestry, S.C., Smith, P.K., (2000) Current status of cardiac surgery in the abciximab-treated patient. *Ann Thorac Surg*, 70(2 Suppl):S12–19.

[38] Dyke, C.M., Bhatia, D., Lorenz, T.J., *et al.*, (2000) Immediate coronary artery bypass surgery after platelet inhibition with eptifibatide: results from PURSUIT. Platelet Glycoprotein IIb/IIIa in Unstable Angina: Receptor Suppression Using Integrelin Therapy. *Ann Thorac Surg*., 70(3): 866–71.

[39] Singh, M., Nuttall, G.A., Ballman, K.V., *et al.*, (2001) Effect of abciximab on the outcome of emergency coronary artery bypass grafting after failed percutaneous coronary intervention. *Mayo Clin Proc*, 76(8):784–8.

[40] The ESPRIT investigators, (2002) Long-term efficacy of platelet glycoprotein IIb/IIIa integrin blockade with eptifibatide in coronary stent intervention. *JAMA*, 287(5):618–21.

[41] Karvouni, E., Katritsis, D.G., Ioannidis, J.P., (2003) Intravenous glycoprotein IIb/IIIa receptor antagonists reduce mortality after percutaneous coronary interventions. *J Am Coll Cardiol*, 41(1):26–32.

[42] Roffi, M., Mukherjee, D., Chew, D.P., *et al.*, (2002) Lack of benefit from intravenous platelet glycoprotein IIb/IIIa receptor inhibition as adjunctive treatment for percutaneous interventions of aortocoronary bypass grafts: a pooled analysis of five randomized clinical trials. *Circulation*, 106(24):3063–7.

[43] Topol, E.J., Yadav, J.S., (2000) Recognition of the importance of embolization in atherosclerotic vascular disease. *Circulation*, 101(5):570–80.

[44] Kandzari, D.E., Hasselblad, V., Tcheng, J.E., *et al.*, (2004) Improved clinical outcomes with abciximab therapy in acute myocardial infarction: a systematic overview of randomized clinical trials. *Am Heart J*, 147(3):457–62.

[45] Madan, M., Radhakrishnan, S., Reis, M., *et al.*, (2005) Comparison of enoxaparin versus heparin during elective percutaneous coronary intervention performed with either eptifibatide or tirofiban (the ACTION Trial). *Am J Cardiol*, 95(11):1295–301.

[46] The GUSTO IV-ACS investigators, (2001) Effect of glycoprotein IIb/IIIa receptor blocker abciximab on outcome in patients with acute coronary syndromes without early coronary revascularisation: the GUSTO IV-ACS randomised trial. *Lancet*, 357(9272):1915–24.

[47] James, S., Armstrong, P., Califf, R., *et al.*, (2002) Safety and efficacy of abciximab combined with dalteparin in treatment of acute coronary syndromes. *Eur Heart J*, 23(19):1538–45.

[48] Lim, M.J., Eagle, K.A., Gore, J.M., *et al.*, (2005) Treating patients with acute coronary syndromes with aggressive antiplatelet therapy (from the Global Registry of Acute Coronary Events). *Am J Cardiol*, 96(7):917–21.

[49] Hirsh, J., (1991) Heparin. *N Eng J Med*, 324:1565–74.

[50] Kaluski, E., Krakover, R., Cotter, C., *et al.*, (2000) Minimal heparinization in coronary angioplasty—how much heparin is really warranted? *Am J Cardiol*, 85(8):953–6.

[51] Denardo, S.J., Davis, K.E., Reid, P.R., Tcheng JE, (2003) Efficacy and safety of minimal dose (< or = 1,000 units) unfractionated heparin with abciximab in percutaneous coronary intervention. *Am J Cardiol*, 91(1):1–5.

[52] Denardo, S.J., Davis, K.E., Tcheng, J.E., (2005) Elective percutaneous coronary intervention using broad-spectrum antiplatelet therapy (eptifibatide, clopidogrel, and aspirin) alone, without scheduled unfractionated heparin or other antithrombin therapy. *Am Heart J*, 149(1):138–44.

[53] Chew, D.P., Bhatt, D.L., Lincoff, A.M., *et al.*, (2001) Defining the optimal activated clotting time during percutaneous coronary intervention: aggregate results from 6 randomized, controlled trials. *Circulation*, 103(7):961–6.

[54] Tolleson, T.R., O'Shea, J.C., Bittl, J.A., *et al.*, (2003) Relationship between heparin anticoagulation and clinical outcomes in coronary stent intervention: observations from the ESPRIT trial. *J Am Coll Cardiol*, 41(3):386–93.

[55] Hirsh, J., Levine, M., (1992) Low molecular weight heparin. *Blood*, 79:1–17.

[56] Goodman, S.G., Cohen, M., Bigonzi, F., *et al.*, (2000) Randomized trial of low molecular weight heparin (enoxaparin) versus unfractionated heparin for unstable coronary artery disease: one-year results of the ESSENCE Study. Efficacy and Safety of Subcutaneous Enoxaparin in Non-Q-Wave Coronary Events. *J Am Coll Cardiol*, 36(3):693–8.

[57] Antman, E.M., McCabe, C.H., Gurfinkel, E.P., *et al.*, (1999) Enoxaparin prevents death and cardiac ischemic events in unstable angina/non-Q-wave myocardial infarction. Results of the thrombolysis in myocardial infarction (TIMI) 11B trial. *Circulation*, 100(15):1593–601.

[58] Mahaffey, K.W., Cohen, M., Garg, J., *et al.*, (2005) High-risk patients with acute coronary syndromes treated with low-molecular-weight or unfractionated heparin: outcomes at 6 months and 1 year in the SYNERGY trial. *JAMA*, 294(20):2594–600.

[59] Blazing, M.A., de Lemos, J.A., White, H.D., *et al.*, (2004) Safety and efficacy of enoxaparin vs unfractionated heparin in patients with non-ST-segment elevation acute coronary syndromes who receive tirofiban and aspirin: a randomized controlled trial. *JAMA*, 292(1): 55–64.

[60] Petersen, J.L., Mahaffey, K.W., Hasselblad, V., *et al.*, (2004) Efficacy and bleeding complications among patients randomized to enoxaparin or unfractionated heparin for antithrombin therapy in non-ST-Segment elevation acute coronary syndromes: a systematic overview. *JAMA*, 292(1): 89–96.

[61] The NICE-3 investigators, (2003) Combining enoxaparin and glycoprotein IIb/IIIa antagonists for the treatment of acute coronary syndromes: final results of the National Investigators Collaborating on Enoxaparin-3 (NICE-3) study. *Am Heart J*, 146(4):628–34.

[62] Collet, J.P., Montalescot, G., Lison, L., *et al.*, (2001) Percutaneous coronary intervention after subcutaneous enoxaparin pretreatment in patients with unstable angina pectoris. *Circulation*, 103(5):658–63.

[63] Karsch, K.R., Preisack, M.B., Baildon, R., *et al.*, (1996) Low molecular weight heparin (reviparin) in percutaneous transluminal coronary angioplasty. Results of a randomized, double-blind, unfractionated heparin and placebo-controlled, multicenter trial (REDUCE trial). Reduction of Restenosis After PTCA, Early Administration of Reviparin in a Double-Blind Unfractionated Heparin and Placebo-Controlled Evaluation. *J Am Coll Cardiol*, 28(6): 1437–43.

[64] Choussat, R., Montalescot, G., Collet, J.P., *et al.*, (2002) A unique, low dose of intravenous enoxaparin in elective percutaneous coronary intervention. *J Am Coll Cardiol*, 40(11):1943–50.

[65] Borentain, M., Montalescot, G., Bouzamondo, A., *et al.*, (2005) Low-molecular-weight heparin vs. unfractionated heparin in percutaneous coronary intervention: a combined analysis. *Catheter Cardiovasc Interv*, 65(2):212–21.

[66] Montalescot, G., STEEPLE Investigators, (2005) Safety and efficacy of enoxaparin in elective percutaneous coronary intervention: an international randomized evaluation. Presentation: European Society of Cardiology Congress, Stockholm, September 2005.

[67] Weitz, J., (1996) Biologic rationale for the therapeutic role of specific antithrombins. *Coron Artery Dis*, 7:409–19.

[68] Weitz, J.L., (2002) Crowther M. Direct thrombin inhibitors. *Thromb Res*, 106:V275–84.

[69] Bittl, J.A., Chaitman, B.R., Feit, F., *et al.*, (2001) Bivalirudin versus heparin during coronary angioplasty for unstable or postinfarction angina: Final report reanalysis of the Bivalirudin Angioplasty Study. *Am Heart J*, 142(6):952–9.

[70] Lincoff, A.M., Bittl, J.A., Harrington, R.A., *et al.*, (2003) Bivalirudin and provisional glycoprotein IIb/IIIa blockade compared with heparin and planned glycoprotein IIb/IIIa blockade during percutaneous coronary intervention. The REPLACE-2 trial. *JAMA*, 289:853–63.

[71] Stone, G.W., Bertrand, M., Colombo, A., *et al.*, (2004) Acute Catheterization and Urgent Intervention Triage strategY (ACUITY) trial: study design and rationale. *Am Heart J*, 148(5):764–75.

[72] Stone, G.W., ACUITY Investigators, (2006) Acute catheterization and urgent intervention triage strategy (ACUITY) trial: preliminary results, in *American College of Cardiology Scientific Sessions*, March 2006, Atlanta, GA.

[73] White, C.M., (2005) Thrombin-directed inhibitors: pharmacology and clinical use. *Am Heart J*, 149(1 Suppl):S54–60.

[74] Dang, C.H., Durkalski, V.L., Nappi, J.M., (2006) Evaluation of treatment with direct thrombin inhibitors in patients with heparin-induced thrombocytopenia. *Pharmacotherapy*, 26(4):461–8.

[75] Mahaffey, K.W., Lewis, B.E., Wildermann N.M., *et al.*, (2003) The anticoagulant therapy with bivalirudin to assist in the performance of percutaneous coronary intervention in patients

with heparin-induced thrombocytopenia (ATBAT) study: main results. *J Invasive Cardiol*, 15(11):611–16.

[76] American Heart Association, (2004) Heart Disease and Stroke Statistics—2005 Update. American Heart Association, Dallas, TX.

[77] Ayanian, J.Z., Epstein, A.M., (1991) Differences in the use of procedures between men and women hospitalized for coronary disease. *N Eng J Med*, 325:221–5.

[78] Mehilli, J., Kastrati, A., Dirschinger, J., *et al.*, (2000) Differences in prognostic factors and outcomes between women and men undergoing coronary artery stenting. *JAMA*, 284:1799–1805.

[79] Watanabe, C.T., Maynard, C., Ritchie, J.L., (2001) Comparison of short-term outcomes following coronary artery stenting in men versus women. *Am J Cardiol*, 88:848–52.

[80] Mehilli, J., Kastrati, A., Dirschinger, J., *et al.*, (2002) Sex-based analysis of outcome in patients with acute myocardial infarction treated predominantly with percutaneous coronary intervention. *JAMA*, 287:210–15.

[81] Glaser, R., Herrmann, H.C., Murphy, S.A., *et al.*, (2002) Benefit of an early invasive management strategy in women with acute coronary syndromes. *JAMA*, 288:3124–9.

[82] Mueller, C., Neumann, F.J., Roskamm, H., *et al.*, (2002) Women do have an improved long-term outcome after non-ST-elevation acute coronary syndromes treated very early and predominantly with percutaneous coronary intervention: a prospective study in 1,450 consecutive patients. *J Am Coll Cardiol*, 40:245–50.

[83] Peterson, E.D., Lansky, A.J., Kramer, J., *et al.*, National cardiovascular network clinical investigators, (2001) Effect of gender on the outcomes of contemporary percutaneous coronary intervention. *Am J Cardiol*, 88:359–64.

[84] Kong, D.F., Califf, R.M., Miller, D.P., *et al.*, (1998) Clinical outcomes of therapeutic agents that block the platelet glycoprotein IIb/IIIa integrin in ischemic heart disease. *Circulation*, 98:2829–35.

[85] Cho, L., Topol, E.J., Balog, C., *et al.*, (2000) Clinical benefit of glycoprotein IIb/IIIa blockade with Abciximab is independent of gender: pooled analysis from EPIC, EPILOG and EPISTENT trials. Evaluation of 7E3 for the Prevention of Ischemic Complications. Evaluation in Percutaneous Transluminal Coronary Angioplasty to Improve Long-Term Outcome with Abciximab GP IIb/IIIa blockade. Evaluation of Platelet IIb/IIIa Inhibitor for Stent. *J Am Coll Cardiol*, 36:381–6.

[86] The ESPRIT investigators, (2002) Is glycoprotein IIb/IIIa antagonism as effective in women as in men following percutaneous coronary intervention? Lessons from the ESPRIT study. *J Am Coll Cardiol*, 40:1085–91.

[87] Billett, H.H., (2006) Antiplatelet agents and arterial thrombosis. *Clin Geriatr Med*, 22(1): 57–74, viii.

[88] Patel, M.R., Roe, M.T., (2002) Pharmacological treatment of elderly patients with acute coronary syndromes without persistent ST segment elevation. *Drugs Aging*, 19(9):633–46.

[89] Attallah, N., Yassine, L., Fisher, K., Yee, J., (2005) Risk of bleeding and restenosis among chronic kidney disease patients undergoing percutaneous coronary intervention. *Clin Nephrol*, 64(6):412–18.

[90] Wu, C., Hannan, E.L., Walford, G., *et al.*, (2006) A risk score to predict in-hospital mortality for percutaneous coronary interventions. *J Am Coll Cardiol*, 47(3):654–60.

[91] Han, J.H., Chandra, A., Mulgund, J., *et al.*, (2006) Chronic kidney disease in patients with non-ST-segment elevation acute coronary syndromes. *Am J Med*, 119(3):248–54.

[92] Collet, J.P., Montalescot, G., Agnelli, G., *et al.*, (2005) Non-ST-segment elevation acute coronary syndrome in patients with renal dysfunction: benefit of low-molecular-weight heparin alone or with glycoprotein IIb/IIIa inhibitors on outcomes. The Global Registry of Acute Coronary Events. *Eur Heart J*, 26(21):2285–93.

[93] Mosenkis, A., Berns, J.S., (2004) Use of low molecular weight heparins and glycoprotein IIb/IIIa inhibitors in patients with chronic kidney disease. *Semin Dial*, 17(5):411–15.

[94] Kruse, M.W., Lee, J.J., (2005) Retrospective evaluation of a pharmacokinetic program for adjusting enoxaparin in renal impairment. *Am Heart J*, 149(3):567.

[95] Best, P.J., Lennon, R., Gersh, B.J., *et al.*, (2003) Safety of abciximab in patients with chronic renal insufficiency who are undergoing percutaneous coronary interventions. *Am Heart J*, 146(2): 345–50.

[96] MICHELANGELO OASIS 5 Steering Committee, (2005) Design and rationale of the MICHELANGELO Organization to Assess Strategies in Acute Ischemic Syndromes (OASIS)-5 trial program evaluating fondaparinux, a synthetic factor Xa inhibitor, in patients with non-ST-segment elevation acute coronary syndromes. *Am Heart J*, 150(6):1107.

[97] Alexander, J.H., Singh, K.P., (2005) Inhibition of Factor Xa: a potential target for the development of new anticoagulants. *Am J Cardiovasc Drugs*, 5(5):279–90.

[98] XaNADU-1B investigators, (2006) Effect of the novel direct factor Xa inhibitor DX-9065a on thrombin generation and inhibition among patients with stable atherosclerotic coronary artery disease. *Thromb Res*, 117(4):439–46.

[99] Vlasuk, G.P., Bradbury, A., Lopez-Kinninger, L., *et al.*, (2003) Pharmacokinetics and anticoagulant properties of the factor VIIa-tissue factor inhibitor recombinant Nematode Anticoagulant Protein c2 following subcutaneous administration in man. Dependence on the stoichiometric binding to circulating factor X. *Thromb Haemost*, 90(5):803–12.

[100] Chew, D.P., Bhatt, D.L., Sapp, S., Topol EJ, (2001) Increased mortality with oral platelet glycoprotein IIb/IIIa antagonists: a meta-analysis of phase III multicenter randomized trials. *Circulation*, 103(2):201–6.

12 Venous Thromboembolic Disease

12.1 INTRODUCTION

VTE, including both DVT and PE, accounts for substantial morbidity and mortality. Despite significant advances in prevention and treatment, VTE is responsible for approximately 150,000 to 200,000 deaths per year in the United States alone [1]. It is important to emphasize that approximately 50% of the patients do not present any symptoms [2]. In addition, PE remains the most common preventable cause of hospital death, affecting patients across the spectrum of diseases and illness severity. Thus, it is imperative that optimal measures aimed at both the treatment and, more importantly, the prevention of VTE continue to be pursued and perfected.

Several variables need to be considered before optimal prevention and treatment of VTE can be implemented. These include the underlying clinical disease state, severity of illness, concomitant co-morbidities (i.e. chronic kidney disease, pregnancy, morbid obesity, etc.), and characteristics of the currently available antithrombotic agents. In addition, the optimal timing and duration of each antithrombotic agent for the purposes of prevention and treatment of VTE is essential. An understanding of these issues will better arm the clinician with ammunition to prevent and treat the formidable foe of VTE. This chapter will briefly review the risk factors associated with VTE and describe the available antithrombotic agents for prevention and treatment.

12.2 RISK OF VTE

That VTE is a multifactorial disease state is made evident by the associated numerous predisposing risk factors that have been identified (Table 12.1). With the majority of the data regarding the risk of VTE being accrued from the surgical literature, VTE has historically been viewed as a surgical complication. However, recent data suggest that VTE is equally prevalent in medical patients [3, 4]. Furthermore, a substantial proportion of ambulatory patients without major illness experience a venous thrombembolic event. This enhanced appreciation of the population at risk mandates scrutiny of risk factors for VTE to identify high-risk patients who could benefit from prophylaxis [5]. Although several factors, including major surgery, multiple trauma, hip fracture or lower extremity paralysis because of spinal cord injury, are individually sufficient to prompt VTE prophylaxis, risk factors are generally cumulative and additional factors such as previous VTE, increasing age, pregnancy, cardiac or respiratory failure, prolonged immobility, presence of central venous lines, estrogens and a wide variety of inherited and acquired hematological conditions contribute to the overall VTE risk [6].

Management Strategies in Antithrombotic Therapy Arman T. Askari, Adrian W. Messerli and A. Michael Lincoff

Table 12.1 Risk factors for VTE

Age >40 years [185]
History of VTE [150]
Surgery with >30 min anesthesia [61, 186]
Trauma [23, 187]
Prolonged immobilization [185]
Congestive heart failure [188–190]
Cancer [125, 126]
Acute medical illness [3, 191]
Stroke [192]
Pregnancy and the postpartum period [7]
Major orthopedic fracture [193–195]
Pelvis
Femur
Tibia
Obesity
Central venous catheters [196]
Estrogen therapy [197]
Selective estrogen receptor modulators [198]
Inflammatory bowel disease [199, 200]
Nephrotic syndrome [201]
The Thrombophilias (genetic and acquired) [202]
Factor V Leiden [203]
Prothrombin G20210A mutation [204]
Anticardiolipin antibody syndrome [205, 206]
Protein C deficiency [207]
Protein S deficiency [208]
AT III deficiency [209]

PREGNANCY

Thromboembolic disease is a rare, but important, complication of pregnancy that remains a leading non-obstetric cause of maternal death. The risk of VTE is five to six times higher during pregnancy and the puerperium [7]. Risk factors include age greater than 35, antiphospholipid antibodies, inherited thrombophilias, operative delivery, increased parity, obesity, mechanical heart valves and family history. The phenomenon is also partially explained by the increased resistance to activated protein C seen in the second and third trimesters [8]. Given the increased risk of VTE associated with pregnancy and the puerperium, an elevated vigilance and a lower threshold for initiating prophylaxis and, if needed, treatment, should be exercised.

SURGICAL PATIENTS

Patients undergoing surgical procedures can be divided into various risk categories for developing VTE (Table 12.2).

Low risk

Patients in this category are young (<40 years of age) with no additional risk factors for the development of VTE. These patients have a risk of developing a proximal DVT that is less than 1% and of developing a fatal PE of 0.002% without prophylaxis.

Table 12.2 Risk Categories for VTE. Modified from ref [210]

Risk category	Risk of VTE(%)		
	Calf vein thrombosis	Proximal vein thrombosis	Fatal pulmonary embolism
High Risk General surgery in patients >40 years with recent history of DVT or PE Extensive pelvic or abdominal surgery for malignant disease Major orthopedic surgery on lower limbs	40–80	10–20	1–5
Moderate Risk General surgery in patients >40 years lasting 30 min or more Non-major surgery in patients 40–60 years with no additional risk factors Immobilization with major medical illness, including stroke, cardiac disease, chronic respiratory disease, bowel disease, and malignancy	10–40	2–10	0.1–0.7
Low Risk Minor surgery in patients <40 years with no additional risk factors	2	0.4	0.002

Intermediate risk

Intermediate-risk patients are over the age of 40, will require general anesthesia for more than 30 min, and have one or more additional risk factors (Table 12.1). Without prophylaxis, their risk of proximal vein thrombosis is 2–10%, and their risk of fatal pulmonary embolism is 0.1–0.7%.

High risk

High-risk patients include those over the age of 40 who are having surgery for malignancy or an orthopedic procedure of the lower extremity lasting more than 30 min, and those who have an inhibitor deficiency state or other risk factors. The risk of proximal vein thrombosis and fatal PE in this group is 10–20% and 1.0–5.0%, respectively.

Patients undergoing orthopedic procedures comprise a particular group of patients at high risk for development of VTE. Asymptomatic DVT is common and occurs in a substantial proportion of patients without thromboprophylaxis [9]. Although the majority of these DVTs are clinically silent, several risk factors associated with orthopedic procedures, including persistent venous injury, stasis due to prolonged immobility, impairment of the endogenous fibrinolytic system and prolonged impairment of venous function, may contribute to thrombus propagation and the development of overt clinical symptoms [10–12]. Furthermore, the development of symptomatic VTE often occurs following hospital discharge [13]. Given the limitation in identifying patients who will develop VTE, thromboprophylaxis is currently recommended for all major orthopedic procedures.

HOSPITALIZATION

Hospitalization for reasons other than a venous thromboembolic event imparts a substantial risk for the development of VTE. For example, a review of residents of Olmstead County for the period from 1980 through 1990, revealed that the age- and sex-adjusted incidence of VTE was more than 130 times greater among hospitalized patients (960 per 10,000 person-years) than among community residents (7.1 per 10,000 person-years) [14]. Furthermore, approximately one-half of community-based VTE cases occur in patients who developed VTE while residing in a nursing home or within 90 days of hospital discharge [15]. The net result is that approximately 60% of all cases of VTE occur in recently institutionalized patients.

Although VTE is most often considered to be associated with recent surgery or trauma, 50–70% of symptomatic thromboembolic events [16] and 70–80% of fatal PEs [17, 18] occur in non-surgical patients. Understanding that VTE develops in a significant proportion of patients hospitalized with medical conditions, it is disconcerting to realize that these patients, unlike their surgical counterparts, do not uniformly receive VTE prophylaxis [19]. The problem of inadequate and omitted prophylaxis in hospitalized patients with medical illness appears to be widespread. A prospective registry of 5451 patients with ultrasound-confirmed DVT conducted at 183 United States hospitals revealed that 3894 (71%) had not received prophylaxis before they developed DVT [20]. Of these 3894 patients, 2295 (59%) were non-surgical, with the most common medical co-morbidities being hypertension (50%), immobility (34%), cancer (32%), previous DVT (22%) and neurological disease (22%). Given the important improvement in outcomes with primary preventive measures in this group of patients, this risk factor alone should strongly influence the use of prophylactic measures.

Patients recovering from multiple trauma compose a group of hospitalized patients at particularly high risk of developing VTE [21, 22]. Without prophylaxis these patients have a high risk of developing a DVT. In a prospective study of 443 major trauma patients not receiving any thromboprophylaxis who had undergone routine bilateral contrast venography, the rates of DVT and proximal DVT were 58% and 18%, respectively [23]. Ominously, dying from a PE is not uncommon in this patient cohort, as it represents the third leading cause of death in those surviving past the first day [24, 25]. Factors that are independently associated with the risk of VTE in this population include spinal cord injury, lower extremity or pelvic fracture, need for a surgical procedure, increasing age, femoral venous line insertion or major venous repair, prolonged immobility and longer duration of hospital stay [23, 26]. It is important to recognize the necessity of VTE prophylaxis in the patient population and individualized on a patient-by-patient basis.

12.3 PREVENTION OF VTE

The majority of the recommendations regarding thromboprophylaxis has been accrued in the surgical patient population and takes into consideration the risk of bleeding complications and the risk of VTE in the various surgical risk categories (Table 12.2). The heterogeneity of non-surgical populations and the lack of high-quality evidence to support specific thromboprophylactic measures has resulted in less uniform recommendations in this patient population. However, a meta-analysis of trials utilizing LMWH or UH for VTE prophylaxis alluded to the necessity and safety of these agents for this indication [27]. Ultimately, the goal of thromboprophylaxis should be one of primary prevention unless contraindicated.

TIMING OF PROPHYLAXIS

Issues pertaining to the initiation and duration of thromboprophylaxis particularly pertain to the peri-operative setting and remain somewhat controversial. The optimal timing of initiation and maintenance of thromboprophylaxis in medical patients remains largely unknown.

Initiation of prophylaxis

The optimal timing of initiation of thromboprophylactic measures depends on the clinical situation as well as on the specific antithrombotic agent utilized. Several characteristics of an ideal agent for this indication include its safety, efficacy, ease of administration, a lack of a need for monitoring and its cost-effectiveness. Although several classes of antithrombotic agents are currently available for thromboprophylaxis, the LMWHs have emerged as the class of antithrombotic agents that most closely approximates the above-stated characteristics and have evolved into the agents of choice for this indication.

Historically, thromboprophylaxis with UH was initiated 2 h prior to general surgery [28, 29]. With the development of LMWH, however, administration of these agents this early pre-operatively was associated with significant increases in bleeding complications [30, 31]. Fortunately, more-recent clinical trials of LMWH and of newer anticoagulants have provided information on the relationship between the timing of the first anticoagulant dose and the efficacy and safety of thromboprophylaxis after major (primarily orthopedic) surgery [32–35]. The data on the optimal timing of initiating prophylaxis come from limited direct randomized comparisons of different timing with the same anticoagulant [31], subgroup analysis of large studies with a single anticoagulant, indirect comparisons across studies in systematic reviews [36–39] and single randomized trials comparing different anticoagulants [31, 34, 35, 40–42].

Of the available LMWH agents, dalteparin and enoxaparin have the best, although limited, data regarding timing of initiation of thromboprophylaxis. In a direct comparison of the timing of initiation, pre-operative initiation of the same regimen of LMWH (dalteparin) increased major bleeding, without improved antithrombotic efficacy compared to the early post operative regimen [31]. In addition, trials comparing enoxaparin with placebo [32, 33] and comparing enoxaparin with warfarin [34, 35] helped to establish that the optimal timing of this LMWH for thromboprophylaxis appears to be 12 h or 12–24 h post-operatively.

Emerging data suggests that a synthetic factor Xa inhibitor, fondaparinux, may be more efficacious than the LMWH enoxaparin. Fondaparinux 2.5 mg, begun 6 h post-operatively is more effective and as safe as the currently approved regimens of enoxaparin begun either 12 h pre-operatively, or 12–4 h post-operatively, in patients undergoing major orthopedic surgery [40–45]. In a subgroup analysis of several large randomized trials, fondaparinux, 2.5 mg, begun <6 h post-operatively was associated with increased major bleeding, without improved efficacy [46]. The results of indirect comparisons also favor the use of a 6-h post-operative starting time for the first dose of fondaparinux [45, 46], while the single randomized trials comparing different anticoagulants performed to date are not helpful in establishing an optimal time for the first dose.

The aggregate clinical research evidence supports the following general conclusions about the relationship between the timing of the first anticoagulant dose and the efficacy and safety of prophylaxis:

- Pre-operative initiation is not required for good efficacy and, when begun within 2 h of surgery, increases major bleeding.
- Although the initiation of thromboprophylaxis early (within 4–6 h post-operatively) is more efficacious, it is associated with increased hemorrhagic complications.
- Initiation of fondaparinux at 6 h post-operatively is effective and not associated with increased major bleeding.
- Initiation of fondaparinux <6 h post-operatively increases major bleeding, without improved efficacy; thus, 6 h appears to be the threshold for early post-operative administration.
- Initiation of enoxaparin 12 to 24 h post-operatively, although more efficacious than oral warfarin, may be less effective than initiation of fondaparinux at 6 h, but further randomized trials comparing the same anticoagulant initiated at different times post-operatively (e.g. 6 h vs 12 h) are required to establish definitively the optimal timing of the first anticoagulant dose.

Duration of prophylaxis

Depending on the clinical situation, thromboprophylaxis is usually continued until the patient becomes fully ambulatory. Certain high-risk situations, such as surgery in cancer patients [47] and major orthopedic procedures [48–54], mandate the use of extended thromboprophylaxis for varying durations of time. In a double-blind, multicenter trial of 332 patients undergoing surgery for abdominal or pelvic cancer, enoxaparin (40 mg subcutaneously daily) administered for 21 days significantly decreased the incidence of VTE at 21 days (4.8% vs 12.0% with placebo, p-value $= 0.02$) and at 3 months (5.5% vs 13.8%, p-value $= 0.01$) without an increase in hemorrhagic complications [47].

The beneficial effect of prolonged thromboprophylaxis has been demonstrated following high-risk orthopedic procedures, with a longer duration of prophylaxis required following total hip replacement than following total knee replacement [49, 51]. Following total knee replacement, thromboprophylaxis with either warfarin or LMWH for 7–10 days appears to be sufficient without a significant benefit seen with more prolonged administration of these agents. On the other hand, trials of prolonged thromboprophylaxis with LMWH following hip replacement have demonstrated decreased rates of VTE at durations of 28 days [52], 35 days [48, 50, 54] and 42 days [49, 51] following surgery without an increased risk of bleeding complications.

PHARMACOLOGIC PROPHYLAXIS

Aspirin

Aspirin has demonstrated some efficacy in preventing VTE events when combined with other thromboprophylactic measures in patients undergoing surgery for hip fracture or elective hip or knee arthroplasty [55]. In this multinational trial of 13,356 patients undergoing surgery for hip fracture and 4088 patients undergoing elective arthroplasty, aspirin (160 mg/day for 35 days) reduced the risk of PE and DVT by at least one-third throughout a period of increased risk [55]. However, the inferior efficacy of aspirin alone compared with other means of VTE prophylaxis [56, 57], and the increased rates of hemorrhagic complications, [55] preclude the recommendation of aspirin for primary thromboprophylaxis.

UH

UH is indicated for prophylaxis of VTE. However, with the demonstration that LMWHs are easier to administer, do not require monitoring, are associated with fewer bleeding complications and impart a lower risk for developing HIT, these agents have become the antithrombotic of choice for this indication. Nevertheless, a role for UH remains.

Low-dose UH

Low dose UH is usually administered at a dose of 5000 U subcutaneously twice to three times daily. This regimen has been demonstrated to be effective for the prophylaxis of VTE peri-operatively in patients undergoing moderate-risk general surgery and in medical patients. A prospective randomized study found that low-dose UH decreased the incidence of venous thrombosis in patients undergoing a moderate risk surgical procedure from 16% to 4% and, more importantly, the risk of proximal DVT from 2.9% to 1.0% [58]. In a larger study of 4121 patients, low-dose UH decreased the incidence of fatal low-dose from 0.7 to 0.1% [59]. These data have been confirmed by meta-analyses that have demonstrated a reduction in all DVT, proximal DVT and PE, including fatal PE, with low-dose UH in the peri-operative setting [60, 61]. Although shown to be effective in patients undergoing elective hip surgery, it is less effective than warfarin, adjusted-dose UH [61] and LMWH [62].

The utility of low-dose UH for prophylaxis of VTE has also been demonstrated across a broad range of medical patients [63]. When administered to patients following MI, heart failure or central nervous system disorders including stroke, and to patients admitted to the medical intensive care unit, low-dose UH was associated with a decrease in venous thromboembolic events [64].

Benefits of this regimen for the prophylaxis of VTE include safety, low associated cost and ease of administration. Whereas minor bleeding events such as wound hematomas occur with slightly increased frequency, the incidence of major bleeding has not been seen with this regimen [61]. In addition, this regimen does not require monitoring of the level of anticoagulation.

Adjusted-dose UH

The concept of adjusted-dose UH for VTE prophylaxis entails administering SC doses to maintain the aPTT in the high normal range. Although this has been shown to be efficacious in patients following total hip arthroplasty, the benefit seen was not as great as that achieved with LMWH [65]. Furthermore, this method of VTE prophylaxis has failed to gain favor, as a result of its labor-intensive nature and the associated costs.

LMWH

LMWHs have been shown to be efficacious in the prophylaxis of VTE and a number of these agents are approved for this indication (Table 12.3). The attraction of LMWHs for VTE prophylaxis is that they can be administered once or twice daily at a constant dose without laboratory monitoring. In addition, a substantially lower risk of HIT with LMWH compared with UH has been suggested [66].

LMWHs have been evaluated for prophylaxis of VTE in several, primarily surgical, situations (Table 12.4). LMWHs have been shown to be as or more efficacious than UH for this indication. It should be noted, however, that comparison across trials of patients treated with LMWH prophylaxis is difficult owing to the variability of the dosing schedules used. Chapter 6 contains details regarding data on LMWH for prophylaxis of VTE.

Oral anticoagulation

The utility of oral anticoagulation for the prophylaxis of VTE has been primarily assessed in the orthopedic surgery literature. Warfarin was historically the primary agent utilized in the peri-operative setting and compared with mechanical thromboprophylaxis [67] or placebo, aspirin [68] or dextran [69], was an effective agent in reducing the incidence of VTE and its associated complications. However, more-recent data suggests that the LMWH class of agents is more effective at preventing VTE following orthopedic surgery [31, 70–72]. One trial demonstrated an absolute reduction in the incidence of VTE of 6% with peri-operative LMWH (31.4% vs 37.4% with warfarin) [70]. In addition, a randomized clinical trial comparing in-hospital LMWH with warfarin in patients undergoing total hip replacement revealed a decreased incidence of symptomatic VTE in the LMWH group [73].

VTE prophylaxis with warfarin can be commenced pre-operatively, at the time of surgery or in the early post-operative period. However, therapy started pre-operatively may be associated with excess bleeding whereas therapy started at the time of surgery or in the early post-operative period may not prevent small venous thrombi from forming during or soon after surgery, because the anticoagulant effect is not achieved until the third or fourth post-operative day [74]. In an attempt to address the limitations of warfarin therapy a 'two-step' method was developed to avoid bleeding complications while maintaining its efficacy in preventing VTE [69]. However, when further analyzed the 'two-step' warfarin protocol appeared to be no more effective than warfarin started the night before surgery in patients undergoing total knee replacement [75].

Given the limitations of warfarin administration, the need for monitoring, and the availability of more efficacious agents, the use of warfarin for the prophylaxis of VTE should be reserved for patients who have contraindications to the alternative agents (i.e. LMWH or Fondaparinux).

Table 12.3 Selected LMWHs

Generic name	Trade name	Manufacturer	Molecular weight (Da)	Xa:IIa	$t_{1/2}$ (after SC dosing)	FDA approved Indications
Ardeparin	Normiflo	Wyeth-Ayerst	6000	1.9	3–4 h	Yes DVT prophylaxis
Dalteparin	Fragmin, Fragmine, Fragmin P Forte	Pfizer	6000	2.7	3–5 h	Yes 3) Prophylaxis and treatment of DVT in patients undergoing hip replacement surgery, in patients undergoing abdominal surgery, and in medical patients with acute illness. 4) Prevention of ischemic complications in UA and NSTEMI
Enoxaparin	Lovenox, Clexane 40, Clexane Forte, Klexane	Aventis Pharmaceuticals	4200	3.8	4.5 h	Yes 5) Prophylaxis and treatment of DVT in patients undergoing hip or knee replacement surgery, in patients undergoing abdominal surgery, and in medical patients with acute illness 6) Inpatient treatment DVT with or without PE, when administered in conjunction with warfarin 7) Outpatient treatment of acute DVT without PE 8) Prophylaxis of ischemic complications of UA and NSTEMI when administered with aspirin
Nadroparin	Fraxiparine	Sanofi	4500	3.6	3–5 h	Not commercially available in US
Tinzaparin	Innohep or Logiparin	Pharmion Corporation	4500	1.9	3–4 h	Yes Treatment of DVT with or without PE (inpatient), when administered in conjunction with warfarin

DVT = deep vein thrombosis; FDA = food and drug administration; h = hour; NSTEMI = non-ST-segment elevation myocardial infarction; PE = pulmonary embolism. SC = subcutaneous; UA = UA; US = United States

Table 12.4 Advantages of LMWH and recommended doses for prevention of VTE

Indication	Advantages of LMWH	Recommended doses*
General surgery	At least as effective as low-dose UH but can be given once daily and cause fewer hematomas at injection site	Low Risk Dalteparin. 2500 U 1–2 h before surgery and qd after surgery Enoxaparin. 4000 U (40 mg) SC qd 12 h after surgery Tinzaparin. 3,500 U 2 h before surgery then qd after surgery Nadroparin. 3,100 U 2 h before surgery then qd after surgery High Risk Dalteparin. 5000 U 10–12 h before surgery then qd after surgery Enoxaparin. 40 mg SC qd
Orthopedic surgery	More effective than low-dose UH; more effective than warfarin in patients undergoing TKR; no monitoring required	Ardreparin. 50 U/kg bid starting 12–14 h after surgery Dalteparin. 5000 U 8–12 h before then once daily starting 12 h after surgery Enoxaparin. 3000 U (30 mg) bid starting 12–24 h after surgery or 4000 U (40 mg) qd starting 10–12 h before surgery Nadroparin. 40 U/kg starting 2 h before and qd after surgery for 3 days; the dose is then increased to 60 U/kg qd Tinzaparin. 50 U/kg 2 h before and qd after surgery or 75 U/kg qd starting 12–24 h after surgery
Acute spinal injury	Apparently effective whereas low-dose UH is not, and higher doses of UH cause excessive bleeding	Enoxaparin. 3000 U (30 mg) q12h
Multiple trauma	More effective than UH	Enoxaparin. 3000 U (30 mg) q12h
Medical conditions	As effective as low-dose UH but can be given once daily	Dalteparin. 5000 U qd Enoxaparin. 4000 U (40 mg) qd

*Doses are given in anti-factor Xa units
bid = twice daily; q12h = every 12 hours; qd = once daily; TKR = total knee replacement

Fondaparinux

Fondaparinux is a synthetic pentasaccharide that selectively binds to AT III, inducing a conformational change that increases anti-factor Xa activity without inhibiting thrombin. It has a favorable and predictable pharmacokinetic profile when administered subcutaneously, and a long half-life, allowing once-daily dosing. Fondaparinux lacks *in vitro* cross-reactivity with heparin-induced antibodies. Major phase III studies have demonstrated that SC fondaparinux sodium 2.5 mg given at least 6 h post-operatively resulted in a 56.4% reduction in the risk of VTE in patients undergoing hip fracture surgery [44], a 55.9% reduction in the risk of VTE in patients undergoing total hip replacement surgery [42] and a 55.2% reduction in the risk of VTE in patients undergoing knee replacement surgery [43] compared with standard enoxaparin (30 mg subcutaneously twice daily) therapy with a similar safety profile [37]. In addition, the use of fondaparinux for prolonged prophylaxis after hip fracture has demonstrated further reduction in VTE events without increasing the risk of bleeding [76]. Thus, fondaparinux is the first of a new class of synthetic factor Xa inhibitors that has demonstrated greater efficacy compared with enoxaparin for the prevention of VTE in major orthopedic surgery without an increase in clinically relevant bleeding. Given the favorable cost-effectiveness analyses [77–79] and improved efficacy profile, fondaparinux should be considered an alternative to warfarin and LMWH for DVT prophylaxis in patients undergoing hip and knee replacement surgery. In patients undergoing hip fracture surgery, fondaparinux should be considered the DVT prophylaxis of choice. Extended thromboprophylaxis up to 28 days resulted in additional reduction in VTE (both symptomatic and venography-proven DVT) in patients with hip fracture surgery. Fondaparinux was approved by the FDA for the prophylaxis of DVT in patients undergoing surgery for hip fracture, hip replacement or knee replacement in December 2001.

DTIs

The beneficial effects of recombinant hirudin (desirudin) for VTE prophylaxis has been demonstrated in patients undergoing total hip replacement. When administered 30 min prior to total hip replacement, desirudin (15 mg subcutaneously twice daily) decreased the relative risk of VTE by 28% compared with enoxaparin (40 mg subcutaneously once daily) initiated the evening prior to surgery [80]. This regimen offers the advantage that VTE prophylaxis may be given to patients in close proximity to their procedure without an increased risk of bleeding complications. Similar to the LMWH, this DTI enjoys the lack of a need to monitor dosing. Although approved for the prophylaxis of VTE by the European Union, parenteral DTIs are reserved for the management of patients with HIT in the United States.

The development of new anticoagulants has been pursued with the aim of finding more effective, safer and/or more convenient therapies. Thrombin is a central regulator in the coagulation and inflammation process and several DTIs with distinct pharmacological profiles, as well as pharmacological differences from the conventional anticoagulants, are currently in clinical use for certain indications or are under development. Two oral DTIs, ximelagatran and dabigatran etexilate, are in clinical development. Dabigatran etexilate has recently been evaluated in clinical trials of patients undergoing total hip replacement [81, 82]. Several trials have now demonstrated the efficacy and safety of ximelagatran in the prevention of VTE following total hip or knee replacement [83–87]. The attraction of ximelagatran is that it can be used with an oral fixed dose without the need for coagulation monitoring or dose adjustment. Hence, it offers significant potential to facilitate the management of anticoagulation in or out of hospital. Despite the safety and efficacy of the oral DTIs, these agents currently remain experimental within the United States.

Recommendations

The primary prophylactic measure employed depends on the risk category (Table 12.2) of the individual patient and the clinical situation. In general, LMWHs have become the antithrombotic agents of choice for the prevention of VTE. Effective alternative agents remain low-dose UH (5000 U subcutaneously every 8–12 h) and oral anticoagulation with warfarin (following major orthopedic surgery). The newer agent, fondaparinux, has demonstrated promise as an effective prophylactic agent, especially within the realm of management for patients with hip fractures. It should be noted that the specific recommendations outlined in Table 12.5 relate only to patients without contraindications to antithrombotic agents. In the case of contraindications to the use of antithrombotic agents the use of mechanical methods (i.e. pneumatic compression devices or graduated compression stockings) should be employed as indicated. An exhaustive list of recommendations is beyond the scope of this chapter and can be referenced in the seventh American College of Chest Physicians Consensus Conference on Antithrombotic Therapy [88].

12.4 TREATMENT OF VTE

Antithrombotic therapy remains the principal treatment for DVT and PE. The anticoagulant regimen used to treat these venous thromboembolic disorders has continued to evolve. Whereas therapy for both entities historically has been with IV UH simultaneously initiated with oral warfarin in an inpatient setting, the development of strategies aimed at reducing costs without sacrificing safety and efficacy has challenged this dogma. However, owing to the potential morbidity and mortality associated with PE, initial treatment is delivered in a closely monitored setting in all but the most stable cases. Integral to the move towards a less intensive approach to both DVT and PE has been the appearance of newer antithrombotic agents such as the LMWH class of anticoagulants (Chapter 6). The need for improving the efficacy of antithrombotic therapy for the treatment of VTE without increasing the risk of bleeding has fostered continued expansion of the available antithrombotic agents. In addition, the optimal duration of therapy continues to be elucidated for specific clinical conditions in order to decrease the risk of recurrent VTE while minimizing the risk of bleeding complications.

UH

The goals of treatment for DVT and PE are to stop clot propagation and prevent clot recurrence, recurrent PEs and a potential complication of recurrent PEs, pulmonary hypertension. Anticoagulant therapy is indicated for patients with proximal DVT since PE will occur within weeks in up to 50% of untreated patients [89, 90]. Anticoagulation is usually achieved with UH overlapped with oral warfarin in the early phase of treatment.

The experiences to date have established that the efficacy of UH rests in the ability to achieve therapeutic levels of anticoagulation, defined as an aPTT >1.5 times normal (range 1.5–2 × normal), within the first 24 h of treatment primarily via continuous IV infusion [91–95]. This point was strongly supported by an analysis of three consecutive randomized double-blind trials evaluating initial UH for treatment of proximal vein thrombosis that revealed a recurrent VTE rate of 23.3% in patients with a subtherapeutic aPTT compared with 4–6% in those whose aPTT exceeded the therapeutic threshold within 24 h [92].

Therapeutic anticoagulation has been shown to be achieved earlier and more successfully using protocol-based UH dosing rather than with physician-directed adjustment [96–98]. In a prospective randomized controlled trial of 115 patients with DVT, PE, UA or acute arterial insufficiency, the time to achieve therapeutic aPTT was significantly reduced with a weight-based nomogram (Table 12.6). Ninety-seven percent of patients receiving the weight-based dosing regimen had therapeutic aPTT levels (>1.5 × control) compared with 77% of those

Table 12.5 Recommendations for the prophylaxis of venous thromboembolic events

Indication	Primary agent	Recommended dose	Secondary agent	Recommended dose	Comment
Surgical patients					
Low-risk	NA	NA	NA	NA	Prophylaxis other than early ambulation usually not recommended
Intermediate-risk	LMWH	≤3400 anti-Xa U once daily	UH	5000 U SC bid	LMWH and UH equally efficacious bur LMWH associated with less bleeding Lower risk of HIT with LMWH Consider mechanical methods of prophylaxis for those at high risk of bleeding, at least until bleeding risk decreased
High-risk	LMWH	≥3400 anti-Xa U once daily	UH	5000 U SC tid	For those at higher risk, mechanical plus pharmacologic prophylaxis recommended Adjusted dose UH requires monitoring and is seldom used
Orthopedic Surgery					
Knee arthroplasty	LMWH	≥3400 anti-Xa U per day	Warfarin	Target INR 2.0–3.0	Prophylaxis should be continued for 7–10 days Fondaparinux a viable alternative at 2.5 mg SC daily beginning 6 h after surgery
Hip arthroplasty	LMWH	≥3400 anti-Xa U per day	Warfarin OR Fondaparinux	Target INR 2.0–3.0 2.5 mg SC daily	Start LMWH 12 h before or 12–24 h after surgery. May use half LMWH dose and start 4–6 h after surgery and increase the following day. Continue prophylaxis for at least 7–10 days. Prophylaxis for 27–42 days decreases DVT without increased risk of bleeding Start fondaparinux 6 h after surgery Start warfarin preoperatively or evening after surgery
HFS	Fondaparinux	2.5 mg SC daily	LMWH OR Warfarin	≥3400 anti-Xa U per day Target INR 2.0–3.0	Start fondaparinux 6 h after surgery. Continue prophylaxis for 28–35 days after surgery. Mechanical prophylaxis if high risk of bleeding

Table 12.5 *(Continued)*

Indication	Primary agent	Recommended dose	Secondary agent	Recommended dose	Comment
Multiple Trauma	LMWH	Enoxaparin 30 mg SC bid	NA	NA	Initiated once active bleeding issues controlled Continue until hospital discharge If prolonged immobility or ongoing risk >2 weeks, continue LMWH or switch to warfarin (INR 2.0–3.0)
ASCI	LMWH	Enoxaparin 30 mg SC bid	NA	NA	Initiated once active bleeding issues controlled Continue until hospital discharge During rehabilitation continue LMWH or switch to warfarin (INR 2.0–3.0)
Medical patients	LMWH	Enoxaparin 40 mg SC daily OR Dalteparin 5000 U SC daily	UH	5000 U SC tid	In acutely ill medical patients with: congestive heart failure, severe respiratory disease, or who are confined to bed and have one or more additional risk factors, including active cancer, previous VTE, sepsis, acute neurologic disease, or inflammatory bowel disease LMWH and UH equally efficacious
nPregnancy	LDUH	5000 U SC bid	LMWH	≥3400 anti-Xa U per day	For pregnant women at intermediate risk of VTE

ASCI = acute spinal cord injury; bid = twice daily; HFS = hip fracture surgery; LDUH = low dose UH; NA = not applicable; tid = three times daily

Table 12.6 A weight-based dosing nomogram for VTE. Adapted from Raschke *et al.* [98]

aPTT	UH dose
Initial dose	80 U/kg bolus, then 18 U/kg per h
<35 s	80 U/kg bolus, then increase by 4 U/kg per h
35–45 s	40 U/kg bolus, then increase by 2 U/kg per h
46–70 s	Therapeutic range *
71–90 s	Decrease infusion by 2 U/kg per h
>90 s	Hold infusion × 1 h, then decrease infusion by 3 U/kg per h

* The therapeutic range should be assessed at every institution by correlation with anti-factor Xa levels between 0.3 and 0.7 U/mL

receiving the standard dosing regimen [98]. This translated into a significantly decreased risk of recurrent VTE among the patients with DVT or PE without an increased risk of bleeding.

For patients with submassive DVT or PE, the administration of UH for 5 days appears to be equivalent in efficacy and safety to 10 days of therapy. A randomized double-blind trial of 199 patients with documented acute proximal DVT compared a 5-day course of IV UH, with warfarin begun on the first day with a conventional 10-day course of IV UH, with warfarin begun on the fifth day. There was no significant difference in the risk of recurrent VTE between the two groups [99]. The adherence to the shorter duration of therapy can facilitate more expeditious anticoagulation and shorten hospitalization times, and cost, without increased adverse event rates.

LMWH

Given the advantageous pharmacologic profile of LMWH, once or twice daily dosing without the need for monitoring, the attraction for using these agents for the treatment of VTE is quite apparent. Numerous trials have demonstrated the safety and efficacy of LMWH for the treatment of VTE. Based on these safety and efficacy trials, four LMWH preparations have received FDA approval for this indication (Table 12.3). LMWH may facilitate outpatient therapy for patients with uncomplicated DVT [100, 101]. LMWHs have also demonstrated utility for use as long-term therapy in elderly patients [102, 103], in patients with cancer [104] and in patients with recurrent VTE despite therapy with warfarin [105, 106].

Residual thrombus imparts a substantial hazard for the recurrence of VTE [107]. Thus, an increased likelihood of facilitating thrombus regression and preventing recurrent thromboembolism in patients with documented DVT would be beneficial and has been shown with the LMWH reviparin compared with IV UH [108].

With a high degree of consistency, several LMWH preparations have shown efficacy for the initial treatment of DVT [109–112]. These trials, comparing LMWH with UH for the treatment of DVT, have demonstrated similar efficacy of LMWH and UH with comparable rates of hemorrhagic complications. In addition, a recent meta-analysis suggested that LMWHs are associated with an improvement in mortality [113].

These agents appear to be cost-effective when utilized as initial therapy for DVT, and become cost-saving even if only a minority of patients are treated in the outpatient setting [114]. The ease of administration of LMWH make the outpatient management of patients with uncomplicated DVT feasible and effective as an initial therapy until warfarin is at a therapeutic level. This approach results in both an improved quality of life and patient satisfaction, and may also result in a substantial cost saving to the healthcare system [114, 115].

Long-term therapy for the treatment of DVT with LMWH also appears to be efficacious and safe. Although therapy with warfarin has traditionally been utilized, the need for monitoring and dose adjustments as well as treatment failures with warfarin have made LMWHs an attractive alternative. One study demonstrated that LMWH is highly effective and safe when used as long-term therapy for secondary prevention in selected prothrombotic disorders in a series of patients with conditions associated with prior warfarin failure or potential resistance to warfarin therapy (antiphospholipid syndrome) [106]. The feasibility and safety of LMWH for long-term treatment of DVT has also been seen in patients with cancer [105, 116–118] as well as in elderly patients [102]. Thus, LMWH offer a viable alternative with potential cost savings to traditional management of DVT.

Owing to the potential morbidity and mortality associated with PE, initial treatment is delivered in a closely monitored setting. However, similar to one of the benefits of LMWH in patients with DVT, the outpatient treatment of select patients with PE is made feasible with LMWH [119]. Until further data support this initial study, the outpatient treatment of PE can not be advocated.

LMWHs have recently been shown to be as effective as UH for the initial treatment of PE [120–122]. One study randomly assigned 1021 patients with symptomatic DVT, low-dose or both to treatment with fixed-dose, twice daily, SC reviparin, or adjusted-dose, IV UH [122]. Low-dose was present in approximately one-third of patients, and all patients started therapy with an oral coumarin derivative on the first hospital day. No significant differences in recurrent thromboembolic events, major bleeding or mortality were found between the two treatment groups. Two additional studies demonstrated that the LMWH tinzaparin was equivalent to UH in patients with symptomatic and submassive PE [120, 121]. Although one meta-analysis suggested a mortality benefit with LMWH compared to UH in patients with a PE [123], the superiority of LMWH has not been demonstrated in prospective randomized trials.

FONDAPARINUX

The efficacy and safety of the synthetic antithrombotic agent fondaparinux was compared with UH in a recent randomized open-label non-inferiority trial involving 2213 patients with acute symptomatic PE [124]. Patients received either fondaparinux (weight-adjusted subcutaneously once daily) or a continuous IV infusion of UH (activated partial-thromboplastin time $1.5-2.5\times$ control), both given for at least five days and until the use of vitamin K antagonists resulted in an international normalized ratio above 2.0. With respect to the primary efficacy outcome (symptomatic, recurrent low-dose (non-fatal or fatal) and new or recurrent DVT at 3 months) fondaparinux was found to be at least as effective and as safe as UH in the initial treatment of hemodynamically stable patients with PE. The possibility of the outpatient use of this agent was alluded to as 14.5% of patients in the fondaparinux group received the drug in part on an outpatient basis. Despite these encouraging results, the use of fondaparinux for the treatment of PE is not recommended until its efficacy and safety in a broader range of patients has been demonstrated.

DTIs

Although these agents provide a viable alternative to UH and LMWH for the treatment of VTE, they are currently not FDA approved for this purpose outside of treatment of patients with HIT complicated by thrombosis. Therefore, the reader is referred to Chapter 13, which deals specifically with HIT.

ORAL ANTICOAGULANT THERAPY

Patients with VTE require long-term anticoagulant treatment to prevent a high frequency of symptomatic extension of thrombosis and/or recurrent venous thromboembolic events. Treatment with a vitamin K antagonist (VKA) such as warfarin is the current preferred approach unless contraindicated (e.g. pregnancy) or indications for which an alternative agent such as LMWH have proved safer and more efficacious (e.g. cancer patients with VTE) [104, 117, 125, 126]. Issues regarding the use of oral anticoagulants such as warfarin pertain to its intrinsic limitations, including the need for laboratory monitoring and dose adjustments due to wide interpatient variation in the anticoagulant response, and the influence of drug interactions and diet on the anticoagulant effect of VKA. Furthermore, the intensity of the anticoagulant effect and the duration of anticoagulant therapy with a VKA remain important issues that are handled on a patient-by-patient basis. Nevertheless, data addressing these issues continue to accrue and assist the clinician in more optimally managing patients with VTE.

The anticoagulant effect of warfarin, which is mediated by inhibition of the vitamin K-dependent gamma-carboxylation of coagulation factors II, VII, IX and X, is delayed until the normal clotting factors are cleared from the circulation; the peak effect does not occur until 36–72 h after drug administration [127]. During the first few days of warfarin therapy, the prothrombin time mainly reflects the depression of factor VII, which has a half-life of 5–7 h. This does not represent adequate anticoagulation, because the intrinsic clotting pathway remains intact until factors II, IX and X are sufficiently reduced, which takes about 5 days with adequate dosing. Therefore, warfarin treatment should overlap that of either UH or LMWH by at least 5 days when warfarin is initiated in patients with thrombotic disease.

Intensity of oral anticoagulation

Although warfarin has proved its worth in the treatment of patients with VTE, its 'Achilles' heel' remains the associated increased risk of bleeding. The intensity of anticoagulation which provides the optimal benefit with the lowest risk of hemorrhagic complications has been suggested to be an INR between 2.0 and 3.0 across a broad range of patient populations [128–130]. In a randomized double-blind study of 738 patients who had completed three or more months of warfarin therapy for unprovoked VTE, those that continued therapy with low intensity (INR 1.5 to 1.9) experienced a significantly greater risk of recurrent VTE without a decreased risk of bleeding over a mean of 2.4 years compared with those assigned to conventional intensity warfarin (INR 2.0 to 3.0) [129].

That an INR between 2.0 and 3.0 is a sufficient level of intensity is further demonstrated by its efficacy in patients with antiphospholipid antibody syndrome and recurrent thrombosis. Customarily, patients with antiphospholipid antibody syndrome and recurrent thrombosis receive doses of warfarin adjusted to achieve an INR of more than 3.0 despite the lack of prospective data to support this approach to thromboprophylaxis. In a randomized, double-blind trial of 114 patients, achieving an INR of 2.0 to 3.0 resulted in a similar rate of recurrent thrombosis over an average follow up of 2.7 years to that experienced in patients with an INR of 3.1 to 4.0 [130]. This is an important observation especially with the observed increased risk of hemorrhagic complications in trials that assessed the higher intensity regimen of warfarin [131–133]. Based on these data, the currently recommended intensity of VKA therapy for VTE is an INR of 2.0 to 3.0.

The precise route taken to achieve an INR of 2.0 to 3.0 remains a process in evolution. Until recently, it was suggested that 5 mg initiation was as effective as 10 mg, without increasing the risk of bleeding [134]. However, the most recent study comparing a 5 mg vs a 10 mg initial dosing nomogram supports an initial dose of 10 mg [135]. These results should be interpreted with caution, however, since patients at high risk for bleeding were excluded from the study. Ultimately, patient-specific factors will affect the maintenance dose, guiding clinicians to start with lower (<5 mg) or higher (>5 mg) doses. Within groups of patients at high risk of bleeding complications (e.g. elderly patients), the adherence to specific dosing nomograms facilitates achievement of therapeutic INR levels while minimizing the risk of over-anticoagulation [136–138].

Duration of oral anticoagulation

That patients with a history of VTE require long-term anticoagulation in order to prevent recurrent events has been indicated by several trials [128, 139–144]. However, it appears that the optimal duration of anticoagulation for specific patient populations continues to evolve. To assist with deciding the duration of oral anticoagulation in patients with VTE, several factors, including the episode of VTE (first or recurrent) [141–143, 145], the presence or absence of transient, reversible risk factors (e.g. immobilization, trauma, surgery, estrogen use) [146], the presence or absence of cancer [147, 148] or prothrombotic gene mutations [149–151] and the presence of residual thrombus [107, 150, 152] need to be taken into consideration.

The outcome of a randomized trial that compared 6 weeks with 6 months of warfarin therapy in 897 patients who had had a first episode of DVT contributed to the standard duration of anticoagulation for most patients with VTE. In that trial, the 6-month course of anticoagulation halved the recurrence rate after 2 years of follow-up compared with a shorter duration of anticoagulation (9.5% vs 18% in the 6-week group) [141]. Since then, several trials have supported the finding that shorter durations of anticoagulation following first idiopathic VTE are associated with increased risk of recurrent events [143, 145]. It is of note, however, that the recurrence of VTE increases following cessation of anticoagulation in the extended duration groups. Furthermore, extended therapy has also been associated with an increased bleeding risk [142]. Thus, the optimal management of patients with idiopathic VTE has not yet been resolved because of the uncertain balance between decreased clotting and increased major bleeding in patients receiving extended-duration anticoagulation.

The standard duration of anticoagulation should be at least 12 months in the following categories of patients: those with anticardiolipin antibody, antithrombin deficiency, malignancy and recurrent VTE. One multicenter clinical trial evaluated the outcome of such patients who received 6 months of oral anticoagulation compared to indefinite therapy after a second episode of VTE [144]. Indefinite therapy for 4 years was associated with a lower rate of recurrent disease (2.6% vs 20.7% in those treated for 6 months, RR, 8.0) and a higher risk of major hemorrhage (8.6 vs 2.7%). Indefinite anticoagulation is recommended for patients with three or more episodes of VTE.

A special group of patients deserves mention when considering anticoagulation with warfarin, those with HIT. Warfarin remains the anticoagulant of choice for the long-term management of patients with HIT and thrombosis (Chapter 13). The DTIs provide overlapping anticoagulation while achieving therapeutic levels of anticoagulation with warfarin.

FIBRINOLYTIC THERAPY

DVT

The use of fibrinolytic therapy for the treatment of DVT remains controversial. Although an improvement in the rate of clot dissolution and of normal follow-up venography compared with UH is seen with these agents, the major benefit of fibrinolytic therapy rests with its ability to decrease the risk of complications of proximal occlusive DVT (i.e. phlegmasia cerulea dolens) and of post-phlebitic syndrome [153–156]. However, given the increased risk of bleeding with fibrinolytic therapy in these patients and the suggestion that most patients would prefer to live with the post-phlebitic syndrome rather than accept the small increased risk of death or disability due to bleeding [157], these agents are reserved for patients with limb-threatening DVT or DVT associated with severe symptoms.

PE

Three fibrinolytic agents with specific regimens have been approved by the FDA for use in patients with an acute PE (Table 12.7). Key issues relating to the use of fibrinolytics for the treatment of PE will be briefly discussed. For a more in-depth discussion of the use of these agents, the reader is referred elsewhere [158–161].

Fibrinolytics vs UH

Whereas a clear role of fibrinolytics for patients with DVT remains to be more optimally defined, the role of fibrinolytics in the management of massive PE appears to be somewhat clearer. Several randomized clinical trials comparing various fibrinolytic agents with UH have demonstrated improvements in angiographic and hemodynamic abnormalities early after treatment [162–168]. However, this advantage appears to be short-lived. Although significant differences in echocardiographic parameters of right ventricular pressure overload were evident within 12 h in patients treated with fibrinolysis compared with those treated

Table 12.7 FDA-approved fibrinolytic regimens for the treatment of PE

AGENT	REGIMEN
SK	250,000 U over 30 min followed by 100,000 U/h for 24 h
Urokinase	4400 U/kg over 10 min followed by 4400 U/kg per h for 24 h
rt-PA	100 mg over 2 h

with UH, these differences were no longer evident at 1 week of follow-up [162]. In addition, a meta-analysis suggested that compared with UH, fibrinolytic therapy does not appear to have therapeutic benefit in unselected patients, but is associated with an increased risk of major hemorrhage [160]. These data mandate the identification of specific patient populations with acute PE in whom the benefits of fibrinolytic therapy clearly outweigh the risks.

Comparative fibrinolytic trials

Several randomized comparative trials have been performed comparing UK with SK [169], UK with rt-PA [170–172], SK with rt-PA [173] and rt-PA with reteplase [174] in patients with PE. These trials again demonstrated a resolution of angiographic, radiographic and echocardiographic abnormalities and a reduction in pulmonary arterial pressures with fibrinolysis. However, no significant differences between the various protocols and regimens were noted.

Characteristics of patients with PE who may benefit from fibrinolysis

Currently, there is consensus that patients with massive PE presenting with overt right ventricular failure (clinical instability and cardiogenic shock) should promptly be treated with fibrinolytic agents, since they are at a particularly high risk for death or life-threatening complications during the acute phase [175]. At the other end of the clinical spectrum, fibrinolysis for PE is not indicated in the absence of right ventricular dysfunction. In fact, the prognosis of patients with small pulmonary emboli (not affecting pulmonary artery pressure and right ventricular afterload) is excellent, and, as a result, the bleeding risks of fibrinolysis may outweigh the potential benefits of this treatment. Where the divergence of opinions occurs is with patients presenting with submassive PE (i.e. presenting with signs of impending right heart failure). While these patients may be difficult to identify, echocardiographic [176, 177] and biomarker abnormalities [178] coupled with clinical factors such as age over 70 years, cancer, congestive heart failure, chronic obstructive lung disease, hypotension and tachypnea [176] may facilitate the recognition of patients with submassive PE who would benefit from fibrinolytic therapy. In a randomized double-blind study of 256 patients presenting with submassive PE, pulmonary hypertension or right ventricular dysfunction without arterial hypotension or shock, a significant decrease in the primary endpoint of in-hospital death or clinical deterioration requiring an escalation of treatment was noted in patients randomized to receive alteplase (100 mg over 2 h) plus UH compared with those who received UH alone (p-value = 0.006) [179]. Despite these encouraging data, the controversy will continue until data from well-designed prospective clinical trials are available.

Timing of fibrinolysis

Several trials of PE fibrinolysis showed that the duration of symptoms did not affect lung scan reperfusion or angiographic clot lysis [170, 171, 180–182]. However, a pooled analysis of 308 patients from these trials demonstrated an inverse relationship between duration of symptoms and improvement on post-treatment lung scan reperfusion scores [183]. For each additional day of symptoms before PE fibrinolysis, there was a decrement of 0.8% of lung tissue reperfusion on lung scanning (95% CI, 0.2% to 1.4%, p-value = 0.008). Similarly, on angiography, less clot lysis immediately following fibrinolysis was observed in the group of patients with the longest duration of symptoms compared with those with the shortest symptom duration. Although fibrinolysis is still useful in patients who have had symptoms for 6–14 days, this inverse relationship between the duration of symptoms and the response to fibrinolysis indicates that fibrinolytic treatment should begin as soon as possible after PE is diagnosed.

RECOMMENDATIONS

In general, the recommendations for the treatment of DVT and PE are similar, given that these two entities are simply different manifestations of the same process along the spectrum of VTE. That anticoagulation remains the cornerstone of treatment for VTE rests with the observation that the vast majority of patients with VTE who receive anticoagulation survive. That said, those with PE are substantially more likely to die within the next year than those with DVT only (1.5% vs 0.4%, respectively) [184]. Therefore, it has been previously recommended that patients with PE be treated for longer durations of anticoagulation than those with DVT. However, it has since been demonstrated that longer durations of anticoagulation simply defers recurrence rather than reducing the number of recurrences [145]. What has been demonstrated is that the presence of characteristics such as reversible risk factors at the time of VTE, the presence of thrombophilias, associated co-morbidities such as cancer, pregnancy or CKD and the number of prior episodes should all be taken into consideration when deciding what the optimal initial and long-term antithrombotic regimens will be (Table 12.8).

12.5 CONCLUSIONS

VTE continues to be an important cause of morbidity and mortality. Improved understanding of the risk factors that predispose patients to the development of VTE has facilitated enhanced rigor not only in the treatment but also in the primary prevention of this disease entity. Research has resulted in antithrombotic regimens that have accounted for improved management of VTE. The LMWHs have secured a role as the preferred agents for the prevention and initial treatment of VTE. Fondaparinux is emerging as a preferred agent in

Table 12.8 Recommendations for the treatment of venous thromboembolic events

Indication	Dose	Duration	Alternative	Comment
Acute DVT				
Initial Treatment				Initial treatment for at least 5 days recommended while initiating a VKA and continued until INR >2.0
UH	Dosed to aPTT	At least 5 days and until VKA INR 2.0–3.0	LMWH	Dose IV UH to aPTT corresponding to plasma heparin levels from 0.3 to 0.7 IU/mL anti-Xa activity Use anti-Xa level for guidance in those requiring large doses
LMWH	Dalteparin. 100 U/kg bid Enoxaparin. 100 U/kg (1 mg/kg) bid Nadroparin. 90 U/kg bid Tinzaparin. 175 U/kg qd	At least 5 days and until VKA INR 2.0–3.0	IV UH	LMWH preferred over UH Outpatient treatment preferred Caution in patients with severe CKD (CrCl <30 mL/min)
Fibrinolytics	Systemic	NA	NA	Not recommended for routine use Recommended for treatment of patients with limb-threatening DVT May use catheter-directed fibrinolysis in selected patients
Long-term treatment				
First episode	VKA targeted to INR 2.0–3.0	Reversible RF – 3 months	LMWH for first 3–6 months in patients with cancer	Consider indefinite anticoagulation in patients with antiphospholipid antibody, Facto V Leidin, prothrombin 20210A gene mutation, AT, protein C or protein S deficiency

		Idiopathic DVT – 6 to 12 months Patient with thrombophilia – 12 months		Dalteparin 200 IU/kg × 1 month then 150 IU/kg daily or tinzaparin 175 IU/kg SC daily are established LMWH regimens for long-term use in patients with cancer
≥2 episodes	VKA targeted to INR 2.0–3.0	Indefinite	NA	
Acute PE *Initial Treatment*				Treatment essentially the same as that for DVT Initial treatment for at least 5 days recommended while initiating a VKA and continued until INR >2.0
UH	Dosed to aPTT	At least 5 days and until VKA INR 2.0–3.0	LMWH preferred in non-massive PE	Preferred in patients with severe CKD (CrCl <30ml/min) Dose IV UH to aPTT corresponding to plasma heparin levels from 0.3 to 0.7 IU/mL anti-Xa activity Use anti-Xa level for guidance in those requiring large doses
LMWH	Dalteparin. 100 U/kg bid Enoxaparin. 100 U/kg (1 mg/kg) bid Nadroparin. 90 U/kg bid Tinzaparin. 175 U/kg qd	At least 5 days and until VKA INR 2.0–3.0	UH preferred in severe CKD	Currently the initial treatment of choice for acute PE Can safely be given in the outpatient setting in low-risk patients
Fibrinolytics	SK – 250,000 U over 30 min followed by 100,000 U/h for 24 h	NA	NA	Suggested in patients who are HD unstable

Table 12.8 (*Continued*)

Indication	Dose	Duration	Alternative	Comment
	UK – 4400 U/kg over 10 min followed by 4400 U/kg per h for 24 h OR 4400 U/kg over 10 min followed by 4400 U/kg per h for 12 h rt-PA – 100 mg over 2 h			May be useful u to 14 days after PE in patients with RV dysfunction
Long-term treatment				
First episode	VKA targeted to INR 2.0–3.0 OR Dalteparin 200 IU/kg × 1 month then 150 IU/kg daily or tinzaparin 175 IU/kg SC daily	Reversible RF – at least 3 months Idiopathic DVT – 6 to 12 months Patient with thrombophilia – 12 months	LMWH for first 3–6 months in patients with cancer	Consider indefinite anticoagulation in patients with first idiopathic PE Consider indefinite anticoagulation in patients with antiphospholipid antibody, Facto V Leidin, prothrombin 20210 gene mutation, AT, protein C or protein S deficiency Consider indefinite anticoagulation in patients following one spontaneous, life-threatening VTE, or a VTE at an unusual site (i.e. mesenteric or cerebral vein)
≥2 episodes	VKA targeted to INR 2.0–3.0	Indefinite	NA	

bid = twice daily; CrCl = creatinine clearance; HD = hemodynamically; NA = not applicable; RF = risk factor; RV = right ventricular; VKA = vitamin K antagonist certain scenarios but further studies remain necessary for it to surpass the role of LMWH. Although warfarin remains the agent of choice for long-term treatment of VTE, the promise of oral DTIs may someday marginalize this antiquated agent. Despite the progress to date, there remains a need for continued pursuit of the optimal preventive and therapeutic strategy to minimize or perhaps eliminate this disease entity all together.

REFERENCES

[1] Horlander, K.T., Mannino, D.M., Leeper, K.V., (2003) Pulmonary embolism mortality in the United States, 1979–1998: an analysis using multiple-cause mortality data. *Arch Intern Med*, 163(14):1711–17.

[2] Gathof, B.S., Picker, S.M., Rojo, J., (2004) Epidemiology, etiology and diagnosis of venous thrombosis. *Eur J Med Res*, 9(3):95–103.

[3] Alikhan, R., *et al.*, (2004) Risk factors for venous thromboembolism in hospitalized patients with acute medical illness: analysis of the MEDENOX Study. *Arch Intern Med*, 164(9):963–8.

[4] Stinnett, J.M., *et al.*, (2005) Venous thromboembolism prophylaxis in medically ill patients and the development of strategies to improve prophylaxis rates. *Am J Hematol*, 78(3):167–72.

[5] Tosetto, A., Frezzato, M., Rodeghiero, F., (2003) Prevalence and risk factors of non-fatal venous thromboembolism in the active population of the VITA Project. *J Thromb Haemost*, 1(8):1724–9.

[6] Rosendaal, F.R., (1999) Venous thrombosis: a multicausal disease. *Lancet*, 353(9159):1167–73.

[7] Doyle, N.M., Monga, M., (2004) Thromboembolic disease in pregnancy. *Obstet Gynecol Clin North Am*, 31(2): 319–44, vi.

[8] Walker, M.C., *et al.*, Changes in activated protein C resistance during normal pregnancy. *Am J Obstet Gynecol*, 177(1):162–9.

[9] Kim, Y.H., Oh, S.H., Kim, J.S., Incidence and natural history of deep-vein thrombosis after total hip arthroplasty. A prospective and randomised clinical study. *J Bone Joint Surg Br*, 85(5):661–5.

[10] Wilson, D., *et al.*, Altered venous function and deep venous thrombosis following proximal femoral fracture. *Injury*, 33(1):33–9.

[11] Westrich, G.H., *et al.*, Correlation of thrombophilia and hypofibrinolysis with pulmonary embolism following total hip arthroplasty: an analysis of genetic factors. *J Bone Joint Surg Am*, 84-A(12):2161–7.

[12] Lindahl, T.L., *et al.*, APC-resistance is a risk factor for post-operative thromboembolism in elective replacement of the hip or knee—a prospective study. *Thromb Haemost*, 81(1):18–21.

[13] White, R.H., *et al.*, (1998) Incidence and time course of thromboembolic outcomes following total hip or knee arthroplasty. *Arch Intern Med*, 158(14):1525–31.

[14] Heit, J.A., *et al.*, (2001) Incidence of venous thromboembolism in hospitalized patients vs community residents. *Mayo Clin Proc*, 76(11):1102–10.

[15] Heit, J.A., *et al.*, (2002) Relative impact of risk factors for deep vein thrombosis and pulmonary embolism: a population-based study. *Arch Intern Med*, 162(11):1245–8.

[16] Goldhaber, S.Z., Dunn, K., MacDougall, R.C., (2000) New onset of venous thromboembolism among hospitalized patients at Brigham and Women's Hospital is caused more often by prophylaxis failure than by withholding treatment. *Chest*, 118(6):1680–4.

[17] Lindblad, B., Sternby, N.H., Bergqvist, D., (1991) Incidence of venous thromboembolism verified by necropsy over 30 years. *Br Med J*, 302(6778):709–11.

[18] Alikhan, R., *et al.*, (2004) Fatal pulmonary embolism in hospitalised patients: a necropsy review. *J Clin Pathol*, 57(12):1254–7.

[19] Menajovsky, L.B., Spandorfer, J., (2004) Benefits of more aggressive VTE prophylaxis in hospitalized medical patients. *Cleve Clin J Med*, 71(12):947–8, 951–3, 956 passim.

[20] Goldhaber, S.Z., Tapson, V.F., (2004) A prospective registry of 5451 patients with ultrasound-confirmed deep vein thrombosis. *Am J Cardiol*, 93(2):259–62.

[21] Rogers, F.B., *et al.*, (2002) Practice management guidelines for the prevention of venous thromboembolism in trauma patients: the EAST practice management guidelines work group. *J Trauma*, 53(1):142–64.

[22] Rogers, F.B., (2001) Venous thromboembolism in trauma patients: a review. *Surgery*, 130(1):1–12.
[23] Geerts, W.H., *et al.*, (1994) A prospective study of venous thromboembolism after major trauma. *N Eng J Med*, 331(24):1601–6.
[24] O'Malley, K.F., Ross, S.E., (1990) Pulmonary embolism in major trauma patients. *J Trauma*, 30(6):748–50.
[25] Acosta, J.A., *et al.*, (1998) Lethal injuries and time to death in a level I trauma center. *J Am Coll Surg*, 186(5):528–33.
[26] Meissner, M.H., Chandler, W.L., Elliott, J.S., (2003) Venous thromboembolism in trauma: a local manifestation of systemic hypercoagulability? *J Trauma*, 54(2):224–31.
[27] Mismetti, P., *et al.*, (2000) Prevention of venous thromboembolism in internal medicine with unfractionated or low-molecular-weight heparins: a meta-analysis of randomised clinical trials. *Thromb Haemost*, 83(1):14–19.
[28] Gallus, A.S., *et al.*, (1973) Small subcutaneous doses of heparin in prevention of venous thrombosis. *N Eng J Med*, 288(11):545–51.
[29] Kakkar, V.V., *et al.*, (1977) Prevention of Fatal Post-operative pulmonary embolism by low doses of heparin. Reappraisal of results of international multicentre trial. *Lancet*, 1(8011):567–9.
[30] Bergqvist, D., *et al.*, (1986) Low molecular weight heparin once daily compared with conventional low-dose heparin twice daily. A prospective double-blind multicentre trial on prevention of post-operative thrombosis. *Br J Surg*, 73(3):204–8.
[31] Hull, R.D., *et al.*, (2000) Low-molecular-weight heparin prophylaxis using dalteparin in close proximity to surgery vs warfarin in hip arthroplasty patients: a double-blind, randomized comparison. The North American Fragmin Trial Investigators. *Arch Intern Med*, 160(14):2199–207.
[32] Turpie, A.G., *et al.*, (1986) A randomized controlled trial of a low-molecular-weight heparin (enoxaparin) to prevent deep-vein thrombosis in patients undergoing elective hip surgery. *N Eng J Med*, 315(15):925–9.
[33] Leclerc, J.R., *et al.*, (1992) Prevention of deep vein thrombosis after major knee surgery—a randomized, double-blind trial comparing a low molecular weight heparin fragment (enoxaparin) to placebo. *Thromb Haemost*, 67(4):417–23.
[34] Leclerc, J.R., *et al.*, (1996) Prevention of venous thromboembolism after knee arthroplasty. A randomized, double-blind trial comparing enoxaparin with warfarin. *Ann Intern Med*, 124(7):619–26.
[35] Fitzgerald, R.H., Jr., *et al.*, (2001) Prevention of venous thromboembolic disease following primary total knee arthroplasty. A randomized, multicenter, open-label, parallel-group comparison of enoxaparin and warfarin. *J Bone Joint Surg Am*, 83-A(6):900–6.
[36] Hull, R.D., *et al.*, (2001) Timing of initial administration of low-molecular-weight heparin prophylaxis against deep vein thrombosis in patients following elective hip arthroplasty: a systematic review. *Arch Intern Med*, 161(16):1952–60.
[37] Turpie, A.G., *et al.*, (2002) Fondaparinux vs enoxaparin for the prevention of venous thromboembolism in major orthopedic surgery: a meta-analysis of 4 randomized double-blind studies. *Arch Intern Med*, 162(16):1833–40.
[38] Strebel, N., *et al.*, (2002) Pre-operative or post-operative start of prophylaxis for venous thromboembolism with low-molecular-weight heparin in elective hip surgery? *Arch Intern Med*, 162(13):1451–6.
[39] Tran, A.H., Lee, G., (2003) Fondaparinux for prevention of venous thromboembolism in major orthopedic surgery. *Ann Pharmacother*, 37(11):1632–43.
[40] Turpie, A.G., Gallus, A.S., Hoek, J.A., (2001) A synthetic pentasaccharide for the prevention of deep-vein thrombosis after total hip replacement. *N Eng J Med*, 344(9): 619–25.
[41] Turpie, A.G., *et al.*, (2002) Post-operative fondaparinux versus post-operative enoxaparin for prevention of venous thromboembolism after elective hip-replacement surgery: a randomised double-blind trial. *Lancet*, 359(9319):1721–6.
[42] Lassen, M.R., *et al.*, (2002) Post-operative fondaparinux versus pre-operative enoxaparin for prevention of venous thromboembolism in elective hip-replacement surgery: a randomised double-blind comparison. *Lancet*, 359(9319):1715–20.

[43] Bauer, K.A., *et al.*, (2001) Fondaparinux compared with enoxaparin for the prevention of venous thromboembolism after elective major knee surgery. *N Eng J Med*, 345(18):1305–10.

[44] Eriksson, B.I., *et al.*, (2001) Fondaparinux compared with enoxaparin for the prevention of venous thromboembolism after hip-fracture surgery. *N Eng J Med*, 345(18): 1298–304.

[45] Turpie, A.G., *et al.*, (2004) Superiority of fondaparinux over enoxaparin in preventing venous thromboembolism in major orthopedic surgery using different efficacy end points. *Chest*, 126(2):501 8.

[46] Turpie, A.G., *et al.*, (2003) New pentasaccharides for the prophylaxis of venous thromboembolism: clinical studies. *Chest*, 124(6 Suppl):371S–378S.

[47] Bergqvist, D., *et al.*, (2002) Duration of prophylaxis against venous thromboembolism with enoxaparin after surgery for cancer. *N Eng J Med*, 346(13):975–80.

[48] Hull, R.D., *et al.*, (2000) Low-molecular-weight heparin prophylaxis using dalteparin extended out-of-hospital vs in-hospital warfarin/out-of-hospital placebo in hip arthroplasty patients: a double-blind, randomized comparison. North American Fragmin Trial Investigators. *Arch Intern Med*, 160(14):2208–15.

[49] Eikelboom, J.W., Quinlan, D.J., Douketis, J.D., (2001) Extended-duration prophylaxis against venous thromboembolism after total hip or knee replacement: a meta-analysis of the randomised trials. *Lancet*, 358(9275):9–15.

[50] Dahl, O.E., *et al.*, (1997) Prolonged thromboprophylaxis following hip replacement surgery—results of a double-blind, prospective, randomised, placebo-controlled study with dalteparin (Fragmin). *Thromb Haemost*, 77(1):26–31.

[51] Comp, P.C., *et al.*, (2001) Prolonged enoxaparin therapy to prevent venous thromboembolism after primary hip or knee replacement. Enoxaparin Clinical Trial Group. *J Bone Joint Surg Am*, 83-A(3):336–45.

[52] Bergqvist, D., *et al.*, (1996) Low-molecular-weight heparin (enoxaparin) as prophylaxis against venous thromboembolism after total hip replacement. *N Eng J Med*, 335(10): 696–700.

[53] Lassen, M.R., *et al.*, (1998) Efficacy and safety of prolonged thromboprophylaxis with a low molecular weight heparin (dalteparin) after total hip arthroplasty—the Danish Prolonged Prophylaxis (DaPP) Study. *Thromb Res*, 89(6):281–7.

[54] Planes, A., *et al.*, (1996) Risk of deep-venous thrombosis after hospital discharge in patients having undergone total hip replacement: double-blind randomised comparison of enoxaparin versus placebo. *Lancet*, 348(9022):224–8.

[55] Prevention of pulmonary embolism and deep vein thrombosis with low dose aspirin: Pulmonary Embolism Prevention (PEP) trial. *Lancet*, 2000. 355(9212):1295–302.

[56] Westrich, G.H., Sculco, T.P., (1996) Prophylaxis against deep venous thrombosis after total knee arthroplasty. Pneumatic plantar compression and aspirin compared with aspirin alone. *J Bone Joint Surg Am*, 78(6):826–34.

[57] Gent, M., *et al.*, (1996) Low-molecular-weight heparinoid orgaran is more effective than aspirin in the prevention of venous thromboembolism after surgery for hip fracture. *Circulation*, 93(1):80–4.

[58] Gallus, A.S., *et al.*, (1976) Prevention of venous thrombosis with small, subcutaneous doses of heparin. *JAMA*, 235(18):1980–2.

[59] Prevention of fatal post-operative pulmonary embolism by low doses of heparin. An international multicentre trial. *Lancet*, 1975. 2(7924):45–51.

[60] Clagett, G.P., Reisch, J.S., (1988) Prevention of venous thromboembolism in general surgical patients. Results of meta-analysis. *Ann Surg*, 208(2):227–40.

[61] Collins, R., *et al.*, (1988) Reduction in fatal pulmonary embolism and venous thrombosis by perioperative administration of subcutaneous heparin. Overview of results of randomized trials in general, orthopedic, and urologic surgery. *N Eng J Med*, 318(18): 1162–73.

[62] Hirsh, J., Levine, M., (1989) Prevention of venous thrombosis in patients undergoing major orthopaedic surgical procedures. *Br J Clin Pract Suppl*, 65:2–8.

[63] Halkin, H., *et al.*, (1982) Reduction of mortality in general medical in-patients by low-dose heparin prophylaxis. *Ann Intern Med*, 96(5):561–5.

[64] Harenberg, J., P. Roebruck, Heene, D.L., (1996) Subcutaneous low-molecular-weight heparin versus standard heparin and the prevention of thromboembolism in medical inpatients. The Heparin Study in Internal Medicine Group. *Haemostasis*, 26(3): p. 127–39.

[65] Leyvraz, P.F., *et al.*, (1991) Prevention of deep vein thrombosis after hip replacement: randomised comparison between unfractionated heparin and low molecular weight heparin. *Br Med J*, 303(6802):543–8.

[66] Warkentin, T.E., *et al.*, (1995) Heparin-induced thrombocytopenia in patients treated with low-molecular-weight heparin or unfractionated heparin. *N Eng J Med*, 332(20):1330–5.

[67] Francis, C.W., *et al.*, (1992) Comparison of warfarin and external pneumatic compression in prevention of venous thrombosis after total hip replacement. *JAMA*, 267(21):2911–5.

[68] Powers, P.J., *et al.*, (1989) A randomized trial of less intense post-operative warfarin or aspirin therapy in the prevention of venous thromboembolism after surgery for fractured hip. *Arch Intern Med*, 149(4):771–4.

[69] Francis, C.W., *et al.*, (1983) Two-step warfarin therapy. Prevention of post-operative venous thrombosis without excessive bleeding. *JAMA*, 249(3):374–8.

[70] Hull, R., *et al.*, (1993) A comparison of subcutaneous low-molecular-weight heparin with warfarin sodium for prophylaxis against deep-vein thrombosis after hip or knee implantation. *N Eng J Med*, 329(19):1370–6.

[71] Francis, C.W., *et al.*, (1997) Prevention of deep-vein thrombosis after total hip arthroplasty. Comparison of warfarin and dalteparin. *J Bone Joint Surg Am*, 79(9):1365–72.

[72] Heit, J.A., *et al.*, (1997) Efficacy and safety of low molecular weight heparin (ardeparin sodium) compared to warfarin for the prevention of venous thromboembolism after total knee replacement surgery: a double-blind, dose-ranging study. Ardeparin Arthroplasty Study Group. *Thromb Haemost*, 77(1):32–8.

[73] Colwell, C.W., Jr., *et al.*, (1999) Comparison of enoxaparin and warfarin for the prevention of venous thromboembolic disease after total hip arthroplasty. Evaluation during hospitalization and three months after discharge. *J Bone Joint Surg Am*, 81(7):932–40.

[74] Brotman, D.J., *et al.*, (2004) Warfarin prophylaxis and venous thromboembolism in the first 5 days following hip and knee arthroplasty. *Thromb Haemost*, 92(5):1012–7.

[75] Francis, C.W., *et al.*, (1996) Comparison of two warfarin regimens in the prevention of venous thrombosis following total knee replacement. *Thromb Haemost*, 75(5):706–11.

[76] Eriksson, B.I., Lassen, M.R., (2003) Duration of prophylaxis against venous thromboembolism with fondaparinux after hip fracture surgery: a multicenter, randomized, placebo-controlled, double-blind study. *Arch Intern Med*, 163(11):1337–42.

[77] Lundkvist, J., Bergqvist, D., Jonsson, B., Cost-effectiveness of fondaparinux vs. enoxaparin as venous thromboembolism prophylaxis in Sweden. *Eur J Health Econ*, 4(4): 254–62.

[78] Annemans, L., *et al.*, (2004) Cost consequence analysis of fondaparinux versus enoxaparin in the prevention of venous thromboembolism after major orthopaedic surgery in Belgium. *Acta Clin Belg*, 59(6):346–57.

[79] Dranitsaris, G., *et al.*, (2004) Pharmacoeconomic analysis of fondaparinux versus enoxaparin for the prevention of thromboembolic events in orthopedic surgery patients. *Am J Cardiovasc Drugs*, 4(5):325–33.

[80] Eriksson, B.I., *et al.*, (1997) A comparison of recombinant hirudin with a low-molecular-weight heparin to prevent thromboembolic complications after total hip replacement. *N Eng J Med*, 337(19):1329–35.

[81] Eriksson, B.I., *et al.*, (2005) A new oral direct thrombin inhibitor, dabigatran etexilate, compared with enoxaparin for prevention of thromboembolic events following total hip or knee replacement: the BISTRO II randomized trial. *J Thromb Haemost*, 3(1): 103–11.

[82] Eriksson, B.I., *et al.*, (2004) Dose escalating safety study of a new oral direct thrombin inhibitor, dabigatran etexilate, in patients undergoing total hip replacement: BISTRO I. *J Thromb Haemost*, 2(9):1573–80.

[83] Eriksson, B.I., *et al.*, (2003) Direct thrombin inhibitor melagatran followed by oral ximelagatran in comparison with enoxaparin for prevention of venous thromboembolism after total hip or knee replacement. *Thromb Haemost*, 89(2):288–96.

[84] Eriksson, B.I., *et al.*, (2002) Ximelagatran and melagatran compared with dalteparin for prevention of venous thromboembolism after total hip or knee replacement: the METHRO II randomised trial. *Lancet*, 360(9344):1441–7.

[85] Eriksson, B.I., *et al.*, (2002) A dose-ranging study of the oral direct thrombin inhibitor, ximelagatran, and its subcutaneous form, melagatran, compared with dalteparin in the prophylaxis of thromboembolism after hip or knee replacement: METHRO I. MElagatran for THRombin inhibition in Orthopaedic surgery. *Thromb Haemost*, 87(2):231–7.

[86] Eriksson, B.I., *et al.*, (2003) The direct thrombin inhibitor melagatran followed by oral ximelagatran compared with enoxaparin for the prevention of venous thromboembolism after total hip or knee replacement: the EXPRESS study. *J Thromb Haemost*, 1(12):2490–6.

[87] Francis, C.W., *et al.*, (2003) Comparison of ximelagatran with warfarin for the prevention of venous thromboembolism after total knee replacement. *N Eng J Med*, 349(18):1703–12.

[88] Geerts, W.H., *et al.*, (2004) Prevention of venous thromboembolism: the Seventh ACCP Conference on Antithrombotic and Thrombolytic Therapy. *Chest*, 126(3 Suppl):338S–400S.

[89] Mannucci, P.M., Poller, L., (2001) Venous thrombosis and anticoagulant therapy. *Br J Haematol*, 114(2):258–70.

[90] Alpert, J.S., Dalen, J.E., (1994) Epidemiology and natural history of venous thromboembolism. *Prog Cardiovasc Dis*, 36(6): p. 417–22.

[91] Hull, R.D., *et al.*, (1997) The importance of initial heparin treatment on long-term clinical outcomes of antithrombotic therapy. The emerging theme of delayed recurrence. *Arch Intern Med*, 157(20):2317–21.

[92] Hull, R.D., *et al.*, (1997) Relation between the time to achieve the lower limit of the APTT therapeutic range and recurrent venous thromboembolism during heparin treatment for deep vein thrombosis. *Arch Intern Med*, 157(22):2562–8.

[93] Hull, R.D., *et al.*, (1986) Continuous intravenous heparin compared with intermittent subcutaneous heparin in the initial treatment of proximal-vein thrombosis. *N Eng J Med*, 315(18): p. 1109–14.

[94] Brandjes, D.P., *et al.*, (1992) Acenocoumarol and heparin compared with acenocoumarol alone in the initial treatment of proximal-vein thrombosis. *N Eng J Med*, 327(21):1485–9.

[95] Raschke, R., Hirsh, J., Guidry, J.R., (2003) Suboptimal monitoring and dosing of unfractionated heparin in comparative studies with low-molecular-weight heparin. *Ann Intern Med*, 138(9): p. 720–3.

[96] Kershaw, B., *et al.*, (1994) Computer-assisted dosing of heparin. Management with a pharmacy-based anticoagulation service. *Arch Intern Med*, 154(9):1005–11.

[97] Elliott, C.G., *et al.*, (1994) Physician-guided treatment compared with a heparin protocol for deep vein thrombosis. *Arch Intern Med*, 154(9):999–1004.

[98] Raschke, R.A., *et al.*, (1993) The weight-based heparin dosing nomogram compared with a 'standard care' nomogram. A randomized controlled trial. *Ann Intern Med*, 119(9): p. 874–81.

[99] Hull, R.D., *et al.*, (1990) Heparin for 5 days as compared with 10 days in the initial treatment of proximal venous thrombosis. *N Eng J Med*, 322(18):1260–4.

[100] Koopman, M.M., *et al.*, (1996) Treatment of venous thrombosis with intravenous unfractionated heparin administered in the hospital as compared with subcutaneous low-molecular-weight heparin administered at home. The Tasman Study Group. *N Eng J Med*, 334(11):682–7.

[101] Levine, M., *et al.*, (1996) A comparison of low-molecular-weight heparin administered primarily at home with unfractionated heparin administered in the hospital for proximal deep-vein thrombosis. *N Eng J Med*, 334(11):677–81.

[102] Veiga, F., *et al.*, (2000) Low molecular weight heparin (enoxaparin) versus oral anticoagulant therapy (acenocoumarol) in the long-term treatment of deep venous thrombosis in the elderly: a randomized trial. *Thromb Haemost*, 84(4):559–64.

[103] Pineo, G.F., Hull, R.D., (2005) Low-molecular-weight heparin for the treatment of venous thromboembolism in the elderly. *Clin Appl Thromb Hemost*, 11(1):15–23.

[104] Lee, A.Y., *et al.*, (2003) Low-molecular-weight heparin versus a coumarin for the prevention of recurrent venous thromboembolism in patients with cancer. *N Eng J Med*, 349(2):146–53.

[105] Luk, C., *et al.*, (2001) Extended outpatient therapy with low molecular weight heparin for the treatment of recurrent venous thromboembolism despite warfarin therapy. *Am J Med*, 111(4): p. 270–3.

[106] Bick, R.L., Rice, J., (1999) Long-term outpatient dalteparin (fragmin) therapy for arterial and venous thrombosis: efficacy and safety—a preliminary report. *Clin Appl Thromb Hemost*, 5 (Suppl 1):S67–71.

[107] Prandoni, P., (2003) Risk factors of recurrent venous thromboembolism: the role of residual vein thrombosis. *Pathophysiol Haemost Thromb*, 33(5–6):351–3.

[108] Breddin, H.K., *et al.*, (2001) Effects of a low-molecular-weight heparin on thrombus regression and recurrent thromboembolism in patients with deep-vein thrombosis. *N Eng J Med*, 344(9): p. 626–31.

[109] Simonneau, G., *et al.*, (1993) Subcutaneous low-molecular-weight heparin compared with continuous intravenous unfractionated heparin in the treatment of proximal deep vein thrombosis. *Arch Intern Med*, 153(13):1541–6.

[110] Prandoni, P., *et al.*, (1992) Comparison of subcutaneous low-molecular-weight heparin with intravenous standard heparin in proximal deep-vein thrombosis. *Lancet*, 339(8791):441–5.

[111] Lindmarker, P., *et al.*, (1994) Comparison of once-daily subcutaneous Fragmin with continuous intravenous unfractionated heparin in the treatment of deep vein thrombosis. *Thromb Haemost*, 72(2):186–90.

[112] Hull, R.D., *et al.*, (1992) Subcutaneous low-molecular-weight heparin compared with continuous intravenous heparin in the treatment of proximal-vein thrombosis. *N Eng J Med*, 326(15): p. 975–82.

[113] Gould, M.K., *et al.*, (1999) Low-molecular-weight heparins compared with unfractionated heparin for treatment of acute deep venous thrombosis. A meta-analysis of randomized, controlled trials. *Ann Intern Med*, 130(10):800–9.

[114] Gould, M.K., *et al.*, (1999) Low-molecular-weight heparins compared with unfractionated heparin for treatment of acute deep venous thrombosis. A cost-effectiveness analysis. *Ann Intern Med*, 130(10):789–99.

[115] O'Brien, B., *et al.*, (2003) Economic evaluation of outpatient treatment with low-molecular-weight heparin for proximal vein thrombosis. *Arch Intern Med*, 159(19):2298–304.

[116] Lee, A.Y., Levine, M.N., (2003) Venous thromboembolism and cancer: risks and outcomes. *Circulation*, 107(23 Suppl 1):I17–21.

[117] Meyer, G., *et al.*, (2002) Comparison of low-molecular-weight heparin and warfarin for the secondary prevention of venous thromboembolism in patients with cancer: a randomized controlled study. *Arch Intern Med*, 162(15):1729–35.

[118] Lee, A.Y., *et al.*, (2005) Randomized Comparison of Low Molecular Weight Heparin and Coumarin Derivatives on the Survival of Patients With Cancer and Venous Thromboembolism. *J Clin Oncol*, 23(10):2123–9

[119] Kovacs, M.J., *et al.*, (2000) Outpatient treatment of pulmonary embolism with dalteparin. *Thromb Haemost*, 83(2):209–11.

[120] Simonneau, G., *et al.*, (1997) A comparison of low-molecular-weight heparin with unfractionated heparin for acute pulmonary embolism. The THESEE Study Group. Tinzaparine ou Heparine Standard: Evaluations dans l'Embolie Pulmonaire. *N Eng J Med*, 337(10): 663–9.

[121] Hull, R.D., *et al.*, (2000) Low-molecular-weight heparin vs heparin in the treatment of patients with pulmonary embolism. American-Canadian Thrombosis Study Group. *Arch Intern Med*, 160(2):229–36.

[122] The Columbus Investigators, (1997) Low-molecular-weight heparin in the treatment of patients with venous thromboembolism. *N Eng J Med*, 337(10):657–62.

[123] Dolovich, L.R., *et al.*, (2000) A meta-analysis comparing low-molecular-weight heparins with unfractionated heparin in the treatment of venous thromboembolism: examining some unanswered questions regarding location of treatment, product type, and dosing frequency. *Arch Intern Med*, 160(2):181–8.

[124] Buller, H.R., *et al.*, (2003) Subcutaneous fondaparinux versus intravenous unfractionated heparin in the initial treatment of pulmonary embolism. *N Eng J Med*, 349(18):1695–702.

[125] Lee, A.Y., (2003) Epidemiology and management of venous thromboembolism in patients with cancer. *Thromb Res*, 110(4):167–72.

[126] Lee, A.Y., (2005) Management of thrombosis in cancer: primary prevention and secondary prophylaxis. *Br J Haematol*, 128(3):291–302.

[127] Hirsh, J., *et al.*, (2001) Oral anticoagulants: mechanism of action, clinical effectiveness, and optimal therapeutic range. *Chest*, 119(1 Suppl):8S–21S.

[128] Ridker, P.M., *et al.*, (2003) Long-term, low-intensity warfarin therapy for the prevention of recurrent venous thromboembolism. *N Eng J Med*, 348(15):1425–34.

[129] Kearon, C., *et al.*, (2003) Comparison of low-intensity warfarin therapy with conventional-intensity warfarin therapy for long-term prevention of recurrent venous thromboembolism. *N Eng J Med*, 349(7):631–9.

[130] Crowther, M.A., *et al.*, (2003) A comparison of two intensities of warfarin for the prevention of recurrent thrombosis in patients with the antiphospholipid antibody syndrome. *N Eng J Med*, 349(12):1133–8.

[131] Hull, R., *et al.*, (1979) Warfarin sodium versus low-dose heparin in the long-term treatment of venous thrombosis. *N Eng J Med*, 301(16):855–8.

[132] Hull, R., *et al.*, (1982) Adjusted subcutaneous heparin versus warfarin sodium in the long-term treatment of venous thrombosis. *N Eng J Med*, 306(4):189–94.

[133] Hull, R., *et al.*, (1982) Different intensities of oral anticoagulant therapy in the treatment of proximal-vein thrombosis. *N Eng J Med*, 307(27):1676–81.

[134] Harrison, L., *et al.*, (1997) Comparison of 5-mg and 10-mg loading doses in initiation of warfarin therapy. *Ann Intern Med*, 126(2):133–6.

[135] Kovacs, M.J., *et al.*, (2003) Comparison of 10-mg and 5-mg warfarin initiation nomograms together with low-molecular-weight heparin for outpatient treatment of acute venous thromboembolism. A randomized, double-blind, controlled trial. *Ann Intern Med*, 138(9): p. 714–9.

[136] Siguret, V., *et al.*, (2005) Initiation of warfarin therapy in elderly medical inpatients: a safe and accurate regimen. *Am J Med*, 118(2):137–42.

[137] Crowther, M.A., (2003) Oral anticoagulant initiation: rationale for the use of warfarin dosing nomograms. *Semin Vasc Med*, 3(3):255–60.

[138] Wilkinson, T.J., R. Sainsbury, (2003) Evaluation of a warfarin initiation protocol for older people. *Intern Med J*, 33(9–10):465–7.

[139] Research Committee of the British Thoracic Society. (1992) Optimum duration of anticoagulation for deep-vein thrombosis and pulmonary embolism. *Lancet*, 340(8824): 873–6.

[140] Levine, M.N., *et al.*, (1995) Optimal duration of oral anticoagulant therapy: a randomized trial comparing four weeks with three months of warfarin in patients with proximal deep vein thrombosis. *Thromb Haemost*, 74(2):606–11.

[141] Schulman, S., *et al.*, (1995) A comparison of six weeks with six months of oral anticoagulant therapy after a first episode of venous thromboembolism. Duration of Anticoagulation Trial Study Group. *N Eng J Med*, 332(25):1661–5.

[142] Kearon, C., *et al.*, (1999) A comparison of three months of anticoagulation with extended anticoagulation for a first episode of idiopathic venous thromboembolism. *N Eng J Med*, 340(12):901–7.

[143] Agnelli, G., *et al.*, (2001) Three months versus one year of oral anticoagulant therapy for idiopathic deep venous thrombosis. Warfarin Optimal Duration Italian Trial Investigators. *N Eng J Med*, 345(3):165–9.

[144] Schulman, S., *et al.*, (1997) The duration of oral anticoagulant therapy after a second episode of venous thromboembolism. The Duration of Anticoagulation Trial Study Group. *N Eng J Med*, 336(6):393–8.

[145] Agnelli, G., *et al.*, (2003) Extended oral anticoagulant therapy after a first episode of pulmonary embolism. *Ann Intern Med*, 139(1):19–25.

[146] Kearon, C., *et al.*, (2004) Comparison of 1 month with 3 months of anticoagulation for a first episode of venous thromboembolism associated with a transient risk factor. *J Thromb Haemost*, 2(5):743–9.

[147] Schulman, S., Lindmarker, P., (2000) Incidence of cancer after prophylaxis with warfarin against recurrent venous thromboembolism. Duration of Anticoagulation Trial. *N Eng J Med*, 342(26):1953–8.

[148] Prandoni, P., Piccioli, A., Pagnan, A., (2003) Recurrent thromboembolism in cancer patients: incidence and risk factors. *Semin Thromb Hemost*, 29 (Suppl 1):3–8.

[149] Simioni, P., *et al.*, (1997) The risk of recurrent venous thromboembolism in patients with an Arg506–>Gln mutation in the gene for factor V (factor V Leiden). *N Eng J Med*, 336(6): p. 399–403.

[150] Palareti, G., Cosmi, B., (2004) Predicting the risk of recurrence of venous thromboembolism. *Curr Opin Hematol*, 11(3): p. 192–7.

[151] Miles, J.S., *et al.*, (2001) G20210A mutation in the prothrombin gene and the risk of recurrent venous thromboembolism. *J Am Coll Cardiol*, 37(1):215–8.

[152] Cosmi, B., Palareti, G., (2003) Oral anticoagulant therapy in venous thromboembolism. *Semin Vasc Med*, 3(3):303–14.

[153] Turpie, A.G., *et al.*, (1990) Tissue plasminogen activator (rt-PA) vs heparin in deep vein thrombosis. Results of a randomized trial. *Chest*, 97(4 Suppl):172S–175S.

[154] Rogers, L.Q., Lutcher, C.L., (1990) Streptokinase therapy for deep vein thrombosis: a comprehensive review of the English literature. *Am J Med*, 88(4):389–95.

[155] Goldhaber, S.Z., *et al.*, (1990) Randomized controlled trial of tissue plasminogen activator in proximal deep venous thrombosis. *Am J Med*, 88(3):235–40.

[156] Mohr, D.N., *et al.*, (2000) The venous stasis syndrome after deep venous thrombosis or pulmonary embolism: a population-based study. *Mayo Clin Proc*, 75(12):1249–56.

[157] O'Meara, J.J., 3rd, *et al.*, (1994) A decision analysis of streptokinase plus heparin as compared with heparin alone for deep-vein thrombosis. *N Eng J Med*, 330(26):1864–9.

[158] Konstantinides, S., (2004) Should thrombolytic therapy be used in patients with pulmonary embolism? *Am J Cardiovasc Drugs*, 4(2):69–74.

[159] Buller, H.R., *et al.*, (2004) Antithrombotic therapy for venous thromboembolic disease: the Seventh ACCP Conference on Antithrombotic and Thrombolytic Therapy. *Chest*, 126(3 Suppl):401S–428S.

[160] Thabut, G., *et al.*, (2002) Thrombolytic therapy of pulmonary embolism: a meta-analysis. *J Am Coll Cardiol*, 40(9): p. 1660–7.

[161] Goldhaber, S.Z., (2002) Thrombolysis for pulmonary embolism. *N Eng J Med*, 347(15): p. 1131–2.

[162] Konstantinides, S., *et al.*, (1998) Comparison of alteplase versus heparin for resolution of major pulmonary embolism. *Am J Cardiol*, 82(8):966–70.

[163] Levine, M., *et al.*, (1990) A randomized trial of a single bolus dosage regimen of recombinant tissue plasminogen activator in patients with acute pulmonary embolism. *Chest*, 98(6): 1473–9.

[164] Tibbutt, D.A., *et al.*, (1974) Comparison by controlled clinical trial of streptokinase and heparin in treatment of life-threatening pulmonay embolism. *Br Med J*, 1(904): p. 343–7.

[165] Dalla-Volta, S., *et al.*, (1992) PAIMS 2: alteplase combined with heparin versus heparin in the treatment of acute pulmonary embolism. Plasminogen activator Italian multicenter study 2. *J Am Coll Cardiol*, 20(3):520–6.

[166] Ly, B., *et al.*, (1978) A controlled clinical trial of streptokinase and heparin in the treatment of major pulmonary embolism. *Acta Med Scand*, 203(6):465–70.

[167] The urokinase pulmonary embolism trial. A national cooperative study. *Circulation*, 1973. 47(2 Suppl):II1–108.

[168] The PIOPED Investigators. (1990) Tissue plasminogen activator for the treatment of acute pulmonary embolism. A collaborative study. *Chest*, 97(3):528–33.

[169] Urokinase-streptokinase embolism trial. Phase 2 results. A cooperative study. *JAMA*, 1974. 229(12):1606–13.

[170] Goldhaber, S.Z., *et al.*, (1988) Randomised controlled trial of recombinant tissue plasminogen activator versus urokinase in the treatment of acute pulmonary embolism. *Lancet*, 2(8606): 293–8.

[171] Goldhaber, S.Z., *et al.*, (1992) Recombinant tissue-type plasminogen activator versus a novel dosing regimen of urokinase in acute pulmonary embolism: a randomized controlled multicenter trial. *J Am Coll Cardiol*, 20(1):24–30.

[172] Meyer, G., *et al.*, (1992) Effects of intravenous urokinase versus alteplase on total pulmonary resistance in acute massive pulmonary embolism: a European multicenter double-blind trial. The European Cooperative Study Group for Pulmonary Embolism. *J Am Coll Cardiol*, 19(2): 239–45.

[173] Meneveau, N., *et al.*, (1998) Comparative efficacy of a two-hour regimen of streptokinase versus alteplase in acute massive pulmonary embolism: immediate clinical and hemodynamic outcome and one-year follow-up. *J Am Coll Cardiol*, 31(5):1057–63.

[174] Tebbe, U., *et al.*, (1999) Hemodynamic effects of double bolus reteplase versus alteplase infusion in massive pulmonary embolism. *Am Heart J*, 138(1 Pt 1):39–44.

[175] Kasper, W., *et al.*, (1997) Management strategies and determinants of outcome in acute major pulmonary embolism: results of a multicenter registry. *J Am Coll Cardiol*, 30(5): 1165–71.

[176] Goldhaber, S.Z., Visani, L., De Rosa, M., (1999) Acute pulmonary embolism: clinical outcomes in the International Cooperative Pulmonary Embolism Registry (ICOPER). *Lancet*, 353(9162):1386–9.

[177] Goldhaber, S.Z., (2002) Echocardiography in the management of pulmonary embolism. *Ann Intern Med*, 136(9):691–700.

[178] Pruszczyk, P., *et al.*, (2003) Cardiac troponin T monitoring identifies high-risk group of normotensive patients with acute pulmonary embolism. *Chest*, 123(6):1947–52.

[179] Konstantinides, S., *et al.*, (1986) Heparin plus alteplase compared with heparin alone in patients with submassive pulmonary embolism. *N Eng J Med*, 347(15):1143–50.

[180] Goldhaber, S.Z., *et al.*, Acute pulmonary embolism treated with tissue plasminogen activator. *Lancet*, 2(8512):886–9.

[181] Goldhaber, S.Z., *et al.*, (1993) Alteplase versus heparin in acute pulmonary embolism: randomised trial assessing right-ventricular function and pulmonary perfusion. *Lancet*, 341(8844):507–11.

[182] Goldhaber, S.Z., Agnelli, G., Levine, M.N., (1994) Reduced dose bolus alteplase vs conventional alteplase infusion for pulmonary embolism thrombolysis. An international multicenter randomized trial. The Bolus Alteplase Pulmonary Embolism Group. *Chest*, 106(3): 718–24.

[183] Daniels, L.B., *et al.*, (1997) Relation of duration of symptoms with response to thrombolytic therapy in pulmonary embolism. *Am J Cardiol*, 80(2):184–8.

[184] Douketis, J.D., *et al.*, (1998) Risk of fatal pulmonary embolism in patients with treated venous thromboembolism. *JAMA*, 279(6):458–62.

[185] Anderson, F.A., Jr., Spencer, F.A., (2003) Risk factors for venous thromboembolism. *Circulation*, 107(23 Suppl 1):I9–16.

[186] Bergqvist, D., (2003) Assessment of the risk and the prophylaxis of venous thromboembolism in surgical patients. *Pathophysiol Haemost Thromb*, 33(5–6):358–61.

[187] Hak, D.J., (2001) Prevention of venous thromboembolism in trauma and long bone fractures. *Curr Opin Pulm Med*, 7(5):338–43.

[188] Samama, M.M., *et al.*, (1999) A comparison of enoxaparin with placebo for the prevention of venous thromboembolism in acutely ill medical patients. Prophylaxis in Medical Patients with Enoxaparin Study Group. *N Eng J Med*, 341(11):793–800.

[189] Howell, M.D., Geraci, J.M., Knowlton, A.A., (2001) Congestive heart failure and outpatient risk of venous thromboembolism: a retrospective, case-control study. *J Clin Epidemiol*, 54(8): 810–6.

[190] Kleber, F.X., *et al.*, (2003) Randomized comparison of enoxaparin with unfractionated heparin for the prevention of venous thromboembolism in medical patients with heart failure or severe respiratory disease. *Am Heart J*, 145(4):614–21.

[191] Alikhan, R., *et al.*, (2003) Prevention of venous thromboembolism in medical patients with enoxaparin: a subgroup analysis of the MEDENOX study. *Blood Coagul Fibrinolysis*, 14(4):341–6.

[192] Kelly, J., *et al.*, (2004) Venous thromboembolism after acute ischemic stroke: a prospective study using magnetic resonance direct thrombus imaging. *Stroke*, 35(10):2320–5.

[193] Abelseth, G., *et al.*, (1996) Incidence of deep-vein thrombosis in patients with fractures of the lower extremity distal to the hip. *J Orthop Trauma*, 10(4):230–5.

[194] Kwong, L.M., (2004) Hip fracture and venous thromboembolism in the elderly. *J Surg Orthop Adv*, 13(3):139–48.

[195] Eriksson, B.I., Lassen, M.R., Colwell, C.W., Jr., (2004) Efficacy of fondaparinux for thromboprophylaxis in hip fracture patients. *J Arthroplasty*, 19(7 Suppl 2):78–81.

[196] Verso, M., *et al.*, (2005) Enoxaparin for the Prevention of Venous Thromboembolism Associated With Central Vein Catheter: A Double-Blind, Placebo-Controlled, Randomized Study in Cancer Patients. *J Clin Oncol*, 23:4057–62

[197] Gomes, M.P., Deitcher, S.R., (2004) Risk of venous thromboembolic disease associated with hormonal contraceptives and hormone replacement therapy: a clinical review. *Arch Intern Med*, 164(18):1965–76.

[198] Cosman, F., (2003) Selective estrogen-receptor modulators. *Clin Geriatr Med*, 19(2):371–9.

[199] Haas, S., (2003) Venous thromboembolism in medical patients—the scope of the problem. *Semin Thromb Hemost*, 29 (Suppl 1):17–21.

[200] Solem, C.A., *et al.*, (2004) Venous thromboembolism in inflammatory bowel disease. *Am J Gastroenterol*, 99(1):97–101.

[201] Ruggeri, M., *et al.*, (1993) Adult patients with the nephrotic syndrome: really at high risk for deep venous thromboembolism? Report of a series and review of the literature. *Haematologica*, 78(6 Suppl 2):47–51.

[202] De Stefano, V., (2004) Inherited thrombophilia and life-time risk of venous thromboembolism: is the burden reducible? *J Thromb Haemost*, 2(9):1522–5.

[203] Juul, K., *et al.*, (2004) Factor V Leiden and the risk for venous thromboembolism in the adult Danish population. *Ann Intern Med*, 140(5):330–7.

[204] Rintelen, C., *et al.*, (2001) Impact of the factor II: G20210A variant on the risk of venous thromboembolism in relatives from families with the factor V: R506Q mutation. *Eur J Haematol*, 67(3):165–9.

[205] Schulman, S., Svenungsson, E., Granqvist, S., (1998) Anticardiolipin antibodies predict early recurrence of thromboembolism and death among patients with venous thromboembolism following anticoagulant therapy. Duration of Anticoagulation Study Group. *Am J Med*, 104(4):332–8.

[206] Neville, C., *et al.*, (2003) Thromboembolic risk in patients with high titre anticardiolipin and multiple antiphospholipid antibodies. *Thromb Haemost*, 90(1):108–15.

[207] Folsom, A.R., *et al.*, (2002) Protein C, antithrombin, and venous thromboembolism incidence: a prospective population-based study. *Arterioscler Thromb Vasc Biol*, 22(6):1018–22.

[208] Engesser, L., *et al.*, (1987) Hereditary protein S deficiency: clinical manifestations. *Ann Intern Med*, 106(5):677–82.

[209] Gallus, A.S., (1987) Antithrombin III deficiency: clinical relevance and replacement therapy. *Dev Biol Stand*, 67:59–66.

[210] Gallus, A.S., Salzman, E.W., Hirsch, J., (1994) Prevention of VTE, in *Hemostasis and Thrombosis: Basic Principles and Clinical Practice*, (eds R.W. Colman, J. Hirsch, V.J. Marder), JB Lippincott: Philadelphia, PA, pp. 1331–45.

13 Heparin-Induced Thrombocytopenia

13.1 INTRODUCTION

UH remains the most widely utilized anticoagulant for the prevention and treatment of arterial and venous thrombotic disorders despite the emergence of effective, alternative agents such as the LMWHs and the DTIs. The central role of UH across the spectrum of CV diseases, ranging from its adjunctive role in patients receiving fibrinolytic therapy for an STEMI to its routine use in patients undergoing PCI and CABG surgery, has been established. Born out of the experience with UH, a number of limitations have been recognized including a risk of hemorrhagic complications, interpatient variability in anticoagulant response and the most feared complication of UH use, HIT [1].

Increased awareness of HIT and its presentation, improved diagnostic tests and an expanding armamentarium of anticoagulants that may be used to treat HIT and its associated thrombotic complications have improved but not eliminated the potentially devastating outcomes of this complication of UH use. Given the severity of immune-mediated HIT (HIT type II), this chapter will primarily focus on the incidence, pathogenesis, diagnosis, clinical manifestations and treatment of HIT type II (hereafter referred to as HIT). Attention will be also given to non-immune HIT (HIT type I) where appropriate.

13.2 INCIDENCE

HIT TYPE I

The reported estimates of the frequency of HIT vary widely. Approximately 10–20% of patients receiving UH will experience a fall in platelet count to less than the normal range or a 50% fall in the platelet count within the normal range beginning within the first few days of therapy and resolving with continued heparin therapy [2]. The majority of these cases are accounted for by a benign form of HIT, termed HIT type I (Table 13.1).

HIT TYPE II

The incidence of true immune-mediated HIT has been variable in the literature and occurs with a frequency of 0.3–3% in patients exposed to heparin for more than four days (Table 13.1) [3–6]. In a trial of 665 patients assigned to therapy with either UH or LMWH for prophylaxis of VTE following hip surgery, HIT developed in 2.7% of patients treated

Management Strategies in Antithrombotic Therapy Arman T. Askari, Adrian W. Messerli and A. Michael Lincoff

Table 13.1 Characteristics of Type I and Type II HIT. Adapted from Brieger *et al.* [138]

	TYPE I	TYPE II
Frequency	10–20%	0.3–3.0%
Timing of onset	1–4 days	5–10 days
Nadir of platelet count	100,000/μL	30,000–60,000/μL
Antibody mediated	No	Yes
Thromboembolic complications	None	Up to 80%
Hemorrhagic complications	None	Rare
Management	Observation	Cessation of heparin Alternative anticoagulation Adjunctive therapies

with UH but in none of those receiving LMWH [3]. The incidence of heparin-dependent IgG antibodies was higher in the patients receiving UH (7.8% vs 2.2% with LMWH). In addition, HIT has been shown to occur in hospitalized medical patients (0.8%) [5], critical care patients (0.39%) [7], and in patients undergoing cardiac surgical procedures (2–5%) [8] among others, with the greatest frequency occurring in surgical followed by medical patients.

The variability in the reported frequency of HIT is strongly influenced by the clinical situation, the heparin formulation used, the frequency of drug use and the test used for detecting heparin-dependent antibodies (Table 13.2). In a study of 305 patients, heparin-dependent IgG antibodies were more likely to form in patients undergoing cardiac surgery than orthopedic patients, as well as in orthopedic patients who received UH instead of LMWH [8]. Paradoxically, among patients in whom antibodies did form, clinical HIT was more frequent in the patients undergoing orthopedic procedures. As part of the syndrome of HIT, approximately 50% of patients who develop HIT will also experience a thrombotic event [9]. Factors associated with an increase risk of HIT with thrombosis include undergoing an orthopedic procedure, a lower nadir of the platelet count and higher titers of the heparin–platelet factor 4 (PF4) antibodies [10]. Issues that may influence the reported incidence of HIT include, but are not limited to, the route of heparin administration (SC vs IV), the heparin formulation (bovine vs porcine; UH vs LMWH), early vs delayed thrombocytopenia and the frequency of thrombotic events in those that develop HIT.

Route of heparin exposure and HIT

That patients receiving IV UH for the treatment of VTE may develop HIT is well established. However, the risk imparted by SC UH for the prophylaxis of VTE is less well defined. In a prospective cohort study of 598 consecutive medical patients receiving subcutaneous UH, the incidence of HIT was 0.8% (95% CI:0.1–1.6%) [5]. All five HIT cases belonged to the subgroup of patients receiving heparin for prophylactic indications; three of the five patients developed thromboembolic complications.

Although most patients developing HIT have received IV or SC UH therapy for the treatment or prophylaxis of a thrombotic event, the amount of heparin required to cause HIT may be quite small. Occasional patients have developed this disorder after exposure to

Table 13.2 Characteristics influencing Type II HIT frequency

Characteristic
Early vs late HIT
Type I HIT usually occurs early
Patient population studied
Related to degree of underlying platelet activation
Surgical >Medical >Obstetric
Route of heparin exposure
IV >SC
Type of heparin
UH >LMWH
Bovine lung heparin >Porcine mucosal heparin
Duration of heparin use
HIT typically begins on days 5–10
Decreased frequency with heparin exposure >10 days
Dose of heparin
Typically larger doses more immunogenic
Small doses (~250 U) may induce HIT (Heparin flushes; CVC associated HIT)

CVC = central venous catheters

minimal amounts of UH (~250 U) during heparin flushes of central venous catheters [11–13] or after the use of heparin-coated central venous catheters [14].

Type of heparin and HIT

Several trials assessed the incidence of HIT following either bovine lung or porcine mucosal heparin administration [15–20]. Taken together, these trials suggest that the risk for developing HIT is higher with bovine lung compared with porcine mucosal heparin. One plausible reason for this finding may relate to the higher sulfate/disaccharide ratio in bovine compared with porcine heparin [21] and the associated greater platelet activation and greater potential for PF4 release [22].

Anecdotal reports indicate that HIT can occur during therapy with LMWH [23, 24]. However, the risk of HIT with LMWH use is substantially lower than that with UH use, in part related to its smaller size and less efficient interaction with PF4 [25]. Despite the development of HIT antibodies in response to LMWH use, clinically evident HIT has been an infrequent occurrence [3, 26, 27]. One study evaluated the differential prevalence and functionality of anti-heparin–PF4 antibodies in plasma samples obtained from 111 clinically suspected HIT patients enrolled in two clinical trials that compared UH with the LMWH clivarin for the treatment or prophylaxis of DVTs [27]. Although anti-heparin–PF4 antibodies were noted in the serum of patients treated with both UH and LMWH, the incidence was greater with UH and the anti-heparin–PF4 antibodies from patients treated with LMWH were deemed non-functional by platelet activation assays. Furthermore, no clinical events consistent with HIT were seen in patients treated with LMWH despite 2.2% of the patients exhibiting serum anti-heparin–PF4 antibodies [3]. A plausible explanation for this 'non-reactivity' may relate to the molecular weight of the various heparin fractions that complex with heparin–PF4, as those less than 5 kDa have been shown to be incapable of inducing platelet activation and thrombocytopenia despite their ability to induce HIT antibodies.

Early- and delayed-onset HIT

The occurrence of thrombocytopenia within the first few days of initiating therapy with heparin can usually distinguish between type I and type II HIT. However, that immune-mediated HIT can occur earlier than the customary 5–10 days following initiation of heparin has been reported [28]. A rapid fall in platelet count may occur upon initiation of heparin therapy in patients with circulating anti-heparin–PF4 antibodies. These antibodies have been shown to fall to undetectable levels at a median time of 50–85 days, depending on the assay used, relating to the risk of HIT following a recent exposure to heparin (about 100 days) [29, 30].

On the other hand, immune-mediated HIT predominantly occurs within 5–10 days following initiation of heparin therapy, with the risk of HIT diminishing during continued heparin administration for longer durations. This may relate to the lower incidence of anti-heparin–PF4 antibody development in patients with more than 10 days of uninterrupted heparin use [3]. Nevertheless, a syndrome of delayed-onset HIT, HIT following cessation of heparin therapy, has been described [31] and can result in devastating consequences if clinically unrecognized [32–34].

Frequency of thrombosis in patients with HIT

Owing to the associated platelet activation and vascular endothelial injury, the development of thrombocytopenia due to HIT is more often associated with thrombotic, rather than hemorrhagic, complications [35]. However, the relationship between the development of HIT and the frequency of thromboembolic events is not absolute. A retrospective analysis of 127 patients with serologically confirmed HIT revealed that approximately two-thirds developed a thrombotic event with more frequent venous (61%) compared with arterial (14%) thromboses.[9] Of the patient cohort with initially recognized thrombocytopenia, the subsequent 30-day risk of thrombosis was approximately 53%. These data were consistent with earlier reports of thrombotic events occurring in patients with HIT [36, 37]. It is of note that the high frequency of thrombotic events reported in these early studies may relate to the retrospective nature of the analyses.

More contemporary prospective reports suggest that the frequency of thrombotic events may be less and is related to the clinical setting, with higher frequencies being observed in clinical conditions associated with more robust platelet activation [8, 35, 38–40]. In a study of 744 patients, the probability of clinically evident HIT was higher in patients following orthopedic surgery (52.6% vs 5% with cardiac surgery, p-value $= 0.001$) despite a lower incidence of HIT antibody formation (3.2% vs 20% with cardiac surgery, p-value $= 0.01$), supporting a dissociation between the frequency of HIT-IgG formation and the risk for HIT that is dependent on the patient population [8]. Consistent with a predisposition for the development of HIT-associated thrombosis, 89.9% of HIT patients receiving heparin for thromboprophylaxis following orthopedic surgery experienced a thrombotic event [3]. A lower frequency of HIT-associated thrombosis (9.7%) has been associated with central venous catheter placement in patients with HIT, suggesting an interaction between local vascular injury and the systemic hypercoagulability of this syndrome [39]. Although less frequent than previously reported, HIT-associated thrombotic events still occur with significant frequency (~30–80%), are related to the underlying clinical situation and are associated with substantial morbidity and mortality.

13.3 PATHOGENESIS

HIT TYPE I

HIT type I is a non-immune-mediated thrombocytopenia resulting from a direct interaction of UH with platelets, inducing platelet activation, aggregation and removal by the reticuloendothelial system [41, 42].

HIT TYPE II

Type II HIT appears to be immune-mediated as evidenced by the formation of antibodies to the heparin–PF4 complex [43]. However, the pathogenesis of HIT is not simply due to the generation of antibodies to the heparin–PF4 complex and subsequent platelet activation, but it also involves endothelial cell activation, interaction with monocytes and inflammation (Table 13.3) [44–46]. The concomitant activation of platelets and endothelial cells coupled with the inflammatory response and enhanced thrombin generation are potential mechanisms for the observed propensity for thrombosis in HIT [46]. Although less common than the more benign form (HIT type I), HIT can result in clinically devastating sequelae [47, 48].

Table 13.3 Components involved in the pathogenesis of HIT. Adapted from Walenga *et al.* [46]

Component	Contribution
Platelets	Platelet activation
	Granule release
	Express P-selectin
	Up-regulate fibrinogen receptor expression
	Platelet aggregation
	Platelet microparticle generation
Endothelial Cells	HIT antibodies bind to ECs
	HIT antibodies activate ECs
	Release coagulation proteins and cytokines
	Up-regulate expression of adhesion molecules
	Increased TF expression
	Increased TM in circulation
	Microvascular ECs directly activated by HIT antibodies
	Platelets bind to ECs
	Monocytes bind to ECs in presence of HIT antibodies
Leukocytes	HIT antibodies induce neutrophil and monocytes interaction with platelets
	HIT antibody activates monocytes
	Release TF – procoagulant state
	Increase expression of IL-8
Inflammation	Monocytes activated in presence of HIT antibody
	Increased circulating cytokines and other inflammatory markers in patients with HIT
HIT antibodies	Heterogeneous in structure and function
	Predominantly IgG
	HIT with IgA and IgM reported

EC = endothelial cell; Ig = immunoglobulin; IL = interleukin; TF = tissue factor; TM = thrombomodulin.

Formation of the heparin–PF4 Complex

Platelet factor 4, a highly positively charged tetrameric glycoprotein found in the α-granules of platelets, is present in low levels in the plasma with its plasma concentration increasing substantially following platelet activation, such as seen with surgery, cardiopulmonary bypass, cancer and IHD [49–52]. When released by platelets, PF4 is a complex of eight tetramers linked to a chondroitin-containing proteoglycan. The PF4 complexes can also bind to endothelial cell proteoglycans. With its greater affinity for the PF4 complexes, heparin binds to and releases PF4 from endothelial cells into the circulation.

Binding of heparin to PF4 also induces a conformational change in PF4 rendering it antigenic [53]. The immunogenicity of heparin–PF4 complexes is strictly dependent on the respective concentrations of heparin and PF4, with optimal interaction occurring at a 1:1 ratio of the two substances [54]. In most clinical circumstances, heparin is present in excess concentrations relative to PF4, resulting in less immunogenicity. However, in certain clinical situations associated with platelet activation, such as orthopedic surgery and cardiopulmonary bypass, the concentration of PF4 may reach stoichiometric levels, spawning antigenic heparin–PF4 complexes and resulting in an increased risk of HIT in these patients [55].

Although the primary antigen recognized by HIT antibodies is the heparin–PF4 complex [56–59], the antibody is not specific for heparin and has been shown to react with other sulfated polysaccharides capable of inducing a similar conformational change in PF4 [60]. The binding of polysaccharides to PF4 is primarily dependent on their chain length and degree of sulfation [61]. For example, the lower risk of HIT with LMWH or the pentasaccharide anticoagulants can be attributed to their minimal interactions with PF4 resulting from their shorter lengths.

Response to the heparin–PF4 Complex

Studies, primarily performed *in vitro,* have demonstrated that the key mediator of HIT is the interaction between HIT antibodies, the heparin–PF4 complex and the Fc receptors on platelets. HIT antibodies bind the heparin–PF4 complex via the Fab portion and cause platelet activation via binding of the Fc portion of the antibody to the platelet FcγRII receptors [62]. Cross-linking of the platelet FcγRII receptors by the antibody–heparin–PF4 complex initiates a cascade of platelet activation, thromboxane biosynthesis, secretion of platelet granular contents including PF4, formation of additional heparin–PF4 complexes, further binding of these complexes by HIT antibody and, ultimately, platelet aggregation (Figure 13.1) [63]. These activated platelet aggregates are removed from the circulation prematurely, resulting in thrombocytopenia and frequently associated thrombosis. That this concept of the pathogenesis of HIT occurs *in vivo* has recently been supported using a transgenic mouse model of HIT [64]. Although platelet activation is integral to the pathogenesis of HIT, it does not occur as an isolated physiologic response. Interactions with endothelial cells and resultant activation may also contribute to the pathogenesis of HIT.

Endothelial cell involvement in HIT

Immune-mediated endothelial cell (EC) injury may play a role in the pathogenesis of HIT. When incubated with human umbilical vein EC (HUVEC), sera from patients with HIT

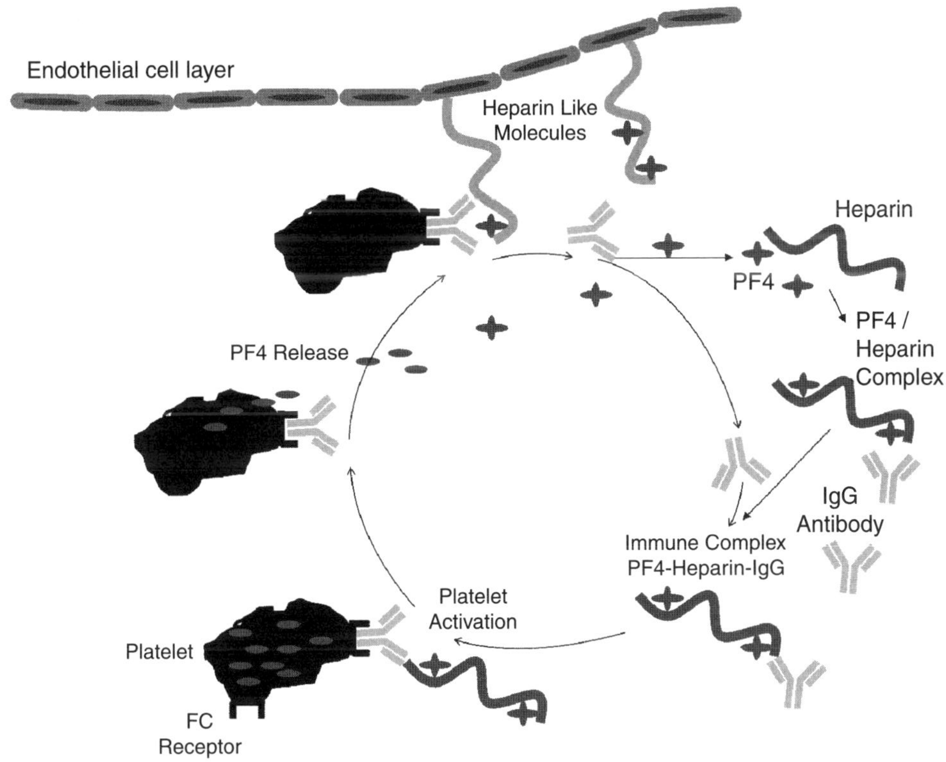

Figure 13.1 Pathogenesis of HIT: Cross-linking of the platelet FcγII receptors by the antibody-heparin/PF4 complex initiates a cascade of platelet activation, thromboxane biosynthesis, secretion of platelet granular contents including PF4, formation of additional heparin/PF4 complexes, further binding of these complexes by HIT antibody, and ultimately, platelet aggregation. A full colour version of this figure can be found in the colour plate section of this book.

deposited higher than normal amounts of IgG and IgA on the HUVEC and stimulated production of tissue factor [65]. In addition, IgG antibodies purified from HIT sera interacted with HUVEC expressing heparin-like glycosaminoglycans only in the presence of PF4 [58]. Furthermore, in the presence of platelets, sera from patients with HIT induced endothelial cell expression of E-selectin, intracellular adhesion molecule (ICAM)-I, vascular adhesion molecule (VCAM)-1, and tissue factor, and the release of IL-1β, IL-6 and PAI-1 [66]. The role endothelial cells play *in vivo*, however, remains to be more clearly elucidated.

Immunoglobulins involved in HIT

In the majority of cases anti-heparin–PF4 antibodies become detectable after 5–7 days of heparin therapy. HIT may also develop sooner than the 'customary' time frame, most often in patients pre-exposed to heparin. The subtype of HIT antibodies implicated in the more than 80% of clinically evident cases is IgG [27, 67]. Although other immunoglobulins (IgA and IgM) have been identified in a minority of cases, the pathogenesis of HIT in this setting remains poorly defined, as platelets do not have receptors for these immunoglobulin subtypes

[68]. Various characteristics including serum concentration, affinity for the heparin–PF4 complex and the specific epitopes on the heparin–PF4 complex may explain, in part, the differential pathogenicity of the different immunoglobulin subtypes [69, 70].

In a substantial minority of patients, pre-existing antibodies to antigens other than the heparin–PF4 complex have been implicated in HIT pathogenesis [71]. Antibodies targeted to PF-4-related chemokines such as interleukin-8 (IL-8) and neutrophil-activating-peptide-2 (NAP-2) may, in the presence of heparin, target these chemokines to platelets, neutrophils and endothelial cells, facilitating immune injury [72]. This could then result in interactions between cells forming cellular aggregates that could lead to vessel occlusion.

13.4 CLINICAL MANIFESTATIONS

It is not uncommon for patients receiving heparin for the treatment or prevention of thrombosis to develop a thrombocytopenia (defined as platelet count <150,000/μL). The difficulty imparted by this clinical scenario lies in the need to decide whether this is related to HIT or arises from an alternative condition. In essence, thrombocytopenia with or without thrombosis during heparin treatment does not necessarily indicate a diagnosis of HIT. A basic understanding of the pleomorphic nature of HIT is integral to differentiating between the two scenarios.

HIT TYPE I

Type I HIT is associated with a mild thrombocytopenia usually within the first few days of heparin therapy. The nadir of the platelet count rarely decreases to a value less than 100,000/μL and usually recovers during continued heparin administration [73]. This type of HIT has not been associated with any untoward clinical consequences.

HIT TYPE II

The hallmark of HIT remains the paradoxic venous and arterial thrombosis in the setting of thrombocytopenia (Table 13.4). As stated above, HIT can be difficult to distinguish from other etiologies of thrombocytopenia. In addition, confirmatory laboratory tests are seldom immediately available. Characteristic features of HIT that may assist in differentiating HIT from other causes of thrombocytopenia include the timing of the onset of thrombocytopenia, the magnitude of the thrombocytopenia and the occurrence of paradoxic thrombosis in the setting of thrombocytopenia. Furthermore, in contrast to other drug-induced immune thrombocytopenia syndromes, HIT is rarely associated with bleeding.

THROMBOCYTOPENIA

Timing of thrombocytopenia

The typical onset of thrombocytopenia, defined as the day the platelet count begins to fall, in the majority of patients with HIT is between days 5 and 10 (inclusive) during an initial exposure to heparin treatment [3, 29]. In a recent study of patients with serologically

Table 13.4 Clinical manifestations of Type II HIT. Adapted from Warkentin [139]

Manifestation	Comment
Thrombocytopenia	
Timing	Typically 5–10 days during heparin therapy May occur earlier in patients with recent (<100 days) exposure Delayed onset (~30 days) after heparin exposure may occur in up to 53%
Severity	Mean nadir platelet count 50,000/μL Rarely <15,000/ μL
Duration	With treatment, platelet count usually recovers in 5–7 days
Venous thrombosis	
DVT	~50% New, progressive, or recurrent Lower limb, often bilateral Upper limb, at site of CVC Phlegmasia cerulea dolens
Warfarin-induced limb gangrene	5–10% of DVT treated with warfarin
PE	~25% With or without r-sided cardiac thrombi
Cerebral dural sinus thrombosis	Rare*
Adrenal hemorrhagic infarction	Rare* Bilateral-acute or chronic adrenal failure Unilateral
Arterial thrombosis	
Aortic or iliofemoral thrombosis	Limb ischemia – 5–10% SC infarction – rare*
Acute stroke	3–5%
MI	3–5%
Miscellaneous thrombosis	Renal, mesenteric, upper limb – rare
Intracardiac thrombosis	Rare*
Miscellaneous syndromes of HIT	
Heparin-induced skin lesions	10–20% At heparin injection sites Erythematous plaques, skin necrosis
Warfarin-induced skin necrosis	Rare* Skin necrosis involving central sites
Acute systemic reactions	~25% Occur following IV heparin bolus in sensitized patients Inflammatory: Fever, chills, flushing CV: Tachycardia, HTN, cardiopulmonary arrest GI: N, V, D Neurological: Transient global amnesia, HA

* <3%

CVC = central venous catheter; D = diarrhea; GI = gastrointestinal; HA = headache; HTN = hypertension; N=nausea; SC = spinal cord, V = vomiting

confirmed HIT, the typical onset of 5 to 10 days was seen in the majority, irrespective of prior heparin exposure [29]. Although previously thought to be related to an anamnestic response, the occurrence of a more rapid thrombocytopenia (within two days of heparin initiation) has since been suggested to be more closely related to the persistence of HIT antibodies [29]. All of the patients that experienced a more rapid fall (median 10.5 h) in platelet count had been exposed to heparin within the prior 100 days. Thus a rapid fall in platelet count following heparin administration is unlikely to represent HIT unless the patient has received heparin within 100 days.

Although not encountered frequently, delayed-onset HIT, HIT after cessation of heparin therapy, has been described [31, 74]. The incidence of this phenomenon is not known, although in a retrospective study of 260 patients with HIT, 14 cases of delayed-onset HIT, occurring at a median time of 14 days (range: 9–40 days) after onset of treatment with UH were identified [74]. Predictors of delayed-onset HIT following cessation of heparin therapy include high titers of anti-heparin–PF4 antibodies and greater IgG-induced heparin-dependent and heparin-independent platelet activation [31].

Severity of thrombocytopenia

In HIT, the thrombocytopenia is usually moderately severe, with platelet counts falling gradually to a mean nadir of 50,000/μL, although platelet counts below 15,000/μL are rare [75]. In the setting of elevated baseline platelet counts, a decrease of more than 50% may occur with overall counts remaining within the normal range. This contrasts with a more 'typical' drug-induced thrombocytopenia during which platelet counts drop precipitously to levels less than 10,000/μL [76].

Duration of thrombocytopenia in HIT

In patients with HIT, platelet counts generally do not recover unless heparin in discontinued. Thereafter, the platelet counts usually recover over 5–7 days. In patients with severe HIT, the platelet counts may take weeks to recover to normal levels.

THROMBOSIS

Timing of thrombosis

HIT is associated with thrombotic rather than hemorrhagic complications, even in the rare case of severe thrombocytopenia [75]. Although thrombotic complications are to some extent related to the severity of the thrombocytopenia [9], the occurrence of any event cannot be predicted from the platelet count alone [77]. Although HIT-related thrombotic events may occur at any time in relation to heparin use, they usually present in the following ways. Thrombosis can be the presenting clinical manifestation of HIT, occurring early during the initial decrease in platelet count [78]. At the other end of the spectrum, HIT-related events may occur after complete recovery of platelet counts and may represent a sub-clinical thrombosis that was present during the thrombocytopenia [9].

Thrombotic complications of HIT may also occur during the phase of platelet recovery despite heparin discontinuation. Discontinuation of heparin therapy in patients with HIT does not eliminate the risk of subsequent thrombotic events. The incidence of thrombosis following heparin cessation in patients with serologically confirmed HIT ranges between, approximately, 38% and 50% at 30 days and does not necessarily diminish with early heparin discontinuation [9, 79]. There is a substantial event rate (6.1% per day) in the interval between the diagnosis of HIT and the initiation of an alternative anticoagulant [80]. The potentially devastating consequences of HIT-related thrombosis and the protracted period of risk despite cessation of heparin advocate the initiation of alternative anticoagulant measures even in isolated HIT.

Localization of thrombosis

The localization of thrombosis in patients with HIT is strongly influenced by clinical factors such as the post-operative state, atherosclerosis and the presence and location of intravascular catheters (injury). For example, arterial thromboses were primarily seen in patients with cardio-vascular disease whereas venous thromboses were primarily seen in post-operative patients [37]. Further supporting the clinical predisposition to thrombus localization in this patient population, central venous catheters are integral to the development of upper limb DVT [39].

Venous thrombosis in HIT

Overall, venous thrombosis appears to occur with greater frequency than arterial thrombosis in patients with HIT. Importantly, the association between HIT and thromboses increases with the severity and atypical nature of thrombosis [3]. The major manifestations of venous thrombosis are DVT and PE [9]. In addition, cerebral sinus thrombosis [81], venous limb gangrene [82] and adrenal hemorrhagic infarction [83] have been seen to complicate HIT.

Arterial thrombosis in HIT

Although less common than venous thrombosis, arterial thrombosis can lead to a variety of clinical manifestations including stroke [40], MI [33], limb ischemia from peripheral arterial occlusion [84] or organ infarction (mesentery, kidney). Micro-vascular thrombosis has also been associated with HIT [85]. The name 'white clot syndrome' arises from the 'white,' platelet-rich thrombi seen in arterial thrombosis.

ADDITIONAL COMPLICATIONS OF HIT

Skin necrosis

Heparin-induced skin necrosis is a well-described complication of either IV or SC UH [82, 86]. Affected areas are usually fat-rich, such as the abdomen, as in warfarin-induced necrosis; however, the distal extremities and the nose can also be involved. The appearance of erythema is followed by purpura and hemorrhage leading to necrosis. Although the lesions appear similar to warfarin-induced skin necrosis, deficiencies of the natural anticoagulants are not present. Affected patients develop heparin-dependent antibodies but most do not experience thrombocytopenia.

Acute systemic reactions

Acute systemic reactions, occurring in ~25% of patients at risk, refers to a variety of symptoms and signs ranging from fevers and chills to tachycardia, tachypnea, chest pain and fatal cardiovascular collapse, or to a transient global amnesia occurring within 5–30 min following an IV heparin bolus in a patient with circulating HIT antibodies [75, 87]. These syndromes are associated with an abrupt transient decrease in the platelet count, mandating a ready evaluation of the platelet count once symptoms occur. These syndromes resemble platelet transfusion reactions [88] and are thought to be related to a cytokine-mediated transient cellular activation.

Heparin resistance

Difficulty in achieving and maintaining therapeutic anticoagulation with heparin may be the result of HIT-associated thrombosis. This occurs in a number of clinical circumstances in which extensive thrombosis exists, and is not specific for HIT [89]. The pathophysiology is thought to be related to neutralization of heparin by PF4 released by activated platelets or related to platelet-derived microparticles [90].

13.5 DIAGNOSIS

Although several tests for HIT are available, there is no absolute 'gold standard' [91]. Therefore, the diagnosis of HIT should initially be made on the basis of clinical grounds, owing to the usual delay in turn-around time of the currently available laboratory tests. HIT is usually suspected in patients on heparin treatment who develop thrombocytopenia, or even a normal platelet count if it has decreased by more than 50% from a prior value, which resolves after discontinuation of heparin and in whom other etiologies have been excluded [92, 93]. Once suspected, the diagnosis of HIT is supported by laboratory testing which can be divided into two types; platelet activation assays and antigen assays (Table 13.5).

FUNCTIONAL (PLATELET ACTIVATION) ASSAYS

Serotonin release assay

The serotonin release assay (SRA) remains the current reference standard for the laboratory diagnosis of HIT [94]. In this assay, radiolabeled, washed platelets from donors with a known positive SRA are incubated with patient sera in the presence of two different doses of heparin. The SRA test is considered positive if platelets release ^{14}C-serotonin at therapeutic (0.1 U/mL) and not high (100 U/mL) heparin concentrations. Although shown to possess a high sensitivity and specificity for HIT, the demanding nature of the test and the need for radioactive material preclude widespread laboratory utilization of this technique. Thus, this assay is primarily employed by reference laboratories to confirm the diagnosis of HIT. Two alternative, non-radioactive, SRAs have been developed that have demonstrated robust sensitivity and specificity [95, 96]; however, the utilization of these tests remains limited.

Heparin-induced platelet aggregation

The heparin-induced platelet aggregation (HIPA) assay remains the most widely used diagnostic test for HIT given its cost, relative ease and readily available results (within 2–3 h). In this assay, the aggregation of either washed donor platelets or platelet-rich

Table 13.5 Laboratory tests utilized in HIT

Functional assays
Serotonin release assay (SRA)
"Gold" Standard
Not widely available
Requires use of radioactive materials
Quantifies platelet activation by assessing amount of ^{14}C-serotonin release from dense granules of activated platelets [94]
Non-radiolabeled techniques of serotonin quantification exist [95, 96]
HIPA
Easier to perform than SRA.
Less costly than SRA
Widely available
Rapid results (~2–3 h)
Visual assessment of platelet aggregation
Specificity >90% [97]
Immunoassays
Target heparin/PF4 complex
Identify presence of HIT antibodies
More sensitive but less specific than platelet activation assays [140]
Widely available
Heparin/PF4 Enzyme immunoassay (EIA)
Surface-bound antigen [99, 100]
Fluid-phase antigen [104]
Particle gel immunoassay [141]
Target PF4-polyvinylsulfonate complexes
PF4-polyvinylsulfonate-EIA [142]

plasma (PRP) is assessed in the presence of patient serum and either low (0.5 U/mL) or high (100 U/mL) doses of heparin. A positive test includes low background aggregation with no added heparin, aggregation with the addition of a low concentration of heparin and absent aggregation with high heparin concentrations. When measured in the setting of appropriate positive and negative controls the HIPA assay demonstrates a specificity greater than 90% [97]. However, HIPA suffers from lack of sensitivity, an issue that can be somewhat ameliorated with the use of washed donor platelets instead of PRP [71].

IMMUNOASSAYS

Several different types of immunoassays exist including the solid-phase enzyme-linked immunosorbent assay (heparin–PF4 ELISA), the PF4-polyvinylsulfonate antigen assay, the fluid-phase enzyme immunoassay and the particle gel immunoassay. Essentially all are based on basic immunoassay techniques with specific nuances. Detailed descriptions of each are beyond the scope of this chapter and the reader is referred to the referenced book chapter for further review [98]. As an example, the heparin–PF4 ELISA will be discussed.

Heparin–PF4 ELISA

The utility of this immunoassay lies in its widespread availability, rapid analysis and greater sensitivity than the platelet activation assays for diagnosing HIT. In this test, heparin–PF4 complexes are coated onto a microtiter plate to which patient serum is added. The presence of HIT antibodies will be determined through the addition of a secondary antibody. Despite its sensitivity, the clinical utility of this assay remains to be determined given its low specificity. A substantial percentage of patients in whom the test is positive do not exhibit clinical characteristics of HIT [99]. However, the specificity may be improved by testing only for the IgG immunoglobulin subtype [100].

Whereas the antigen assays serve to identify patients with HIT antibodies, the platelet activation assays serve to identify patients in whom these HIT antibodies are clinically significant. Thus the two tests can be used to provide additive information in patients at high risk or with clinically evident HIT.

13.6 PREVENTION

The key to preventing the development of HIT and its associated complications is minimizing a patient's exposure to heparin. Often overlooked strategies include limiting heparin duration to less than 5 days and initiating warfarin therapy early in patients requiring long-term anticoagulation. Furthermore, the use of alternative anticoagulants such as LMWH, where appropriate, has been associated with a decreased risk of HIT [26, 101]. Additional measures that may avoid HIT-related complications include avoiding substitution of LMWH for UH after HIT develops and initiating warfarin therapy with an overlapping alternative anticoagulant such as a DTI. Given the substantial risk of thrombosis in patients with HIT, there is a substantial need for alternative anticoagulants in this syndrome.

13.7 TREATMENT

HIT TYPE I

Given the benign nature of this type of HIT, there is no need to discontinue heparin therapy. However, in certain circumstances the differentiation between type I and type II HIT may be difficult. In these cases, heparin should be discontinued and the patient should be managed as if they had type II HIT.

HIT TYPE II

The central dogma for the treatment of HIT is the discontinuation of all forms of heparin exposure, including heparin anticoagulation, heparin line flushes, use of heparin-coated central venous catheters, etc. Absolute heparin avoidance is the rule. However, discontinuation of heparin as the sole method of managing patients with HIT is contraindicated given the high risk of subsequent thrombosis within 30 days in such patients [9]. The use of concomitant anticoagulation with an agent that inhibits thrombin activity or generation is recommended. If patients require long-term anticoagulation, warfarin remains the drug of choice. However, it is important to remember that initiation of warfarin must be overlapped with one of the alternative anticoagulants, given the risk of venous limb gangrene when initiated alone in these patients [82]. The use of LMWHs as alternative anticoagulants in patients with acute HIT should be avoided given the 80–100% *in vitro* cross-reactivity in this situation.

Three agents, danaparoid, lepirudin and argatroban, have been the major treatment options to date for patients with HIT (Table 13.6). Additional agents, such as bivalirudin and the pentasaccharide fondaparinux, may become more important in the future, but data assessing their utility in this situation remain limited 105]. Although no prospective randomized control trial exists comparing the various alternative anticoagulants that are recommended for use in patients with HIT, various pharmacokinetic or pharmacodynamic differences between them may favor the use of one over another depending on the clinical circumstances.

Danaparoid

Danaparoid (Orgaran ®), FDA-approved for the prophylaxis of DVT during hip replacement surgery, is low-molecular-weight heparinoid, and consists of a mixture of heparin (84%), dermatan (12%) and chondroitin (4%) sulfates [106]. Danaparoid exerts its anticoagulant effect primarily by interacting with factor Xa, possesses a low tendency to cause bleeding and has minimal effects on the fibrinolytic system. In addition, danaparoid has a long plasma half-life and is primarily cleared via the kidneys. Danaparoid has a low cross-reactivity rate with heparin-associated antiplatelet antibodies (~10%), representing a significant advantage over LMWH as a potential replacement agent for UH in patients with HIT [107].

Although danaparoid is not FDA-approved for use in patients with HIT, an extensive experience of its use in patients has accrued [107–110]. In the only multicenter randomized comparative trial of alternative anticoagulants in HIT, danaparoid was associated with a greater effective clinical response than dextran in patients with HIT plus thrombosis, without an increased risk of bleeding 111]. In a worldwide compassionate-use program involving a total of 667 patients with HIT, a 93% clinical success rate with an infrequent rate of persistent or recurrent thrombocytopenia or the development of new thromboembolic events was observed [112]. In addition, a lower mortality rate was observed in patients who were treated with danaparoid compared with those who were not (10.4% vs 23.5%). IV therapy with danaparoid sodium is accomplished with an initial bolus dose of 2500 U, followed by a continuous infusion of 400 U/h for 4 h, 300 U/h for 4 h, and then 150 U/h thereafter, with dose adjustment based on serum anti-factor Xa levels.

Limitations of danaparoid include its long half-life, the need to monitor factor Xa levels and the lack of an effective antidote for its anticoagulant effect. Although cross-reactivity with HIT antibodies is infrequent, the phenomenon has been demonstrated. Therefore, it seems prudent to assess for HIT antibody cross-reactivity prior to initiating this therapy in patients. Despite these limitations, danaparoid appears to be an effective and well-tolerated replacement agent for UH in many patients with HIT who require further anticoagulation. Unfortunately, production of danaparoid has ceased owing to a shortage of drug substance in the United States.

Lepirudin

Lepirudin (Refludan ®) is a recombinant DTI that possesses no cross-antigenicity in HIT and is FDA-approved for the treatment of HIT complicated by thrombosis. Lepirudin exerts its anticoagulant effect by binding irreversibly with the active center and substrate recognition site of both clot-bound and soluble thrombin (Chapter 7) [113]. Lepirudin is exclusively cleared by the kidneys, decreasing its utility in patients with CKD.

Table 13.6 Alternative anticoagulants for the treatment of HIT

Anticoagulant	Class of agent	Dosage	Monitoring	$T_{1/2}$	Metabolism	Bleeding risk	FDA approved for HIT	Comment
Danaparoid sodium (Organ)	Low-molecular weight heparinoid	Bolus: 2500 U Infusion: 400 U/h for 4 h; 300 U/h for 4 h; 150 U/h monitoring for anti-factor Xa	Anti-factor Xa levels (0.5–0.8 anti-Xa units/mL)	~25 h	Renal	++	No	Withdrawn from US market due to rare *in vivo* cross-reactivity
Lepirudin (Refludan)	DTI	Bolus: 0.4 mg/kg Infusion: 0.15 mg/kg per h	aPTT (goal 1.5–2.5 × control)	~80 min	Renal	+/++	Yes: for treatment of HIT-related thrombosis	High incidence of anti-hirudin antibodies and risk of anaphylaxis. $T_{1/2}$ rises with renal insufficiency
Argatroban (Novastan)	DTI	2 μg/kg per min; no bolus	aPTT (goal 1.5–3.0 × control)	40–50 min	Hepatic	+/++	Yes: for prevention and treatment of HIT-related thrombosis	Argatroban increases INR. Target higher INR when overlapping with warfarin. No need for dose adjustment in renal insufficiency, but contraindicated with hepatic disease
Investigational Drugs for HIT								
Bivalirudin (Angiomax)	DTI	0.15–0.20 mg/kg per h; no bolus	aPTT (goal 1.5–2.5 × control)	25 min	Enzymatic >renal	+/++	No	Anecdotal reports in HIT. FDA approved for PCI (non-HIT)
Fondaparinux (Arixtra)	Pentasaccharide Factor Xa inhibitor	??	??	17–20 h	Renal	??	No	Approved for DVT prophylaxis following orthopedic surgery

?? = not established

Lepirudin has gained widespread acceptance as an alternative to heparin for numerous indications including the management of HIT [28, 78, 80, 114–116]. Two prospective multicenter studies, HAT-1 [114] and HAT-2 [78], have been performed and have demonstrated the utility of lepirudin for the management of HIT. Normalization of platelet counts occurred in 88.7% and 92.6% in the HAT-1 and HAT-2 trials, respectively. Compared to historical controls, patients who received lepirudin experienced a more favorable clinical outcome. The 35-day event rate (combined endpoint: new thromboembolic complication, limb amputation and death) occurred less frequently in patients in both HAT-1 (25.1%) and HAT-2 (31.9%) than in historic controls (52.1%). Consistent with these data, a meta-analysis of the two trials demonstrated that the combined endpoint was lower in patients who received lepirudin compared with historic controls, primarily as a result of fewer thromboembolic complications [80].

Major hemorrhage remains the primary limitation of lepirudin therapy and has been shown to increase with activated partial thromboplastin times (aPTT) greater than 2.5 × control [80]. Whereas aPTTs <1.5 × control were associated with inferior clinical responses, it appeared that aPTTs between 1.5 and 2.5 × control showed optimal efficacy, with moderate risk of bleeding. Dosing of lepirudin depends both on the indication for use and the renal function of the patient (Table 13.6).

Potentially complicating the use of lepirudin for HIT is the development of anti-hirudin antibodies. The development of these antibodies, present in 44% of patients receiving lepirudin for at least 10 days, was shown to be related to the duration of use [117]. Although the presence of these antibodies was not associated with any untoward clinical events in the randomized trials, the presence of these antibodies was associated with supra-therapeutic levels of anticoagulation and bleeding. Thus, daily aPTT levels should be monitored in patients receiving prolonged (>5 days) lepirudin anticoagulation in order to avoid this complication. Similarly, the lack of an antidote for lepirudin further obligates the need for close monitoring of the level of anticoagulation.

Anaphylaxis to lepirudin therapy has recently been reported as a potential complication of its use in patients with HIT [118]. Although the risk of this complication is rare, (approximately 0.015% on first exposure and 0.16% in reexposed patients), it has been associated with devastating consequences. These reactions primarily occurred within minutes of IV lepirudin administration and were fatal in four of the nine cases identified [118]. In these four cases, a previous uneventful treatment course with lepirudin was identified (1–12 weeks earlier).

Argatroban

Argatroban (Novastan ®) is a synthetic, reversible DTI that is FDA-approved for the prophylaxis or treatment of thrombosis in HIT. It is a small molecule which, in contrast to hirudin, interacts with the active site of thrombin but does not make contact with the substrate recognition sites. The anticoagulant effects of argatroban are easily monitored with aPTT, although dose-dependent increases in the prothrombin time also occur [119]. Given the short plasma half-life, argatroban achieves steady-state concentrations rapidly. Equally, the anticoagulant effects of argatroban are short-lived following discontinuation of the IV infusion [120]. Argatroban is primarily metabolized by the liver. Argatroban does not display any cross-reactivity with UH. In addition, it appears that argatroban does not elicit an immune response [121]. Similar to danaparoid and lepirudin, no specific antidote exists. However, the relatively short half-life of argatroban enhances the attractiveness of this agent.

A recently completed multicenter non-randomized prospective study assessed the efficacy of argatroban in 418 patients with HIT compared to historical controls [122]. Platelet counts recovered more rapidly in argatroban-treated patients than in controls. The composite endpoint (all-cause death, all-cause amputation or new thrombosis in 37 days) was significantly reduced in patients with HIT (28.0% vs 38.8% in controls, p-value $= 0.04$) without an increase in bleeding complications. Argatroban was administered by continuous IV infusion with a target aPTT 1.5 to 3.0 $\times$ control values.

Ancrod

Ancrod is a defibrinogenating agent derived from the venom of the Malayan pit viper. This agent is immunologically distinct from heparin and is not associated with thrombocytopenia. Ancrod has been used safely and effectively in a number of patients with HIT complicated by thrombosis [123, 124]. However, its limited availability, inability to limit thrombin generation and erratic efficacy, especially in patients with HIT complicated by arterial thrombosis, have limited its role in this syndrome [125].

Additional Therapies

Several additional therapies exist for the treatment of patients with HIT. It is important to note, however, that these therapies should not supplant the therapies discussed above, but rather serve an adjunctive role in patients with complicated HIT.

Fibrinolysis

Fibrinolysis is not contraindicated in patients with HIT. SK, UK and tissue plasminogen activator, administered either locally or systemically, have been assessed as adjunctive therapies in patients with HIT [126–129]. The use of fibrinolytics, however, increases local thrombin generation and may perpetuate recurrent thrombotic events. Therefore, a concomitant agent such as lepirudin, danaparoid or argatroban should be given for the duration of the fibrinolytic effect. The administration of fibrinolytics in patients with HIT should be reserved for patients with limb-threatening or life-threatening thromboembolic complications.

Intravenous Gamma Globulin (IVIG)

IVIG may be of benefit in HIT patients with life- or limb-threatening thrombosis. The mechanism of action is felt to be related to inhibition of HIT-antibody-induced platelet activation via occupation of the platelet Fc receptors [130]. The usual dose of IVIG is g/kg body weight for two consecutive days.

Plasma Exchange

Although the mechanism of benefit remains unclear – removal of HIT antibodies and immune complexes; restoration of relative deficiencies of one or more natural anticoagulant proteins; or both – plasma exchange may be another useful adjunct to the treatment of severe HIT [131–133].

Surgical Thromboembolectomy

Vascular surgery may be required to salvage ischemic limbs threatened by HIT-related arterial thrombosis. The thrombocytopenia associated with HIT is not a contraindication to surgery. It is important to remember that an alternative anticoagulant to heparin must be used peri-operatively.

Heparin Re-exposure

Heparin re-exposure in the setting of a positive laboratory test for HIT antibodies is associated with a high risk for thrombocytopenia and thrombosis [134]. However, re-exposure to heparin after the disappearance of HIT antibodies has been demonstrated to be feasible in certain circumstances such as cardiopulmonary bypass [135] and in chronic hemodialysis patients [136]. In these situations the drawbacks of danaparoid, lepirudin and argatroban are well recognized. The possibility of heparin re-exposure would ease the burden of the risk of bleeding in these patients. As described above, circulating HIT antibodies disappear within 100 days following an episode of HIT [29]. In addition, upon re-exposure to heparin a second primary immune response occurs that requires at least 3 days to regenerate HIT antibodies. Therefore, the brief exposure to heparin in these patients may be reasonable in patients with a negative laboratory test for circulating HIT antibodies. This approach, however, should be used with caution, if alternative anticoagulants are unavailable, given that recurrent HIT-related events may occur even after laboratory tests become negative [137].

13.8 CONCLUSIONS

Given that heparin remains the anticoagulant most utilized in the clinical arena, it is not surprising that HIT remains a formidable challenge. With a better understanding of the pathophysiology of HIT and the subtleties of the diagnosis of HIT, the treatment of these patients can be readily initiated in an attempt to minimize the potentially devastating consequences. It is important to remember that the cornerstone of therapy for HIT remains absolute cessation of heparin exposure during the acute episode, with institution of an alternative anticoagulant. A major limitation of the currently available alternative anticoagulants, however, remains the risk of hemorrhage along with the lack of an antidote. Furthermore, a significant risk of adverse events related to HIT exists despite the utilization of the available therapies for these patients. The increasing use of LMWH as a primary anticoagulant, along with the development of additional alternatives such as the pentasaccharide fondaparinux, may lead to HIT becoming a historic clinical entity.

REFERENCES

[1] Hirsh, J., Warkentin, T.E., Shaughnessy, S.G., *et al.*, (2001) Heparin and low-molecular-weight heparin: mechanisms of action, pharmacokinetics, dosing, monitoring, efficacy, and safety. *Chest*, 119:64S–94S.

[2] Harenberg, J., Jorg, I., Fenyvesi T., (2002) Heparin-induced thrombocytopenia: pathophysiology and new treatment options. *Pathophysiol Haemost Thromb*, 32:289–94.

[3] Warkentin, T.E., Levine, M.N., Hirsh, J., *et al.*, (1995) Heparin-induced thrombocytopenia in patients treated with low-molecular-weight heparin or unfractionated heparin. *N Eng J Med*, 332:1330–5.

[4] Shuster, T.A., Silliman, W.R., Coats, R.D., Mureebe, L., Silver D., (2003) Heparin-induced thrombocytopenia: twenty-nine years later. *J Vasc Surg*, 38:1316–22.

[5] Girolami, B., Prandoni, P., Stefani PM, *et al.*, (2003) The incidence of heparin-induced thrombocytopenia in hospitalized medical patients treated with subcutaneous unfractionated heparin: a prospective cohort study. *Blood*, 101:2955–9.

[6] Harbrecht, U., Bastians, B., Kredteck, A., *et al.*, (2004) Heparin-induced thrombocytopenia in neurologic disease treated with unfractionated heparin. *Neurology*, 62:657–9.

[7] Verma, A.K., Levine, M., Shalansky, S.J., *et al.*, (2003) Frequency of heparin-induced thrombocytopenia in critical care patients. *Pharmacotherapy*, 23:745–53.

[8] Warkentin, T.E., Sheppard, J.A., Horsewood, P., *et al.*, (2000) Impact of the patient population on the risk for heparin-induced thrombocytopenia. *Blood*, 96:1703–8.

[9] Warkentin, T.E., Kelton, J.G., (1996) A 14-year study of heparin-induced thrombocytopenia. *Am J Med*, 101:502–7.

[10] Fabris, F., Luzzatto, G., Soini, B., *et al.*, (2002) Risk factors for thrombosis in patients with immune mediated heparin-induced thrombocytopenia. *J Intern Med*, 252:149–54.

[11] Heeger, P.S., Backstrom, J.T., (1986) Heparin flushes and thrombocytopenia. *Ann Intern Med*, 105:143.

[12] Rizzoni, W.E., Miller, K., Rick, M., Lotze, M.T., (1988) Heparin-induced thrombocytopenia and thromboembolism in the postoperative period. *Surgery*, 103:470–6.

[13] Brushwood, D.B., (1992) Hospital liable for allergic reaction to heparin used in injection flush. *Am J Hosp Pharm*, 49:1491–2.

[14] Laster, J., Silver, D., (1988) Heparin-coated catheters and heparin-induced thrombocytopenia. *J Vasc Surg*, 7:667–72.

[15] Bell, W.R., Royall, R.M., (1980) Heparin-associated thrombocytopenia: a comparison of three heparin preparations. *N Eng J Med*, 303:902–7.

[16] Cipolle, R.J., Rodvold, K.A., Seifert, R., Clarens, R., Ramirez-Lassepas, M., (1983) Heparin-associated thrombocytopenia: a prospective evaluation of 211 patients. *Ther Drug Monit*, 5:205–11.

[17] Green, D., Martin, G.J., Shoichet, S.H., DeBacker, N., Bomalaski, J.S., Lind, R.N., (1984) Thrombocytopenia in a prospective, randomized, double-blind trial of bovine and porcine heparin. *Am J Med* Sci, 288:60–4.

[18] Powers, P.J., Kelton, J.G., Carter, C.J., (1984) Studies on the frequency of heparin-associated thrombocytopenia. *Thromb Res*, 33:439–43.

[19] Ansell, J.E., Price, J.M., Shah, S., Beckner, R.R., (1985) Heparin-induced thrombocytopenia. What is its real frequency? *Chest*, 88:878–82.

[20] Bailey, R.T., Jr., Ursick, J.A., Heim, K.L., *et al.*, (1986) Heparin-associated thrombocytopenia: a prospective comparison of bovine lung heparin, manufactured by a new process, and porcine intestinal heparin. *Drug Intell Clin Pharm*, 20:374–8.

[21] Casu, B., Johnson, E.A., Mantovani, M., *et al.*, (1983) Correlation between structure, fat-clearing and anticoagulant properties of heparins and heparan sulphates. *Arzneimittelforschung*, 33:135–42.

[22] Barradas, M.A., Mikhailidis, D.P., Epemolu, O., *et al.*, (1987) Comparison of the platelet pro-aggregatory effect of conventional unfractionated heparins and a low molecular weight heparin fraction (CY 222). *Br J Haematol*, 67:451–7.

[23] Plath, J., Schulze, R., Barz, D., *et al.*, (1997) Necrotizing skin lesions induced by low-molecular-weight heparin after total knee arthroplasty. *Arch Orthop Trauma Surg*, 116:443–5.

[24] Elalamy, I., Lecrubier, C., Horellou, M.H., *et al.*, (2000) Heparin-induced thrombocytopenia: laboratory diagnosis and management. *Ann Med*, 32 (Suppl 1):60–7.

[25] Walenga, J.M., Jeske, W.P., Prechel, M.M., *et al.*, (2004) Decreased prevalence of heparin-induced thrombocytopenia with low-molecular-weight heparin and related drugs. *Semin Thromb Hemost*, 30 (Suppl 1):69–80.

[26] Ahmad, S., Haas, S., Hoppensteadt, D.A., *et al.*, (2002) Differential effects of clivarin and heparin in patients undergoing hip and knee surgery for the generation of anti-heparin-platelet factor 4 antibodies. *Thromb Res*, 108:49–55.
[27] Ahmad, S., Untch, B., Haas, S., *et al.*, (2004) Differential prevalence of anti-heparin-PF4 immunoglobulin subtypes in patients treated with clivarin and heparin: implications in the HIT pathogenesis. *Mol Cell Biochem*, 258:163–70.
[28] Paparella, D., Galeone, A., Micelli, M., *et al.*, (2004) Early onset of heparin-induced thrombocytopenia with thrombosis after open heart surgery: importance of an early diagnosis and Lepirudin treatment. *Blood Coagul Fibrinolysis*, 15:183–5.
[29] Warkentin, T.E., Kelton, J.G., (2001) Temporal aspects of heparin-induced thrombocytopenia. *N Eng J Med*, 344:1286–92.
[30] Lubenow, N., Kempf, R., Eichner, A., *et al.*, (2002) Heparin-induced thrombocytopenia: temporal pattern of thrombocytopenia in relation to initial use or reexposure to heparin. *Chest*, 122:37–42.
[31] Warkentin, T.E., Kelton, J.G., (2001) Delayed-onset heparin-induced thrombocytopenia and thrombosis. *Ann Intern Med*, 135:502–6.
[32] Badmanaban, B., Sachithanandan, A., Hunter, I., *et al.*, (2003) Massive pulmonary embolism due to late-onset heparin-induced thrombocytopenia following coronary artery bypass graft surgery: successful treatment with lepirudin. *J Card Surg*, 18:316–18.
[33] Suzuki, S., Sakamoto, S., Okada, T., *et al.*, (2003) Acute myocardial infarction caused by delayed heparin-induced thrombocytopenia and acute immunoreaction due to re-exposure to heparin in a systemic lupus erythematosus patient with HIT antibodies. *Clin Appl Thromb Hemost*, 9:341–6.
[34] Warkentin, T.E., Bernstein, R.A., (2003) Delayed-onset heparin-induced thrombocytopenia and cerebral thrombosis after a single administration of unfractionated heparin. *N Eng J Med*, 348:1067–9.
[35] Wester, J.P., Haas, F.J., Biesma, D.H., *et al.*, (2004) Thrombosis and hemorrhage in heparin-induced thrombocytopenia in seriously ill patients. *Intensive Care Med*, 30:1927–34.
[36] Silver, D., Kapsch, D.N., Tsoi, E.K., (1983) Heparin-induced thrombocytopenia, thrombosis, and hemorrhage. *Ann Surg*, 198:301–6.
[37] Boshkov, L.K., Warkentin, T.E., Hayward, C.P., *et al.*, (1993) Heparin-induced thrombocytopenia and thrombosis: clinical and laboratory studies. *Br J Haematol*, 84:322–8.
[38] Warkentin, T.E., Elavathil, L.J., Hayward, C.P., *et al.*, (1997) The pathogenesis of venous limb gangrene associated with heparin-induced thrombocytopenia. *Ann Intern Med*, 127:804–12.
[39] Hong, A.P., Cook, D.J., Sigouin, C.S., Warkentin, T.E., (2003) Central venous catheters and upper-extremity deep-vein thrombosis complicating immune heparin-induced thrombocytopenia. *Blood*, 101:3049–51.
[40] LaMonte, M.P., Brown, P.M., Hursting, M.J., (2004) Stroke in patients with heparin-induced thrombocytopenia and the effect of argatroban therapy. *Crit Care Med*, 32:976–80.
[41] Chong, B.H., Castaldi, P.A., (1986) Platelet proaggregating effect of heparin: possible mechanism for non-immune heparin-associated thrombocytopenia. *Aust NZ J Med*, 16:715–16.
[42] Greinacher, A., (1995) Antigen generation in heparin-associated thrombocytopenia: the nonimmunologic type and the immunologic type are closely linked in their pathogenesis. *Semin Thromb Hemost*, 21:106–16.
[43] Chong, B.H., Eisbacher, M., (1998) Pathophysiology and laboratory testing of heparin-induced thrombocytopenia. *Semin Hematol*, 35:3–8; Discussion 35–6.
[44] Blank, M., Shoenfeld, Y., Tavor, S., *et al.*, (2002) Anti-platelet factor 4/heparin antibodies from patients with heparin-induced thrombocytopenia provoke direct activation of microvascular endothelial cells. *Int Immunol*, 14:121–9.
[45] Petersen, F., Bock, L., Flad, H.D., Brandt, E., (1999) Platelet factor 4-induced neutrophil-endothelial cell interaction: involvement of mechanisms and functional consequences different from those elicited by interleukin-8. *Blood*, 94:4020–8.
[46] Walenga, J.M., Jeske, W.P., Prechel, M.M., Bakhos, M., (2004) Newer insights on the mechanism of heparin-induced thrombocytopenia. *Semin Thromb Hemost*, 30 (Suppl 1):57–67.
[47] Deitcher, S.R., Carman, T.L., (2001) Heparin-induced thrombocytopenia: natural history, diagnosis, and management. *Vasc Med*, 6:113–19.

[48] Chong, B.H., (2003) Heparin-induced thrombocytopenia. *J Thromb Haemost*, 1:1471–8.
[49] De Caterina, R., Gazzetti, P., Mazzone, A., Marzilli, M., L'Abbate A., (1988) Platelet activation in angina at rest. Evidence by paired measurement of plasma beta-thromboglobulin and platelet factor 4. *Eur Heart J*, 9:913–22.
[50] Rinder, C.S., Bohnert, J., Rinder, H.M., *et al.*, (1991) Platelet activation and aggregation during cardiopulmonary bypass. *Anesthesiology*, 75:388–93.
[51] Harrison, P., Cramer, E.M., (1993) Platelet alpha-granules. *Blood Rev*, 7:52–62.
[52] Kawamori, R., Imano, E., Watarai, T., *et al.*, (1994) Platelet activation in diabetic patients with asymptomatic atherosclerosis. *Diabetes Res Clin Pract*, 24:89–95.
[53] Greinacher, A., Potzsch, B., Amiral, J., *et al.*, (1994) Heparin-associated thrombocytopenia: isolation of the antibody and characterization of a multimolecular PF4-heparin complex as the major antigen. *Thromb Haemost*, 71:247–51.
[54] Rauova, L., Poncz, M., McKenzie, S.E., *et al.*, (2004) Ultralarge complexes of heparin and PF4 are central to the pathogenesis of heparin-induced thrombocytopenia. *Blood*, 105:131–8.
[55] Visentin, G.P., Malik, M., Cyganiak, K.A., Aster, R.H., (1996) Patients treated with unfractionated heparin during open heart surgery are at high risk to form antibodies reactive with heparin:platelet factor 4 complexes. *J Lab Clin Med*, 128:376–83.
[56] Gruel, Y., Boizard-Boval, B., Wautier, J.L., (1993) Further evidence that alpha-granule components such as platelet factor 4 are involved in platelet-IgG-heparin interactions during heparin-associated thrombocytopenia. *Thromb Haemost*, 70:374–5.
[57] Amiral, J., Bridey, F., Dreyfus, M., *et al.*, (1992) Platelet factor 4 complexed to heparin is the target for antibodies generated in heparin-induced thrombocytopenia. *Thromb Haemost*, 68:95–6.
[58] Visentin, G.P., Ford, S.E., Scott, J.P., Aster, R.H., (1994) Antibodies from patients with heparin-induced thrombocytopenia/thrombosis are specific for platelet factor 4 complexed with heparin or bound to endothelial cells. *J Clin Invest*, 93:81–8.
[59] Horne, M.K., 3rd, Hutchison, K.J., (1998) Simultaneous binding of heparin and platelet factor-4 to platelets: further insights into the mechanism of heparin-induced thrombocytopenia. *Am J Hematol*, 58:24–30.
[60] Visentin, G.P., Moghaddam, M., Beery, S.E., *et al.*, (2001) Heparin is not required for detection of antibodies associated with heparin-induced thrombocytopenia/thrombosis. *J Lab Clin Med*, 138:22–31.
[61] Greinacher, A., Alban, S., Dummel, V., *et al.*, (1995) Characterization of the structural requirements for a carbohydrate based anticoagulant with a reduced risk of inducing the immunological type of heparin-associated thrombocytopenia. *Thromb Haemost*, 74:886–92.
[62] Chong, B.H., Fawaz, I., Chesterman, C.N., Berndt, M.C., (1989) Heparin-induced thrombocytopenia: mechanism of interaction of the heparin-dependent antibody with platelets. *Br J Haematol*, 73:235–40.
[63] Newman, P.M., Chong, B.H., (2000) Heparin-induced thrombocytopenia: new evidence for the dynamic binding of purified anti-PF4-heparin antibodies to platelets and the resultant platelet activation. *Blood*, 96:182–7.
[64] Reilly, M.P., Taylor, S.M., Hartman, N.K., *et al.*, (2001) Heparin-induced thrombocytopenia/thrombosis in a transgenic mouse model requires human platelet factor 4 and platelet activation through FcgammaRIIA. *Blood*, 98:2442–7.
[65] Cines, D.B., Tomaski, A., Tannenbaum, S., (1987) Immune endothelial-cell injury in heparin-associated thrombocytopenia. *N Eng J Med*, 316:581–9.
[66] Herbert, J.M., Savi, P., Jeske, W.P., Walenga, J.M., (1998) Effect of SR121566A, a potent GP IIb-IIIa antagonist, on the HIT serum/heparin-induced platelet mediated activation of human endothelial cells. *Thromb Haemost*, 80:326–31.
[67] Chong, B.H., Pitney, W.R., Castaldi, P.A., (1982) Heparin-induced thrombocytopenia: association of thrombotic complications with heparin-dependent IgG antibody that induces thromboxane synthesis in platelet aggregation. *Lancet*, 2:1246–9.
[68] Amiral, J., Wolf, M., Fischer, A., *et al.*, (1996) Pathogenicity of IgA and/or IgM antibodies to heparin-PF4 complexes in patients with heparin-induced thrombocytopenia. *Br J Haematol*, 92:954–9.

[69] Suh, J.S., Aster, R.H., Visentin, G.P., (1998) Antibodies from patients with heparin-induced thrombocytopenia/thrombosis recognize different epitopes on heparin: platelet factor 4. *Blood*, 91:916–22.

[70] Amiral, J., Pouplard, C., Vissac, A.M., *et al.*, (2000) Affinity purification of heparin-dependent antibodies to platelet factor 4 developed in heparin-induced thrombocytopenia: biological characteristics and effects on platelet activation. *Br J Haematol*, 109:336–41.

[71] Greinacher, A., Amiral, J., Dummel, V., *et al.*, (1994) Laboratory diagnosis of heparin-associated thrombocytopenia and comparison of platelet aggregation test, heparin-induced platelet activation test, and platelet factor 4/heparin enzyme-linked immunosorbent assay. *Transfusion*, 34:381–5.

[72] Amiral, J., Marfaing-Koka, A., Wolf, M., *et al.*, (1996) Presence of autoantibodies to interleukin-8 or neutrophil-activating peptide-2 in patients with heparin-associated thrombocytopenia. *Blood*, 88:410–16.

[73] Warkentin, T.E., Chong, B.H., Greinacher, A., (1998) Heparin-induced thrombocytopenia: towards consensus. *Thromb Haemost*, 79:1–7.

[74] Rice, L., Attisha, W.K., Drexler, A., Francis, J.L., (2002) Delayed-onset heparin-induced thrombocytopenia. *Ann Intern Med*, 136:210–15.

[75] Warkentin, T.E., (1998) Clinical presentation of heparin-induced thrombocytopenia. *Semin Hematol*, 35:9–16; Discussion 35–6.

[76] Pedersen-Bjergaard, U., Andersen, M., Hansen, P.B., (1997) Drug-induced thrombocytopenia: clinical data on 309 cases and the effect of corticosteroid therapy. Eur *J Clin Pharmacol*, 52:183–9.

[77] Hach-Wunderle, V., Kainer, K., Salzmann, G., *et al.*, (1997) Heparin-related thrombosis despite normal platelet counts in vascular surgery. *Am J Surg*, 173:117–19.

[78] Greinacher, A., Janssens, U., Berg, G., *et al.*, (1999) Lepirudin (recombinant hirudin) for parenteral anticoagulation in patients with heparin-induced thrombocytopenia. Heparin-Associated Thrombocytopenia Study (HAT) investigators. *Circulation*, 100: 587–93.

[79] Wallis, D.E., Workman, D.L., Lewis, B.E., *et al.*, (1999) Failure of early heparin cessation as treatment for heparin-induced thrombocytopenia. *Am J Med*, 106:629–35.

[80] Greinacher, A., Eichler, P., Lubenow, N., *et al.*, (2000) Heparin-induced thrombocytopenia with thromboembolic complications: meta-analysis of 2 prospective trials to assess the value of parenteral treatment with lepirudin and its therapeutic aPTT range. *Blood*, 96:846–51.

[81] Pohl, C., Harbrecht, U., Greinacher, A., *et al.*, (2000) Neurologic complications in immune-mediated heparin-induced thrombocytopenia. *Neurology*, 54:1240–5.

[82] Srinivasan, A.F., Rice, L., Bartholomew, J.R., *et al.*, (2004) Warfarin-induced skin necrosis and venous limb gangrene in the setting of heparin-induced thrombocytopenia. *Arch Intern Med*, 164:66–70.

[83] Weyrich, P., Balletshofer, B., Hoeft, S., *et al.*, (2001) Acute adrenocortical insufficiency due to heparin-induced thrombocytopenia with subsequent bilateral haemorrhagic infarction of the adrenal glands. *Vasa*, 30:285–8.

[84] Nand, S., Wong, W., Yuen, B., *et al.*, (1997) Heparin-induced thrombocytopenia with thrombosis: incidence, analysis of risk factors, and clinical outcomes in 108 consecutive patients treated at a single institution. *Am J Hematol*, 56:12–16.

[85] Warkentin, T.E., Whitlock, R.P., Teoh, K.H., (2004) Warfarin-associated multiple digital necrosis complicating heparin-induced thrombocytopenia and Raynaud's phenomenon after aortic valve replacement for adenocarcinoma-associated thrombotic endocarditis. *Am J Hematol*, 75:56–62.

[86] Mar, A.W., Dixon, B., Ibrahim, K., Parkin, J.D., (1995) Skin necrosis following subcutaneous heparin injection. *Australas J Dermatol*, 36:201–3.

[87] Ling, E., Warkentin, T.E., (1998) Intraoperative heparin flushes and subsequent acute heparin-induced thrombocytopenia. *Anesthesiology*, 89:1567–9.

[88] Heddle, N.M., Klama, L., Singer, J., *et al.*, (1994) The role of the plasma from platelet concentrates in transfusion reactions. *N Eng J Med*, 331:625–8.

[89] Deitcher, S.R., (2003) Cancer and thrombosis: mechanisms and treatment. *J Thromb Thrombolysis*, 16:21–31.

[90] Bharadwaj, J., Jayaraman, C., Shrivastava, R., (2003) Heparin resistance. *Lab Hematol*, 9:125–31.

[91] Walenga, J.M., Jeske, W.P., Fasanella, A.R., *et al.*, (1999) Laboratory tests for the diagnosis of heparin-induced thrombocytopenia. *Semin Thromb Hemost*, 25 (Suppl 1):43–9.

[92] Januzzi, J.L., Jr., Jang, I.K., (1999) Heparin induced thrombocytopenia: diagnosis and contemporary antithrombin management. *J Thromb Thrombolysis*, 7:259–64.

[93] Picker, S.M., Gathof, B.S., (2004) Pathophysiology, epidemiology, diagnosis and treatment of heparin-induced thrombocytopenia (HIT). *Eur J Med Res*, 9:180–5.

[94] Sheridan, D., Carter, C., Kelton, J.G., (1986) A diagnostic test for heparin-induced thrombocytopenia. *Blood*, 67:27–30.

[95] Harenberg, J., Huhle, G., Giese, C., *et al.*, (2000) Determination of serotonin release from platelets by enzyme immunoassay in the diagnosis of heparin-induced thrombocytopenia. *Br J Haematol*, 109:182–6.

[96] Gobbi, G., Mirandola, P., Tazzari, P.L., *et al.*, (2003) Flow cytometry detection of serotonin content and release in resting and activated platelets. *Br J Haematol*, 121:892–6.

[97] Chong, B.H., Burgess, J., Ismail, F., (1993) The clinical usefulness of the platelet aggregation test for the diagnosis of heparin-induced thrombocytopenia. *Thromb Haemost*, 69:344–50.

[98] Warkentin, T.E., Greinacher, A., (2001) Laboratory testing for HIT, in *Heparin-Induced Thrombocytopenia*, (eds T.E. Warkentin, A. Greinacher), New York: Marcel Dekker, Inc., New York.

[99] Martinuzzo, M.E., Forastiero, R.R., Adamczuk, Y., *et al.*, (1999) Antiplatelet factor 4–heparin antibodies in patients with antiphospholipid antibodies. *Thromb Res*, 95:271–9.

[100] Lindhoff-Last, E., Gerdsen, F., Ackermann, H., Bauersachs, R., (2001) Determination of heparin-platelet factor 4-IgG antibodies improves diagnosis of heparin-induced thrombocytopenia. *Br J Haematol*, 113:886–90.

[101] Planes, A., Samama, M.M., Lensing, A.W., *et al.*, (1999) Prevention of deep vein thrombosis after hip replacement—comparison between two low-molecular heparins, tinzaparin and enoxaparin. *Thromb Haemost*, 81:22–5.

[102] Greinacher, A., Michels, I., Mueller-Eckhardt, C., (1992) Heparin-associated thrombocytopenia: the antibody is not heparin specific. *Thromb Haemost*, 67:545–9.

[103] Cohen M. (1999) Heparin-induced thrombocytopenia and the clinical use of low molecular weight heparins in acute coronary syndromes. *Semin Hematol*, 36:33–6.

[104] Newman, P.M., Swanson, R.L., Chong, B.H., (1998) Heparin-induced thrombocytopenia: IgG binding to PF4-heparin complexes in the fluid phase and cross-reactivity with low molecular weight heparin and heparinoid. *Thromb Haemost*, 80:292–7.

[105] Harenberg, J., Jorg, I., Fenyvesi, T., (2004) Treatment of heparin-induced thrombocytopenia with fondaparinux. *Haematologica*, 89:1017–8.

[106] Acostamadiedo, J.M., Iyer, U.G., Owen J. (2000) Danaparoid sodium. *Expert Opin Pharmacother*, 1:803–14.

[107] Magnani, H.N., (1993) Heparin-induced thrombocytopenia (HIT): an overview of 230 patients treated with orgaran (Org 10172). *Thromb Haemost*, 70:554–61.

[108] Chong, B.H., Ismail, F., Cade, J., Gallus, A.S., Gordon, S., Chesterman, C.N., (1989) Heparin-induced thrombocytopenia: studies with a new low molecular weight heparinoid, Org 10172. *Blood*, 73:1592–6.

[109] Tardy-Poncet, B., Tardy, B., Reynaud, J., *et al.*, (1999) Efficacy and safety of danaparoid sodium (ORG 10172) in critically ill patients with heparin-associated thrombocytopenia. *Chest*, 115:1616–20.

[110] Lindhoff-Last, E., Betz, C., Bauersachs, R., (2001) Use of a low-molecular-weight heparinoid (danaparoid sodium) for continuous renal replacement therapy in intensive care patients. *Clin Appl Thromb Hemost*, 7:300–4.

[111] Chong, B.H., Gallus, A.S., Cade, J.F., *et al.*, (2001) Prospective randomised open-label comparison of danaparoid with dextran 70 in the treatment of heparin-induced thrombocytopaenia with thrombosis: a clinical outcome study. *Thromb Haemost*, 86:1170–5.

[112] Wilde, M.I., Markham, A., (1997), Danaparoid. A review of its pharmacology and clinical use in the management of heparin-induced thrombocytopenia. *Drugs*, 54:903–24.

[113] Kaplan, K.L., Francis, C.W., (2002) Direct thrombin inhibitors. *Semin Hematol*, 39: 187–96.

[114] Greinacher, A., Volpel, H., Janssens, U., *et al.*, (1999) Recombinant hirudin (lepirudin) provides safe and effective anticoagulation in patients with heparin-induced thrombocytopenia: a prospective study. *Circulation*, 99:73–80.

[115] Becker, R.C., (2000) Hirudin-based anticoagulant strategies for patients with suspected heparin-induced thrombocytopenia undergoing percutaneous coronary interventions and bypass grafting. *J Thromb Thrombolysis*, 10 Suppl 1:59–68.

[116] Cochran, K., DeMartini, T.J., Lewis, B.E., *et al.*, (2003) Use of lepirudin during percutaneous vascular interventions in patients with heparin-induced thrombocytopenia. *J Invasive Cardiol*, 15:617–21.

[117] Eichler, P., Friesen, H.J., Lubenow, N., Jaeger, B., Greinacher A., (2000) Antihirudin antibodies in patients with heparin-induced thrombocytopenia treated with lepirudin: incidence, effects on aPTT, and clinical relevance. *Blood*, 96:2373–8.

[118] Greinacher, A., Lubenow, N., Eichler P., (2003) Anaphylactic and anaphylactoid reactions associated with lepirudin in patients with heparin-induced thrombocytopenia. *Circulation*, 108:2062–5.

[119] Sheth, S.B., DiCicco, R.A., Hursting, M.J., *et al.*, (2001) Interpreting the International Normalized Ratio (INR) in individuals receiving argatroban and warfarin. *Thromb Haemost*, 85:435–40.

[120] Kathiresan, S., Shiomura, J., Jang, I.K., (2002) Argatroban. *J Thromb Thrombolysis*, 13:41–7.

[121] Walenga, J.M., Ahmad, S., Hoppensteadt, D., *et al.*, (2002) Argatroban therapy does not generate antibodies that alter its anticoagulant activity in patients with heparin-induced thrombocytopenia. *Thromb Res*, 105:401–5.

[122] Lewis, B.E., Wallis, D.E., Leya, F., *et al.*, (2003) Argatroban anticoagulation in patients with heparin-induced thrombocytopenia. *Arch Intern Med*, 163:1849–56.

[123] Demers, C., Ginsberg, J.S., Brill-Edwards, P., *et al.*, (1991) Rapid anticoagulation using ancrod for heparin-induced thrombocytopenia. *Blood*, 78:2194–7.

[124] Lathan, L.O., Staggers, S.L., (1996) Ancrod: the use of snake venom in the treatment of patients with heparin-induced thrombocytopenia and thrombosis undergoing coronary artery bypass grafting: nursing management. *Heart Lung*, 25:451–60; quiz 461–2.

[125] Lewis, B.E., Leya, F.S., Wallis, D., Grassman, E., (1994) Failure of ancrod in the treatment of heparin-induced arterial thrombosis. *Can J Cardiol*, 10:559–61.

[126] Cohen, J.I., Cooper, M.R., Greenberg, C.S., (1985) Streptokinase therapy of pulmonary emboli with heparin-associated thrombocytopenia. *Arch Intern Med*, 145:1725–6.

[127] Clifton, G.D., Smith, M.D., Thrombolytic therapy in heparin-associated thrombocytopenia with thrombosis. *Clin Pharm*, 5:597–601.

[128] Janssens, U., Breithardt, O.A., Greinacher, A., (1999) Successful thrombolysis of right atrial and ventricle thrombi encircling a temporary pacemaker lead in a patient with heparin-induced thrombocytopenia type II. *Pacing Clin Electrophysiol*, 22:678–81.

[129] Reilly, M.P., Weiss, R., Askenase, A., *et al.*, (2000) Hirudin therapy during thrombolysis for venous thrombosis in heparin-induced thrombocytopenia. *Vasc Med*, 5:239–42.

[130] Winder, A., Shoenfeld, Y., Hochman, R., *et al.*, (1998) High-dose intravenous gamma-globulins for heparin-induced thrombocytopenia: a prompt response. *J Clin Immunol*, 18:330–4.

[131] Warkentin, T.E., (1997) Heparin-induced thrombocytopenia. Pathogenesis, frequency, avoidance and management. *Drug Saf*, 17:325–41.

[132] Poullin, P., Pietri, P.A., Lefevre, P., (1998) Heparin-induced thrombocytopenia with thrombosis: successful treatment with plasma exchange. *Br J Haematol*, 102:630–1.

[133] Kajitani, M., Aguinaga, M., Johnson, C.E., *et al.*, (2001) Use of plasma exchange and heparin during cardiopulmonary bypass for a patient with heparin induced thrombocytopenia: a case report. *J Card Surg*, 16:313–18.

[134] Laster, J., Elfrink, R., Silver, D., (1989) Reexposure to heparin of patients with heparin-associated antibodies. *J Vasc Surg*, 9:677–81; discussion 681–2.

[135] Potzsch, B., Klovekorn, W.P., Madlener, K., (2000) Use of heparin during cardiopulmonary bypass in patients with a history of heparin-induced thrombocytopenia. *N Eng J Med*, 343:515.

[136] Matsuo, T., Matuo, M., Wanaka, K., Sakai, R., (2003) Heparin re-exposure after heparin-induced thrombocytopenia in a chronic hemodialysis patient. *Clin Lab Haematol*, 25:333–4.

[137] Gruel, Y., Lang, M., Darnige, L., *et al.*, (1990) Fatal effect of re-exposure to heparin after previous heparin-associated thrombocytopenia and thrombosis. *Lancet*, 336:1077–8.

[138] Brieger, D.B., Mak, K.H., Kottke-Marchant, K., Topol, E.J., (1998) Heparin-induced thrombocytopenia. *J Am Coll Cardiol*, 31:1449–59.

[139] Warkentin, T.E., (2001) Clinical picture of HIT, in: *Heparin-Induced Thrombocytopenia*, (eds T.E. Warkentin, A. Greinacher), Marcel Dekker, Inc., New York.

[140] Arepally, G., Reynolds, C., Tomaski, A., *et al.*, (1995) Comparison of PF4/heparin ELISA assay with the 14C-serotonin release assay in the diagnosis of heparin-induced thrombocytopenia. *Am J Clin Pathol*, 104:648–54.

[141] Eichler, P., Raschke, R., Lubenow, N., Meyer, O., Schwind, P., Greinacher, A., (2002) The new ID-heparin/PF4 antibody test for rapid detection of heparin-induced antibodies in comparison with functional and antigenic assays. *Br J Haematol*, 116:887–91.

[142] Warkentin, T.E., Heddle, N.M., (2003) Laboratory diagnosis of immune heparin-induced thrombocytopenia. *Curr Hematol Rep*, 2:148–57.

Index